Trauma and Reconstruction

Editor

DAVID S. PRECIOUS

ORAL AND MAXILLOFACIAL SURGERY CLINICS OF NORTH AMERICA

www.oralmaxsurgery.theclinics.com

Consulting Editor
RICHARD H. HAUG

November 2013 • Volume 25 • Number 4

ELSEVIER

1600 John F. Kennedy Boulevard • Suite 1800 • Philadelphia, Pennsylvania, 19103-2899

http://www.oralmaxsurgery.theclinics.com

ORAL AND MAXILLOFACIAL SURGERY CLINICS OF NORTH AMERICA Volume 25, Number 4
November 2013 ISSN 1042-3699, ISBN-13: 978-0-323-26114-2

Editor: John Vassallo; j.vassallo@elsevier.com
Developmental Editor: Susan Showalter

Oral and Maxillofacial Surgery Clinics of North America (ISSN 1042-3699) is published quarterly by Elsevier Inc., 360 Park Avenue South, New York, NY 10010-1710. Months of issue are February, May, August, and November. Business and Editorial Offices: 1600 John F. Kennedy Blvd., Suite 1800, Philadelphia, PA 19103-2899. Periodicals postage paid at New York, NY and additional mailing offices. Subscription prices are $385.00 per year for US individuals, $567.00 per year for US institutions, $175.00 per year for US students and residents, $455.00 per year for Canadian individuals, $680.00 per year for Canadian institutions, $520.00 per year for international individuals, $680.00 per year for international institutions and $235.00 per year for Canadian and foreign students/residents. To receive student/resident rate, orders must be accompanied by name or affiliated institution, date of term, and the *signature* of program/residency coordinator on institution letterhead. Orders will be billed at individual rate until proof of status is received. Foreign air speed delivery is included in all *Clinics* subscription prices. All prices are subject to change without notice. **POSTMASTER:** Send address changes to *Oral and Maxillofacial Surgery Clinics of North America,* Elsevier Periodicals Customer Service, 11830 Westline Industrial Drive, St. Louis, MO 63146. Tel: 1-800-654-2452 (U.S. and Canada); 314-447-8871 (outside U.S. and Canada). Fax: 314-447-8029. E-mail: journalscustomerservice-usa@elsevier.com (for print support); journalsonlinesupport-usa@elsevier.com (for online support).

Reprints. For copies of 100 or more, of articles in this publication, please contact the Commercial Reprints Department, Elsevier Inc., 360 Park Avenue South, New York, NY 10010-1710. Tel.: 212-633-3874; Fax: 212-633-3820; Email: reprints@elsevier.com.

Oral and Maxillofacial Surgery Clinics of North America is covered in *MEDLINE/PubMed* (*Index Medicus*), *Science Citation Index Expanded (SciSearch®), Journal Citation Reports/Science Edition,* and *Current Contents®/Clinical Medicine.*

Printed and bound by CPI Group (UK) Ltd, Croydon, CR0 4YY

Transferred to digital print 2012

Contributors

CONSULTING EDITOR

RICHARD H. HAUG, DDS
Carolinas Center for Oral Health,
Charlotte, North Carolina

EDITOR

**DAVID S. PRECIOUS, CM, DDS, MSc,
FRCDC, FRCS, Dhc**
Dean Emeritus and Professor, Oral and
Maxillofacial Surgery, Dalhousie University,
Halifax, Nova Scotia, Canada

AUTHORS

A. OMAR ABUBAKER, DMD, PhD
Professor and Chair, Department of Oral and
Maxillofacial Surgery, School of Dentistry, VCU
Medical Center, Virginia Commonwealth
University, Richmond, Virginia

R. BRYAN BELL, DDS, MD, FACS
Medical Director, Oral, Head and Neck
Cancer Program and Clinic, Providence Cancer
Center, Providence Portland Medical Center;
Attending Surgeon, Trauma Service/Oral and
Maxillofacial Surgery Service, Legacy Emanuel
Medical Center; Affiliate Professor, Oregon
Health and Science University, Portland, Oregon

DANIEL CAMERON BRAASCH, DMD
Formerly Chief Resident, Department of Oral
and Maxillofacial Surgery, School of Dentistry,
VCU Medical Center, Virginia Commonwealth
University, Richmond, Virgina; Private Practice,
Nashua, New Hampshire

WILLIAM CURTIS, MD, DMD
Former Craniomaxillofacial Fellow, FACES,
Women and Children's Hospital, Charleston,
West Virginia

**BEN DAVIS, DDS, Dip OMFS and
Anesthesia, FRCD**
Associate Professor and Chair, Department
of Oral and Maxillofacial Sciences, Dalhousie
University, Halifax, Nova Scotia, Canada

**JEAN CHARLES DOUCET, DDS, MD, MSc,
FRCD(C)**
Assistant Professor, Department of Oral and
Maxillofacial Sciences, Dalhousie University,
Halifax, Nova Scotia, Canada

KYLE S. ETTINGER, DDS
Resident, Oral and Maxillofacial
Surgery, Division of Oral and Maxillofacial
Surgery, Department of Surgery, Mayo
College of Medicine, Rochester,
Minnesota

W. JONATHAN FILLMORE, DMD, MD
Resident, Oral and Maxillofacial
Surgery, Division of Oral and Maxillofacial
Surgery, Department of Surgery, Mayo
College of Medicine, Rochester,
Minnesota

BELINI FREIRE-MAIA, DDS, MSc
Head of Department Oral Surgery, School of
Dentistry, Pontifícia Universidade Católica de
Minas Gerais; Consultant and Coordinator,
Oral and Maxillofacial Surgery, Hospital da
Baleia; Consultant, Oral and Maxillofacial
Surgery, Hospital Lifecenter, Belo Horizonte,
Minas Gerais, Brazil

SAVANNAH GELESKO, DDS, MD
Resident, Department of Oral and
Maxillofacial Surgery, Oregon Health and
Science University, Portland, Oregon

**REGINALD H.B. GOODDAY, DDS, MSc,
FRCD(C), FICD, FACD**
Professor and Chair, Department of Oral and
Maxillofacial Sciences, Faculty of Dentistry,
Dalhousie University, Halifax, Nova Scotia,
Canada

**CURTIS E. GREGOIRE, BSc, DDS, MS, MD,
FRCD(C)**
Active Staff, Department of Oral and
Maxillofacial Surgery, QEII Health Sciences
Centre; Associate Professor, Department of
Oral and Maxillofacial Sciences, Faculty of
Dentistry, Dalhousie University, Halifax, Nova
Scotia, Canada

BRUCE B. HORSWELL, MD, DDS, MS, FACS
Director of FACES, Associate Clinical
Professor of Surgery, Women and Children's
Hospital, Charleston, West Virginia

VESA T. KAINULAINEN, DDS, PhD
Assistant Professor, Institute of Dentistry, Oulu
University Hospital, University of Oulu, Oulu,
Finland

REHA KISNISCI, DDS, PhD
Professor, Department of Oral and
Maxillofacial Surgery, School of Dentistry,
Ankara University, Ankara, Turkey

ANTTI-VEIKKO KOIVUMÄKI, DDS
Staff Surgeon, Oral and Maxillofacial Unit,
Department of Otorhinolaryngology, Tampere
University Hospital, Tampere, Finland

DEEPAK G. KRISHNAN, DDS
Department of Surgery, Division of Oral and
Maxillofacial Surgery, University of Cincinnati
College of Medicine, University of Cincinnati
Medical Center, Cincinnati, Ohio

**RODRIGO OTÁVIO MOREIRA MARINHO,
DDS, MSc, FDSRCS**
Consultant and Coordinator, Oral and
Maxillofacial Surgery, Hospital Lifecenter;
Consultant, Oral and Maxillofacial Surgery,
Hospital HGIP/IPSEMG, Belo Horizonte, Minas
Gerais, Brazil

MICHAEL R. MARKIEWICZ, DDS, MPH, MD
Resident, Department of Oral and
Maxillofacial Surgery, Oregon Health and
Science University, Portland, Oregon

AIMO MIETTINEN, DDS
Senior Surgeon, Oral and Maxillofacial Unit,
Department of Otorhinolaryngology, Tampere
University Hospital, Tampere, Finland

**ARCHIBALD D. MORRISON, DDS, MS,
FRCD(C)**
Active Staff, Department of Oral and
Maxillofacial Surgery, QEII Health Sciences
Centre; Assistant Professor, Department of
Oral and Maxillofacial Sciences, Faculty of
Dentistry, Dalhousie University, Halifax, Nova
Scotia, Canada

MIKKO PYYSALO, DDS
Staff Surgeon, Oral and Maxillofacial Unit,
Department of Otorhinolaryngology, Tampere
University Hospital, Tampere, Finland

KEVIN L. RIECK, DDS, MD
Assistant Professor of Surgery, Division of Oral
and Maxillofacial Surgery, Department of
Surgery, Mayo College of Medicine,
Rochester, Minnesota

**CHAD G. ROBERTSON, DDS, MD, MSc,
FRCD(C)**
Assistant Professor and Director of Graduate
Training, Department of Oral and Maxillofacial
Sciences, Dalhousie University, Halifax, Nova
Scotia, Canada

**GEORGE K.B. SÁNDOR, MD, DDS, PhD,
Dr Habil**
Professor of Tissue Engineering, Regea-
BioMediTech, University of Tampere,
Tampere; Professor of Oral and Maxillofacial
Surgery, Institute of Dentistry, University of
Oulu, Oulu, Finland

JAN WOLFF, DDS, PhD
Senior Researcher, Tissue Engineering,
Regea-BioMediTech, University of Tampere;
Senior Surgeon, Oral and Maxillofacial Unit,
Department of Otorhinolaryngology, Tampere
University Hospital, Tampere, Finland

Contents

The systematic assessment of patients with facial injuries is the culmination of wisdom from trials and errors, audits of failures and successes, careful and mindful reflection of current practice, and a willingness to change. Emerging technology has positively impacted the practice of management of facial trauma. A systematic evaluation and physical examination of the trauma victim remain the gold standard and the first step toward effective care.

This article reviews the current standard of care in imaging considerations for the diagnosis and management of craniomaxillofacial trauma. Injury-specific imaging techniques and options for computer-aided surgery as related to craniomaxillofacial trauma are reviewed, including preoperative planning, intraoperative navigation, and intraoperative computed tomography. Specific imaging considerations by anatomic region include frontal sinus fractures, temporal bone fractures, midfacial fractures, mandible fractures, laryngotracheal injuries, and vascular injuries. Imaging considerations in the pediatric trauma patient are also discussed. Responsible postoperative imaging as it relates to facial trauma management and outcomes assessment is reviewed.

Injuries to the oral and maxillofacial region are commonly encountered, and the appropriate management of patients with these injuries frequently requires the expertise of an anesthesiologist. Injuries to this region may involve any combination of soft tissue, bone, and teeth. Injuries to these structures often produce anesthesia-related challenges, which must be overcome to achieve optimal outcomes. This article addresses the common challenges faced by anesthesiologists specific to patients with facial fractures.

Proper anatomic reduction of the fracture and accelerated complete recovery are desirable goals after trauma reconstruction. Over the recent decades, significant headway in craniomaxillofacial trauma care has been achieved and advancements in the management for the injuries of the mandibular condyle have also proved to be no exception. A trend in operative and reconstructive options for proper anatomic reduction and internal fixation has become notable as a result of newly introduced technology, surgical techniques, and operative expertise.

Fractures through the angle of the mandible are one of the most common facial fractures. The management of such fractures has been controversial, however. This controversy is related to the anatomic relations and complex biomechanical aspects of the mandibular angle. The debate has become even more heated since the evolution of rigid fixation and the ability to provide adequate stability of the fractured segments. This article provides an overview of the special anatomic and biomechanical features of the mandibular angle and their impact on the management of these fractures.

Mandibular fracture, specifically in the symphysis and body regions combined, is the most common facial fracture requiring hospitalization in North America. The primary treatment objective is to restore form and function by achieving anatomic reduction and placing fixation that eliminates mobility of the bone fragments. Several treatment options and surgical techniques are available for performing closed or open reduction. Special considerations are necessary when treating pediatric patients and fractures of the edentulous mandible. Complications relating to the tooth and denture-bearing regions of the mandible include infection, nonunion, and neurosensory changes.

The zygomaticomaxillary complex (ZMC) has important aesthetic, structural, and functional roles that need to be preserved and/or restored during treatment of facial fractures. Surgical treatment of ZMC fractures is indicated when there is displacement of the bony fragments, and open reduction and internal fixation is the treatment of choice in cases of comminution or fracture instability. The surgical approaches used for fracture reduction as well as the type, number, and location of the fixation will be determined by the pattern of the fracture and the surgeon's preference. This article discusses the main points of the management of ZMC fractures.

Repair of fractures involving the nasofrontal region remains a mainstay of contemporary oral and maxillofacial surgery. This article discusses the epidemiology of these injuries, anatomy of the area, and management of these fractures with insight into potential complications. These include fractures of the frontal sinus, naso-orbital-ethmoidal region, root of the nose, and associated adjacent structures.

Panfacial fractures are defined as fractures involving the lower, middle, and upper face. Treatment can be challenging and requires an individualized treatment plan. A firm understanding of the treatment principles of each individual fracture is necessary before attempting to tackle the patient with panfacial fractures. Advances in rigid fixation, wide exposure, primary bone grafting, and attention to soft tissue reattachment have significantly improved the treatment of the patient with panfacial fractures.

Late Reconstruction of Condylar Neck and Head Fractures

Ben Davis

Condyle fractures are a common injury, but only a few of these injuries require immediate or late reconstruction. The complications that most frequently necessitate condylar reconstruction include proximal segment degeneration, malunion, and ankylosis. Costochondral grafts and total joint prostheses, both stock and custom, remain the most common methods of reconstruction. Reconstruction plates with condylar extensions should only be used temporarily as an unacceptable number cause serious complications. Distraction osteogenesis may have an occasional role in reconstructing the posttraumatic condyle.

Late Reconstruction of Orbital and Naso-orbital Deformities

Jan Wolff, George K.B. Sándor, Mikko Pyysalo, Aimo Miettinen, Antti-Veikko Koivumäki, and Vesa T. Kainulainen

Acute orbital fractures and naso-orbital ethmoid fractures can result in chronic orbital and naso-orbital deformities. Understanding the acute injury is the first step in reconstructing the established late deformity. The best management strategy for reconstruction of orbital hypertelorism is to avoid late complications by repairing these deformities early near the time of the original fractures. New technologies from computer-guided surgical planning and additive manufacturing technology produce passive fitting implants tailored for patient-specific needs.

Late Revision or Correction of Facial Trauma–Related Soft-Tissue Deformities

Kevin L. Rieck, W. Jonathan Fillmore, and Kyle S. Ettinger

Surgical approaches used in accessing the facial skeleton for fracture repair are often the same as or similar to those used for cosmetic enhancement of the face. Rarely does facial trauma result in injuries that do not in some way affect the facial soft-tissue envelope either directly or as sequelae of the surgical repair. Knowledge of both skeletal and facial soft-tissue anatomy is paramount to successful clinical outcomes. Facial soft-tissue deformities can arise that require specific evaluation and management for correction. This article focuses on revision and correction of these soft-tissue–related injuries secondary to facial trauma.

ORAL AND MAXILLOFACIAL SURGERY CLINICS OF NORTH AMERICA

RELATED INTEREST

Surgical Clinics of North America August 2012 (Vol. 92, No. 4)
Recent Advances and Future Directions in Trauma Care
Jeremy W. Cannon, MD, SM, *Editor*

THE CLINICS ARE NOW AVAILABLE ONLINE!
Access your subscription at:
www.theclinics.com

Preface

Trauma and Reconstruction: It is in Our DNA

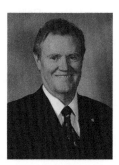

David S. Precious, CM, DDS, MSc, FRCDC, FRCS, Dhc
Editor

The management of facial trauma and subsequent reconstruction of associated residual stigmata is part of the very "DNA" of oral and maxillofacial surgery (OMS) in both substance and history. There is good reason for this. The best results of treatment of facial injuries require that the treating clinicians have not only a profound depth of knowledge of relevant functional anatomy, but also, in the case of pediatric and adolescent patients, an in-depth understanding and familiarity with facial growth and development.

Facial trauma is relatively common and can be serious. An American Association of Oral and Maxillofacial Surgeons' news release in 2013 states that nearly half of children 14 and under who are hospitalized for bicycle-related injuries are diagnosed with brain injuries, and helmets can reduce the risk of a head injury by 85% and brain injury by 88%. Nalliah et al, using the Nationwide Inpatient Sample of 39.88 million total admissions in the United States, estimated that 21,244

of these had primary procedure diagnoses germane to facial fractures.[1] "The total hospitalization charges were about $1.06 billion, and total hospitalization days was 93,808. About 80% of all hospitalizations occurred among men. The frequently occurring external causes of injuries leading to hospitalization for reduction in facial fractures include assault (36.5% of all hospitalizations), motor vehicle traffic accidents (16%), falls (15%), and other transportation accidents (3.5%). The frequently performed procedures were open reduction in mandibular fractures (52.2%), open reduction in facial fractures including those of orbital rim or wall (14.7%), closed reduction in mandibular fractures (12.1%), and open reduction in malar and zygomatic fractures (11.8%)."

It is my opinion that there are a number of reasons the management of facial fractures must remain an integral part of OMS. First (and, in my view, the most important), the quality of patient care is optimized, operating times are generally

Oral Maxillofacial Surg Clin N Am 25 (2013) ix–x
http://dx.doi.org/10.1016/j.coms.2013.07.012
1042-3699/13/$ – see front matter © 2013 Published by Elsevier Inc.

shorter, discharge rates from hospital (duration of stay) are enhanced, the requirement for revision surgery is minimized, and favorable long-term functional and esthetic results are the rule, not the exception to the rule. Second, this real expertise possessed and demonstrated by OMS serves as the foundation on which our specialty builds and maintains strong professional relationships with other important hospital colleagues, such as emergency room physicians, operating room nurses, surgical specialists, and, importantly, hospital administrators and government health authorities, to name only a few.

When taken as an ensemble, all of these facts reflect favorably on oral and maxillofacial surgeons in their role as providers of core specialty surgical services as part of the modern global health care team. Accordingly, this is one aspect of our scope of specialty that we must never abandon, if only for the sake of the patients that we serve.

David S. Precious, CM, DDS, MSc, FRCDC, FRCS, Dhc
Oral and Maxillofacial Surgery
Dalhousie University
5981 University Avenue, PO Box 15000
Halifax, Nova Scotia, Canada B3H 4R2

E-mail address:
d.s.precious@dal.ca

REFERENCE

1. Nalliah RP, Allareddy V, Kim MK, et al. Economics of facial fracture reductions in the United States over 12 months. Dent Traumatol 2013;29(2):115–20.

Systematic Assessment of the Patient with Facial Trauma

Deepak G. Krishnan, DDS

KEYWORDS

• Facial injury • Trauma • Assessment • Treatment • Intervention

KEY POINTS

• The systematic assessment of patients with facial injuries is the culmination of wisdom from trials and errors, audits of failures and successes, careful and mindful reflection of current practice, and a willingness to change.
• Emerging technology has positively impacted the practice of management of facial trauma.
• A systematic evaluation and physical examination of the trauma victim remain the gold standard and the first step toward effective care.

Traumatic injuries affect thousands of individuals and account for billions of dollars in direct and indirect expenditures annually. More than 9 people die every minute from injuries and violence according to the World Health Organization. In the last 2 decades or so, a system-wide improvement in assessment, resuscitation, and management of trauma has improved overall outcomes, thus reducing the impact of traumatic injuries on the society as a whole. Dissemination of this information from the developed to the developing world has had a positive impact.[1]

The committee on Trauma of the American College of Surgeons established Advanced Trauma Life Support (ATLS) in 1980 and has since developed, refined, and defined a system for accurate and systematic assessment of injury based on protocols. Approximately 25% to 30% of deaths caused by trauma can be prevented when this systematic and organized approach is used.[2–5]

The main goal of a systematic initial assessment of a trauma patient is to recognize the patient with severe life-threatening injuries, establish treatment priorities, and manage them efficiently and aggressively. Toward this, at presentation, all trauma injuries can generally be divided into the 3 following categories:

• Severe injuries: pose an immediate threat to life. These injuries represent more than 50% of traumatic deaths. These patients will present with a major disruption of their vital physiologic function and will benefit from acute intervention.
• Urgent injuries: these patients usually present with stable vital signs but have injuries grave enough that require an intervention, but are not usually life-threatening.
• Nonurgent injuries: most common injuries, fortunately. These patients do not present with an immediate threat to life, but generally require an intervention after a thorough evaluation and possibly observation.

ASSESSMENT PRINCIPLES IN TRAUMA

The principles in systematic assessment of the trauma patients as outlined by the ATLS protocols are as follows[1]:

• Preparation and transport
• Triage
• Primary survey (ABCDEs)
• Resuscitation
• Adjuncts to primary survey and resuscitation including monitoring and radiography

Disclosures: The author has nothing to disclose.
Department of Surgery, Division of Oral/Maxillofacial Surgery, University of Cincinnati College of Medicine, University of Cincinnati Medical Center, 200 Albert Sabin Way, ML 0461, Cincinnati, OH 45219, USA
E-mail address: gopaladk@ucmail.uc.edu

Oral Maxillofacial Surg Clin N Am 25 (2013) 537–544
http://dx.doi.org/10.1016/j.coms.2013.07.009
1042-3699/13/$ — see front matter Published by Elsevier Inc.

- Consideration for the need for patient transfer
- Secondary survey—head-to-toe evaluation, patient history
- Adjuncts to secondary survey—special investigations, such as computed tomographic (CT) scanning or angiography
- Continued postresuscitation monitoring and ongoing reevaluation
- Definitive care

Over time, this system of assessment and intervention has seen the development of trauma scores, identification of factors highly correlated with life-threatening injuries, identification of anatomic factors correlated with high mortality, simple reproducible systems of assessment, and development of protocols of treatment based on collective wisdom, experience, and observational studies. All aspects of treatment both clinical and medico-legal have had a positive evolution within this system. Despite this systematic reproducible methodology of assessment, the incidence of missed injuries following trauma continues to be reported as between 4% and 65%.

Although most maxillofacial injuries (other than penetrating wounds to neck or other life-threatening injuries) are identified and addressed following the primary survey and resuscitation efforts following the ATLS protocol, the same principles of this protocol are often applied in the early assessment and treatment planning of these injuries as well.[6]

Accordingly, facial injuries could be addressed based on the urgency to treat.

- Severe facial injuries: those that require immediate and often resuscitative treatment. These injuries could include injuries to the airway, injuries causing severe hemorrhage, cranial injuries including facial injuries, ophthalmologic traumatic emergencies, and severe facial soft tissue injuries, including special structures such as ducts or nerves whereby acute intervention would presumably yield better outcomes.
- Urgent facial injuries: facial injuries that can often wait a few hours until the trauma team has completed their primary survey and successful resuscitation. These injuries are often soft tissue injuries or contaminated wounds.
- Nonurgent facial injuries: injuries that may be addressed safely in a delayed manner, such as most facial fractures.

It is not the goal of this article to summarize the detailed ATLS protocol for the multisystem evaluation in a trauma patient. However, polytrauma patients often present with maxillofacial injuries that may or may not be readily apparent at primary survey. The ATLS approach is applied regardless of the anatomic presentation. For instance, a patient that presents with a gunshot wound to the face and neck would have his maxillofacial injuries addressed on presentation to the trauma bay according to ABCDEs of primary survey: Airway maintenance with cervical spine protection, Breathing and ventilation, Circulation with hemorrhage control, Disability and neurologic status, and Exposure, environmental control.

Similarly, a patient with multiple injuries, including long-bone injuries, sternal and possibly intracranial injuries, may not have a nasal fracture identified until the secondary survey is completed and adjunctive investigations are completed.

If the patient's maxillofacial injuries are secondary and the patient has been stabilized, it always helps to obtain a history of the presenting condition and a brief review of systems from either the patient or a representative.

The pneumonic AMPLE serves as an easy template while obtaining the history of the patient:

- A, Allergies
- M, Medications
- P, Pregnancy, past illnesses
- L, Last meal
- E, Events related to admission

In the alert patient, it also helps immensely to obtain a review of pertinent systems: continued headache, nausea, and vomiting following the injury may suggest neuro-trauma; double vision, blurry vision, headache, and so on might suggest ocular or orbital injuries; a clear discharge from nose or ears may suggest a base of skull fracture; complaints of lack of sensation on the face may indicate an underlying facial skeleton; a change in bite and limited mouth opening suggest a fracture of the maxilla or mandible, and hoarseness or stridor may suggest laryngeal fracture.

The systematic assessment of the patient with facial trauma should follow the same principles of primary survey, intervention, secondary survey, and definitive care.

AIRWAY WITH CERVICAL SPINE PROTECTION

Penetrating neck trauma, complex multiple facial soft tissue, and bony injuries of the maxillofacial skeleton necessitate immediate intervention to protect the anatomic airway. Foreign bodies, gastric content regurgitation, and tracheal or laryngeal fractures may not be dramatically apparent. Whenever possible, an endotracheal intubation is preferred and attempted and a surgical airway is sought only when the endotracheal intubation is not practical or possible.

Bilateral mandibular body or parasymphysis fractures causing a flail segment that is pulled back by the genial musculature in a supine patient can also cause airway embarrassment. Positioning the patient properly, and in dentate patients, simply bridling a wire between teeth stabilizing these segments may be simple and effective interventions that assist in keeping the airway patent.

A typical chin lift or jaw thrust maneuver may not be easy in patients with mandibular fractures. Pain, dislodgment of loose teeth into the airway, a new hematoma formation,and so forth may be risked when a broken jaw is manipulated.

Although laryngeal fractures are rare, pain, stridor, odynophagia, hoarseness, hemoptysis, and subcutaneous emphysema are the common presenting symptoms in these injuries. The presence of stridor and hemoptysis are suggestive of major injury. Early surgical intervention is recommended for all major injuries to ensure a good outcome.[7,8] Not all of these patients require airway intervention, but many do.

Examination for a direct airway injury or a major vascular injury in the neck is important before intubation in patients with facial trauma.

Endotracheal intubation is often performed orally with a rapid sequence tracheal intubation. Care must be taken to applying cricoid pressure to prevent aspiration.

When routine intubation is not possible because of profuse hemorrhage, severe edema, or other inability to intubate, a surgical airway must be established. In the emergency setting, in an adult, a cricothyroidotomy is preferred over a tracheotomy because of its ease of performance and reduced bleeding. Cricothyroidotomies however often need to be converted to formal tracheotomies for the prolonged airway maintenance in a nonacute setting.

Anesthesiologists may be reluctant to pass nasotracheal tubes for intubating patients with mid face fractures. This reluctance is based on the prudence of causing an inadvertent passage of tubes (nasogastric or suction catheters) intracranially through an undetected skull base fracture. A careful evaluation of the patient's CT scan for these skull base fractures are important to alleviate such unfounded fear.

Care must be taken in ensuring that the cervical spine is stable in these patients while attempting airway stabilization. Many epidemiologic studies have looked at the prevalence of cervical injury in patients with maxillofacial trauma. In the setting of an isolated mandible, nasal, orbital floor, malar/maxilla, or frontal/parietal bone fracture, cervical spine injury ranged from 4.9% to 8.0%. In the setting of 2 or more facial fractures, the prevalence of cervical spine injury ranged from 7.0% to 10.8%.[9] All patients that require airway intervention, regardless of concomitant maxillofacial injuries, must be assumed to have an undetected cervical injury, and care must be taken to avoid hyperflexion or hyperextension of the neck. Excessive movement of the neck can result in neuronal deficit and paralysis. The presence of distracting injuries, especially in the head and neck, can often lead to missed cervical injuries. A cervical collar is placed until a cervical injury is definitively cleared in secondary survey or during the hospital stay.

In patients with a cervical injury that has not been cleared, a trip to the operating theater for surgery of the maxillofacial region would mean that this cervical collar should be temporarily relieved, which is done by stabilizing the neck on either side with sandbags and taping the patient's head tightly to the operating table. Tilting the table is often needed instead of turning the patient's head, should that be required.

BREATHING AND VENTILATION

ATLS suggests exposure of the neck and chest and ensuring immobilization of the head and neck. Tracheal deviation, signs of airway obstruction, and subtle signs such as cyanosis of the lips suggestive of hypoperfusion are not to be missed. Transient brain hypoxia can cause severe secondary brain injury. Simple maneuvers such as stabilizing the mandible can improve breathing and ventilation, preventing long-term hypoxia-related neuro-deficits.

CIRCULATION WITH HEMORRHAGE CONTROL

As in primary survey for polysystem trauma, circulation is a priority only following stabilization of airway and ensuring breathing and ventilation.

Structures of the head and neck are extremely vascular and can often cause significant extravasation of blood that can contribute to shock. An assessment for bleeding should be systematic, complete, and thorough, addressing all evident and occult bleeding from vessels of the maxillofacial region.

Occult bleeding could occur acutely or in a chronic manner from blood vessels of the neck, especially at the base of the skull. The neck is divided into horizontal zones to help manage penetrating injuries (**Fig. 1**):

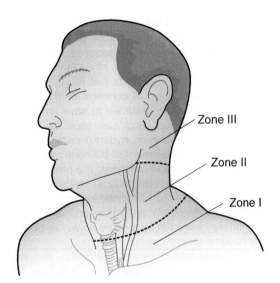

Fig. 1. Zones of the neck. (*From* Townsend CM, Beauchamp RD, Evers BM, et al. Sabiston textbook of surgery. Philadelphia: Elsevier; 2008. p. 490; with permission.)

- Zone 1: horizontal zone extending superiorly from sternal notch to cricoid cartilage.
- Zone 2: horizontal zone extending from cricoid cartilage to inferior border of mandible.
- Zone 3: horizontal zone from inferior border of mandible to base of skull.

Traditionally, the platysma had been considered the barrier for penetrating neck injuries. The standard of care was neck exploration for those injuries that penetrated the platysma. However, improvements in imaging technology, particularly CT angiography, have altered the management of patients with penetrating neck injuries. Although some centers still advocate routine exploration for all zone 2 neck injuries penetrating the platysma, many civilian centers in the United States have adopted a policy of selective exploration based on clinical and radiographic examination.[10]

Occasionally, closed tight spaces in the base of the skull, infratemporal region, and so forth, can cause delayed bleeding or formation of pseudo-aneurysms that can cause a shunting effect and hemodynamic instability. Interventional radiology techniques have again become the treatment modality of choice for these.[11]

Lacerations of the face are hard to miss and are often superficial and, if deep, readily accessible to repair and control of bleeding. Scalp lacerations, especially of the posterior scalp, are notoriously missed and, if left exposed to bleed or form large hematomas, can cause future infection. A systematic examination of the patient's scalp often reveals a missed occult source of serious bleeding that requires immediate attention. Large scalp lacerations could cause significant blood loss and must be stabilized expeditiously.[12] Repaired scalp lacerations often require a pressure dressing to prevent a hematoma in the acute after-repair phase. This is especially true in patients who are pharmacologically anti-coagulated or have a bleeding disorder.

Lacerations to the muscles of the cheek and tongue cause a significant amount of blood loss. Pressure application, primary repair, and temporary packing help to reduce the blood loss. Bleeding from broken ends of bones, especially of the mandible, can be stopped by pressure packing or by placing a bridle wire or temporary maxilla-mandibular fixation until the definitive treatment.

Epistaxis in facial trauma can impair visualization of the airway, impede a proper examination, cause obstruction of airway, and lead to shock and aspiration. Epistaxis can be fatal. Mid facial trauma can cause significant epistaxis that needs to be recognized and managed efficaciously. Most emergency rooms are equipped with packing materials for both anterior and posterior nose. Packs are at risk of being left in for prolonged periods of time and can cause serious infections. Posterior nasal packs can be inadvertently shoved into the cranial cavity if the patient has a skull base fracture. Often, the reduction of facial fractures will allow for control of the perinasal hemorrhage.

Proper visualization of facial lacerations often requires concomitant control of bleeding. Simple injections of local anesthetic solution with vasoconstrictors or pressure packing help stop most bleeding. In addition, small hand-held mono-polar cautery devices assist in hemostasis. Most emergency rooms also carry silver nitrate sticks that could be useful in intra-oral bleeding (**Fig. 2**).

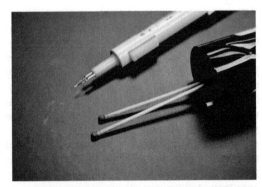

Fig. 2. Hand-held electro-cautery unit and silver nitrate sticks—good local measures for control of bleeding in the acute trauma setting.

DISABILITY (NEUROLOGIC AND FUNCTIONAL EVALUATION)

During the primary survey, a Glasgow Coma Scale establishes a baseline neurologic status for the patient. During the secondary survey and later, this is reassessed constantly using a simple *AVPU* method:

A—Patient is awake, alert, and *a*ppropriate
V—Patient responds to *v*oice
P—Patient responds to *p*ain
U—Patient is *u*nresponsive

Pupillary examination is a quick assessment of the cerebral function. Any changes in pupillary response indicates cerebral damage, optic nerve damage, or changes in intracranial pressure. In patients with facial trauma, the ocular examination goes beyond pupillary response. A palpation of the globe for pressure, hard or soft, and ruling out an afferent pupillary defect, is an imperative part of assessment.

Facial injuries often cause cranial nerve trauma. Facial lacerations can cause trauma to the facial nerve and its branches. Distal branches are often not amenable to repair but the larger proximal branches could be attempted to be primarily anastomosed with micro-neuro-surgical repair. Lacerations of the face lateral to a line drawn perpendicular to the outer canthus of the eye should be examined for parotid duct injury. Primary repair of this must be attempted on detection of the same.

EXPOSURE

Patients that present with a helmet (sports-related or motorcycle-related) should have the helmet removed while the head and neck are held in a neutral position using a 2-person technique. The American College of Surgeons provides a poster entitled, "Techniques of Helmet Removal from Injured Patients" (www.facs.org/trauma/publications/helmet.pdf).

Dentures and other removable appliances that may not have caught the attention of the resuscitating team may become evident on secondary survey by the practitioner assessing facial injuries. These devices must be removed, preserved, and could be potentially used in repair of fractures when patient is stable. Avulsed teeth must be accounted for. Aspiration should be considered a potential in the unconscious patient and the routine chest radiograph must be checked for aspirated teeth. Subluxed teeth must be considered a potential aspirate and must be stabilized or removed.

Patients that wear contact lenses must have them removed at examination. Prolonged retention of these in patients that are intubated or with low levels of consciousness can cause severe corneal injuries.

The skin of the scalp and face and neck must be inspected for embedded foreign bodies and dirt or debris. These foreign bodies could become future sources for infection.

SYSTEMATIC CLINICAL EXAMINATION OF THE FACIAL TRAUMA PATIENT

To minimize not finding injuries, and optimizing the assessment in a busy trauma bay, a systematic assessment pattern is recommended in examining patients with facial trauma. It is best to examine every patient the same way every time and record the findings comprehensively every time to ensure a thorough examination.

For purposes of the physical examination, the face and neck are divided into different zones and structures in each zone will be inspected and palpated and then correlated with findings of adjuncts such as a CT scan to formulate a diagnosis of the patient's injuries.

Soft Tissues

Injuries to the soft tissues of the face may be the most apparent trauma on the patient as the examiner begins assessment. The soft tissue wounds must be qualified and quantified by location, depth, and layers of involvement, involvement of vital or crucial structures, and treatment rendered. Superficial wounds often do not require any more treatment than cleansing and dressing. Deeper wounds might require repair with varying levels of complexity either in the emergency room setting or in an operation theater. Scalp wounds may be easy to miss in patients with thick hair or if the wounds are in the back of the head on a patient lying supine. Oral wounds require special attention; muscles may require reapproximation before mucosa. Bleeding control is an essential part of wound repair, as discussed earlier.

Often facial lacerations serve as excellent access for repair of underlying fractures. Definitive repair of such lacerations may be deferred until fracture repair; however, cleaning and decontaminating these wounds serve better results in the future.

Soft tissue injuries involving eyelids, external ear, lacrimal system, parotid duct, nerves, and vessels require specialized attention and repair. If the laceration is in the vicinity of such structures, careful attention must be paid during assessment to the patency and integrity of these structures.

Tetanus vaccination status should be checked and dosing regimen followed.

Frontal Region

Inspection
The forehead and frontal region are inspected for lacerations, contusions, or step deformities. In an awake and alert patient, loss of sensation of the skin over the forehead must be checked. In patients with thick hair, lacerations in the scalp or within the eyebrows must be inspected. Previous injuries such as scars should also be inspected.

Palpation
Obvious or subtle step deformities should be palpated. In an awake or responsive patient, pain on palpation should be checked as well as for crepitus.

Ear

Inspection
Obvious signs of lacerations or deformities should be inspected and also signs of previous injuries, such as a cauliflower ear deformity. A speculum examination following cleaning of the external auditory canal for blood, debris, and cerumen will allow for inspection of the tympanic membrane. Hemorrhage or cerebrospinal fluid (CSF) otorrhea may indicate base of skull or temporal bone fractures. Integrity of the tympanic membrane is important to record.

Battle sign or postauricular ecchymosis may be suggestive of temporal or skull base fractures (**Fig. 3**).

Formal conductive and neurosensory examination may not be practical in a busy trauma bay. However, an ear examination is not complete without at least a cursory whispering test and loss of hearing may indicate cranial nerve VIII damage.

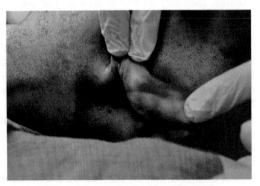

Fig. 3. Battle's sign: postauricular ecchymosis.

Eyes and Orbit

Inspection
Inspection of the orbit and the eyes can be challenging in patients with facial injuries. Early edema in the peri-orbital area and neurologic impairment may make a thorough examination difficult.

The inspection of position and alignment of eyes must be grossly examined. Increased orbital volume from orbital fractures can cause the sinking of the contents of the orbit, causing enophthalmos and vertical dystopia. An increase in orbital volume can cause exophthalmos, suggestive of a foreign body or a retrobulbar hematoma. Edema might obscure these findings in an acute setting.

The eyelids should be inspected for evident lacerations, or previous scarring, in addition to ectropion, entropion, or ptosis. Inspection of the conjunctiva and sclera will disclose conjunctivitis, chemosis, and subconjunctival hemorrhage, all indicatiing orbital and/or ocular trauma. In addition, blood in the anterior chamber of the eye or hyphema is an important finding.

Inspection of the pupils is important to test due to the pathways involved. They are innervated by both the sympathetic and the parasympathetic systems and can give a general indication of the neurologic condition. Normal pupillary response and reactivity to light tests sensory and motor function of the eyes. Afferent pupillary defects or Marcus Gunn pupil is tested with the swinging flashlight test. Pupillary size is noted. Miosis refers to pupillary diameter less than 2 mm and mydriasis or a "blown pupil" may be suggestive of orbital trauma, head injury, or drugs. Anisocoria or unequal pupillary diameter may be suggestive of actual globe injury. Epiphora in the medial canthus may suggest injury or disruption of the lacrimal drainage apparatus.

In patients who are awake and responsive to commands, it helps to check range of motion of the extraocular muscles of the eyes. Extraocular muscles are tested for movement in an H pattern. Examination would reveal entrapment of muscles in between fracture fragments of the orbit. In addition to causing diplopia, prolonged entrapment may lead to necrosis and permanent mobility restriction.

Palpation
Palpation of the globes for pressure of the contents can often reveal retro-bulbar hematoma, or other causes for proptosis. Palpation of the orbital rims will elicit step deformities suggestive of fracture and displacement of the orbital skeleton. Edema may confound findings initially and, as with anything in trauma, repeated examination

and secondary surveys may help unfold injuries that were not apparent at first presentation.

Naso-orbito-ethmoid Region

The naso-orbito-ethmoid (NOE) region must be included in the examination, right after examining the eyes and orbits.

Inspection

Peri-orbital ecchymosis and circumorbital edema giving the patient an appearance of raccoon eyes is a hallmark of NOE fractures. Subconjunctival hemorrhage is often seen as well. NOE fractures with displacement can cause depression of the nasal projection. Disruption of the medial canthal ligament attachments can cause telecanthus and blunting of the medial palpebral fissures. Intercanthal distance measurement is an imperative part of the examination. Racial differences in norms should be considered for this measurement but, in general, the intercanthal distance should be about 50% of the interpupillary distance. Loss of volume of the orbit from the medial orbital/ethmoid fractures can cause enophthalmos.

Palpation

Mobility and crepitus of the NOE complex is the hallmark of this fracture. Mobility may be tested with an instrument inserted in the nose with its tip placed deep to the medial orbital area and the fingers and thumbs of the other hand supporting the NOE region. Moving the instrument will then generate movement of the medial canthal and NOE complex. In addition, a "bowstring" test can elicit movement of medial tendon when tugging on the lateral canthal tendon.

Nasal Skeleton

The nasal skeleton would be the next logical area on the face to examine. Nasal complex requires good lighting, suction, and a nasal speculum to illuminate and examine properly.

Inspection

Obvious deformities and lacerations are noted; the depth of these lacerations must be examined, and involvement of cartilage must be noted. Nasal deformities must be examined facing the patient, from a worm's eye view and from a bird's eye view. Intranasal examination must be performed after cleaning out dried blood, CSF, and debris, with good lighting and using a nasal speculum. Intranasal examination should focus on obvious lacerations, septal fractures, perforations or hematomas, and sources of bleeding. Septal hematomas require early recognition and management. These septal hematomas can detach the perichondrium from the septal cartilage, thus strangulating its blood supply, and can possibly cause septal necrosis, leading to loss of septal support and resulting in a saddle nose esthetic deformity. A simple lance and drain or needle decompression with or without packing or splinting will help manage this problem when identified. Active CSF rhinorrhea must be examined when base of skull fractures are suspected.

Palpation

Nasal bones must be palpated for obvious mobility and crepitus.

Zygomatic o-maxillary Complex

Inspection

Peri-orbital edema and ecchymosis, obvious facial asymmetry, and malar depression with or without difficulty to open the mandible wide may be hallmarks of zygomatico-maxillary complex fractures. Acute edema may obscure malar flattening. Malar depression and asymmetry may be more evident when examined from a bird's eye view as opposed to frontal view.

Palpation

Step deformities at the orbital rim may be part of the zygomatico-maxillary complex fracture. Examination from the bird's eye view along with palpation of the arches may demonstrate malar depression and asymmetry more readily, even in the face of mild to moderate edema of the region.

Maxillo-mandibular Structures

Oral examination and examination of the maxilla, mandible, and dento-alveolar structures should be performed last in the systematic evaluation to avoid contamination of saliva to other facial wounds.

Inspection

Obvious lacerations in the peri-oral region or within the oral cavity must be examined for debris, contaminants, and loose teeth. In awake and responsive patients, the maximum incisal opening should be checked with the patient opening voluntarily; any deviations while opening may be suggestive of location of fractures of the mandible.

Ecchymosis in the buccal vestibules or floor of the mouth often indicates a fracture of a bone nearby.

Evaluation of the occlusion is performed with care and can often be suggestive of the location of the fracture as well, which could be a challenge in orally intubated patients.

Palpation

Palpation for step deformities and obvious tenderness and mobility indicate fractures. Mobility of the maxillary complex indicates a disjunction of the maxilla from the remaining facial skeleton. Depending on the level of this disjunction, the area of mobility may vary. For instance, in Le Fort I level fractures, only the dento-alveolar segments of the maxilla may elicit mobility, whereas in Le Fort II and III level fractures, the area of mobility would be higher up on the face according to the pattern of fracture sustained. It is useful to Gently support the nasal complex while checking for mobility of the maxilla. Manual stretching of the mandible may cause coronoid impingement on a displaced zygomatic arch.

Correlating Physical Examination to Radiographic Findings

The gold standard for radiographic evaluation of facial injuries has become the helical CT with its multiplanar reconstructions. It has largely replaced single-view plain radiographs in almost all instances except perhaps the isolated mandible fracture in an ambulatory patient. The added ability to obtain a 3-dimensional reformatted image not only helps to plan treatment but also to obtain stereolithographic models from 3-dimensional printing and virtual surgical planning. Advanced imaging technology now allows better resolution, rapid scanning time, and added ability to use navigation and involves lesser radiation.

CT, however, remains an adjunct to diagnosis and is never to be replaced by the act of the systematic physical examination and assessment. Correlation of the findings of the physical examination with the radiographic assessment would lead to an accurate diagnosis and assistance with treatment planning.

Axial, coronal, and sagittal views on a CT scan of the face all provide different perspectives of the same injury. In addition, CT angiography has an increased role in both diagnosis and management of maxillofacial vascular injuries, as discussed earlier.

SUMMARY

The systematic assessment of the patient with facial injuries as practiced today is the culmination of the collective wisdom from trials and errors, audits of failures and successes, careful and mindful reflection of current practice, and a willingness to change. Emerging technology has positively impacted the practice of management of facial trauma. Regardless, a systematic evaluation and physical examination of the trauma victim remain the gold standard and the first step toward effective care.

REFERENCES

1. Advanced trauma life support Student Course Manual. 9th edition. Chicago: American College of Surgeons; 2012.
2. Cales RH, Trunkey DD. Preventable trauma deaths. A review of trauma care systems development. JAMA 1985;254(8):1059–63.
3. Teixeira PG, Inaba K, Hadjizacharia P, et al. Preventable or potentially preventable mortality at a mature trauma center. J Trauma 2007;63(6):1338–46 [discussion: 1346–7].
4. Thomson CB, Greaves I. Missed injury and the tertiary trauma survey. Injury 2008;9(1):107–14.
5. Brooks A, Holroyd B, Riley B. Missed injury in major trauma patients. Injury 2004;35(4):407–10.
6. Cunningham LL Jr, Khader R. Early assessment and treatment planning of the maxillofacial trauma patient in Oral and Maxillofacial Trauma. Fonseca, Walker, Barber, Powers, Frost. 4th edition. Elsevier; 2013.
7. Kim JP, Cho SJ, Son HY, et al. Analysis of clinical feature and management of laryngeal fracture: recent 22 case review. Yonsei Med J 2012;53(5):992–8.
8. Akhtar S, Awan S. Laryngotracheal trauma: its management and Sequelae. J Pak Med Assoc 2008;58(5):241–3.
9. Mulligan RP, Mahabir RC. The prevalence of cervical spine injury, head injury, or both with isolated and multiple craniomaxillofacial fractures. Plast Reconstr Surg 2010;126(5):1647–51.
10. Bell RB, Osborn T, Dierks EJ, et al. Management of penetrating neck injuries: a new paradigm for civilian trauma. J Oral Maxillofac Surg 2007;65(4):691–705.
11. Krishnan DG, Marashi A, Malik A. Pseudoaneurysm of internal maxillary artery secondary to gunshot wound managed by endovascular technique. J Oral Maxillofac Surg 2004;2(4):500–2.
12. Turnage B, Maull KI. Scalp laceration: an obvious 'occult' cause of shock. South Med J 2000;93(3):265–6.

Responsible and Prudent Imaging in the Diagnosis and Management of Facial Fractures

Savannah Gelesko, DDS, MD[a],*,
Michael R. Markiewicz, DDS, MPH, MD[a],
R. Bryan Bell, DDS, MD[b,c,d]

KEYWORDS

- Maxillofacial trauma • Computer planning • Navigation • Computer-aided surgery • Facial fracture

KEY POINTS

- Every effort should be made to optimize treatment outcome during the initial operative treatment.
- Judicious use of computed tomographic (CT) imaging is required, tempered by the potential risks associated with repeated radiation exposure.
- Until optimal radiation thresholds are established, the surgeon must use their best judgment, in consultation with an informed patient, to obtain enough preoperative, intraoperative, and postoperative data.
- Computer-aided surgery, utilizing preoperative planning, intraoperative navigation, and intraoperative CT scanning, appears to favorably improve outcomes in the treatment of complex posttraumatic craniomaxillofacial deformities.

INTRODUCTION

The past century has seen a dramatic change in the type, quality, and method of diagnostic imaging techniques used for craniomaxillofacial traumatic injuries. This article systematically reviews the current standard of care in imaging considerations for the diagnosis and management of craniomaxillofacial trauma. In addition, injury-specific imaging techniques and options for computer-aided surgery as related to craniomaxillofacial trauma are reviewed, including preoperative planning, intraoperative navigation, and intraoperative computed tomography (CT) scanning. Specific imaging considerations by anatomic region include frontal sinus fractures, temporal bone fractures, midfacial fractures, mandible fractures, laryngotracheal injuries, and vascular injuries. Imaging considerations in the pediatric trauma patient are also discussed. Responsible postoperative imaging as it relates to facial trauma management and outcomes assessment is reviewed.

Disclosures: R.B. Bell is a consultant for Stryker.
Conflicts of interest: none.
[a] Department of Oral and Maxillofacial Surgery, Oregon Health and Science University, Mail code: SDOMS, 611 Southwest Campus Drive, Portland, OR 97239, USA; [b] Oral, Head and Neck Cancer Program and Clinic, Providence Cancer Center, Providence Portland Medical Center, 4805 Northeast Glisan Street, Suite 6N50, Portland, OR 97213, USA; [c] Trauma Service/Oral and Maxillofacial Surgery Service, Legacy Emanuel Medical Center, 2801 North Gantenbein Avenue, Portland, OR 97227, USA; [d] Oregon Health and Science University, Mail code: SDOMS, 611 Southwest Campus Drive, Portland, OR 97239, USA
* Corresponding author. Department of Oral and Maxillofacial Surgery, Oregon Health and Science University, Mail code: SDOMS, 611 Southwest Campus Drive, Portland, OR 97239.
E-mail address: gelesko@ohsu.edu

Oral Maxillofacial Surg Clin N Am 25 (2013) 545–560
http://dx.doi.org/10.1016/j.coms.2013.07.001
1042-3699/13/$ – see front matter © 2013 Published by Elsevier Inc

COMPUTER-AIDED SURGERY

Virtual, or computer-aided, surgery encompasses 3 forms of computer-assistance for the maxillofacial surgeon: (1) presurgical planning, (2) intraoperative navigation, and (3) intraoperative CT scanning.

Virtual surgery can be divided into 4 broad phases: (1) data acquisition phase, (2) planning phase, (3) surgical phase, and (4) assessment phase. These phases are modified based on which maxillofacial procedures are being performed. In this article, each phase is reviewed with regard to the treatment of maxillofacial trauma. A thorough discussion on implementing virtual surgery into practice with a step-by-step case review of a panfacial trauma case has recently been described by our institution.[1]

Data Acquisition Phase

A careful clinical examination is an essential portion of the data acquisition phase, because the bony evaluation must be balanced with the soft tissue, focusing on the character of the tissue and any traumatic defects, as well as the dentition, which plays a large role in establishing final occlusion and reduction of most maxillofacial injuries involving the maxilla and mandible. In terms of imaging for maxillofacial trauma, high-resolution CT (HRCT) scanning is imperative, because low-resolution CT scans offer a poor representation of the thin-walled orbits and paranasal sinuses. The HRCT scan data are taken in DICOM (digital information and communications in medicine) format. These DICOM data are then imported into a proprietary CAD-CAM (computer-aided design, computer-aided manufacturing) software program. The investigators recommend choosing a proprietary software program that allows for back-conversion, discussed later, which is essentially the opposite of the initial data translation from DICOM format to the virtual proprietary software format.

Presurgical Planning Phase

The presurgical planning phase consists of analyzing the newly formatted CT data in 3 dimensions, segmenting out the traumatized portions of the facial skeleton, and using the mirror image of the unaffected side to overlay the defected portions of the facial skeleton. The planning phase differs greatly depending on the portions of the maxillofacial skeleton that are deformed and the type of reconstruction planned.[2] For instance, in orbital fractures a critical measure of successful reconstruction is restoration of orbital volume, whereas in isolated zygomaticomaxillary complex fractures, successful reconstruction is largely based on restoration of bizygomatic width and facial projection, and in comminuted mandibular fractures, restoration of dental occlusion as well as mandibular width are key goals. In general, the mirror image of the unaffected side, or standardized measurements, can be used to segment out the fractured portions of the facial skeleton and plan the reconstruction. This portion of the surgical planning can either be performed by the surgeon, or as is our preference, a Web meeting can be set up with the proprietary software company, in which a computer planning specialist assists the surgeon in manipulating the CT data for the planned reconstruction. Once the surgical plan is finalized, the proprietary software data plan should be back-converted. Back-conversion specifically refers to translating the surgical data plan created by the proprietary software back to the standard DICOM format. This DICOM format may then be viewed on work stations not loaded with the proprietary software, and it allows interoperability between the planning software and intraoperative navigation systems.

Surgical Phase

During the surgical phase, the virtual surgical plan is translated to the patient using a combination of stereolithographic models, cutting guide stents, or intraoperative navigation (**Fig. 1**). Stereolithographic models are particularly useful for severely comminuted fractures and panfacial fractures, because they allow for preoperative plate bending and decreased time in the operating room. Cutting guide stents in maxillofacial trauma surgery are most useful in the secondary reconstruction of posttraumatic deformities, and less useful in the acute setting, in which the bones can still be mobilized for adequate reduction. Intraoperative navigation is particularly useful for real-time assessment of facial width and projection when repairing zygomaticomaxillary complex fractures, and for evaluation of plate placement during repair of orbital floor and medial orbital wall fractures.[3]

Assessment Phase

The assessment phase has historically consisted of clinical examination with or without conventional postoperative CT imaging. Now, this phase can begin in the operating room with an intraoperative CT scan verifying the accuracy of the presurgical plan compared with the surgical result, and allowing for immediate surgical modification if indicated. Intraoperative clinical assessment of facial

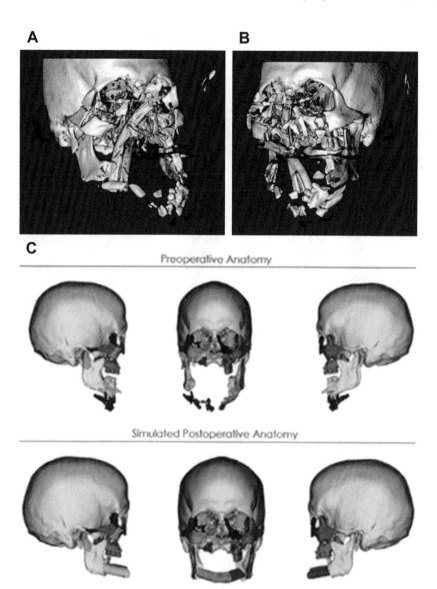

Fig. 1. Computer planning, navigation, and intraoperative CT scan to aid in treatment of a self-inflicted facial gunshot wound: (*A, B*) three-dimensional (3D) reconstruction of initial high-resolution CT scan taken in DICOM (digital information and communications in medicine) format on initial presentation. (*C*) 3D CT scan after being imported into the proprietary software with segmentation of the fractured preoperative anatomy, and simulated fibular free flap reconstruction. (*D*) Mandibular cutting guides. (*E*) Fibular cutting guides. (*F*) Simulated fibular reconstruction of the mandible with custom plate. (*G*) Preoperative planning for second-phase surgery with preoperative fibular reconstruction of mandible and simulated fibular reconstruction of the maxilla.

projection, facial width, and orbital volume in severely displaced fractures is difficult given the typical swelling and soft tissue deformities that accompany severe panfacial and midfacial fractures. The authors have found intraoperative CT imaging to be particularly useful in the treatment of panfacial fractures, naso-orbitoethmoid fractures, zygomaticomaxillary complex fractures, and orbital fractures (**Fig. 2**).

IMAGING CONSIDERATIONS BY ANATOMIC REGION

Frontal Sinus and Frontobasilar Skull Fractures

Mechanism of injury

Frontal sinus fractures occur as a result of high-velocity blunt trauma to the frontal bone, most commonly from motor vehicle collisions. More than one-third of patients with frontal sinus fractures are likely to have concomitant intracranial

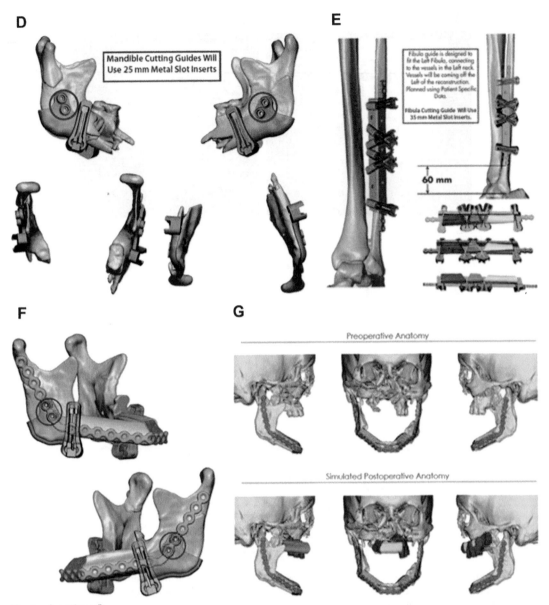

D

Mandible Cutting Guides Will Use 25 mm Metal Slot Inserts

E

Fibula guide is designed to fit the Left Fibula, connecting to the vessels in the Left neck. Vessels will be coming off the Left of the reconstruction. Planned using Patient Specific Data.

Fibula Cutting Guide Will Use 35 mm Metal Slot Inserts.

60 mm

F

G

Preoperative Anatomy

Simulated Postoperative Anatomy

Fig. 1. (*continued*)

injury.[4–6] Most of these patients have already been evaluated by the trauma team and received a head and maxillofacial CT scan before the maxillofacial surgeon is consulted.[7]

Clinical signs and symptoms

Except frontal depression with severe anterior table fractures, and leak of cerebrospinal fluid (CSF) with posterior table fractures, clinical signs of frontal sinus injury may not be apparent until later.

Diagnostic imaging

Fracture to the upper face and midface are poorly diagnosed by plain films. The CT scan should be evaluated in the axial views for identification of anterior and posterior frontal sinus fractures, and in the coronal and sagittal views for evaluation of the orbital apex and frontonasal ducts. Three-dimensional CT scan reconstruction is helpful and allows for evaluation of basilar skull fractures from all angles. The clear sinus sign, or absence of fluid in any paranasal sinus cavity, is a reliable indicator to exclude fracture of the sinus wall.[7–13] However, presence of fluid does not indicate fracture, because bleeding can result from injury to the vascular mucoperiosteum lining the sinus walls. Intraoperative CT scanning can be used to confirm minimally invasive reduction of minor anterior table

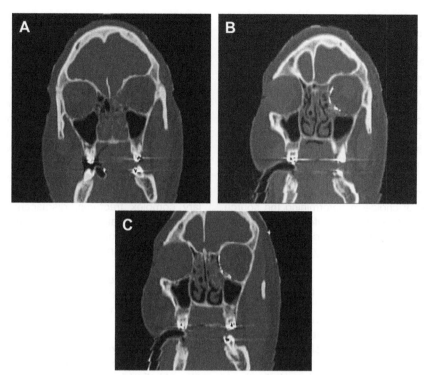

Fig. 2. Medial orbital wall fracture revision after intraoperative CT scan. (*A*) Preoperative CT taken in operating room before surgery, for registration purposes. (*B*) Intraoperative CT taken to assess repair of medial orbital wall showing plate within the orbit adjacent to the medial rectus. (*C*) Intraoperative CT after revision of the medial orbital plate showing excellent adaptation to the remaining orbital walls. The scan is slightly angled, but shows good contour of the repaired medial orbital wall.

fractures.[1,14] Imaging considerations for CSF leaks are discussed later.

Treatment overview

Careful evaluation of the CT scan with regards to frontonasal outflow tract injury, anterior versus posterior table fracture, and amount of displacement, is critical in treatment planning and determination of the need for neurosurgical support.[15] Fractures isolated to the anterior table and nasoethmoid region may be managed by the maxillofacial surgeon alone.[16] Intraoperative CT scanning is useful to confirm adequate reduction, particularly in cases when plating is not used. Fractures involving the posterior table, orbital roof, and sphenoidal-parasellar are commonly associated with dural tears and significant neurologic injury, necessitating a team approach with the neurologic surgeon if transfrontal access is planned.[17]

Temporal Bone Fractures

Mechanism of injury

Temporal bone fractures most commonly result from high-energy blunt trauma to the temporoparietal region. They are often found incidentally in combination with other facial and cranial injuries.[18]

Traumatic temporal bone injuries are typically unilateral, and can result in temporal bone fracture, unilateral labyrinthitis, or exacerbation of already present temporal bone lesions.[19]

Clinical signs and symptoms

Hearing loss, of both sensorineural and conductive origin, vertigo, balance disturbance, dizziness, tinnitus, hemorrhagic otorrhea, hemotympanum, facial weakness, and Battle sign are common findings in temporal bone injury.[4] Facial nerve weakness and CSF rhinorrhea or otorrhea are of particular importance because they are highly associated with otic capsule disruption and possible need for surgical intervention, depending on timing of clinical course.[20]

Diagnostic imaging

Proper evaluation requires high-resolution specific temporal bone CT scanning, with cuts less than or equal to 1.5 mm, which is often obtained after the patient has been stabilized and not in the acute trauma setting.[4,8,9,11–13,15] Evaluation by magnetic resonance imaging (MRI) is indicated only in cases of facial nerve injury not explained by HRCT, or for evaluation of intracranial contents in preparation for surgical intervention.[21] Radiographic description of bone fractures was historically described as a combination of either longitudinal, transverse, or mixed, then later oblique based on fracture geometry.[22] However, more clinically useful radiographic descriptions have since been proposed, including otic capsule (cochlear and vestibular system)–sparing versus otic capsule–violating fractures, petrous versus nonpetrous fractures, and subclassifications of mastoid or middle ear involvement.[23,24] Persistent CSF leaks requiring surgical intervention necessitate locating the source of the leak. HRCT scanning without intrathecal contrast has repeatedly proved to be the imaging of choice in determining the source location of CSF leakage. It is preferred over CT cisternography, magnetic resonance cisternography, and radionuclide cisternography.[5,25,26]

Treatment overview

Immediate onset of facial nerve paralysis typically requires surgical intervention.[20] Temporal bone fracture–associated CSF fistulas most often resolve with conservative treatment. Refractory cases may require lumbar drainage or surgical intervention.[27] Hearing loss necessitates an audiology evaluation.[18] Other than these indications, surgical management is often unnecessary.

Midfacial Fractures

Mechanism of injury

Midfacial fractures can occur as a result of blunt or penetrating facial trauma from motor vehicle accidents, gunshot wounds, assault, or falls. A detailed history including whether there was penetration of glass or other fragments into the wound, whether the patient was wearing eyewear at the time of injury, and the patient's baseline vision are key historical points.[28]

Clinical signs and symptoms

Severe and comminuted midfacial trauma results in a rounded, flattened face with increase of the bizygomatic width and medial canthal distance, and depression of the malar eminences and nasal complex. Minor midfacial trauma can often be localized based on clinical examination with maxillary mobility pointing to LeFort fracture; severe subconjunctival hemorrhage, hyphema, poor ocular motility, and change in visual acuity are suggestive of orbital fractures; malar and temporal depression are suggestive of zygomaticomaxillary complex fractures; epistaxis and nasal crepitus are suggestive of nasal fractures.

Diagnostic imaging

Midfacial fractures are included in 1 section of this article, because the recommended initial CT imaging is the same for all midfacial fractures except isolated nasal fractures, which do not always require imaging.[29]

In orbital fractures, key findings on coronal and sagittal cuts include orbital contents in the ethmoid or maxillary sinuses for medial orbital wall and orbital floor fractures, respectively. Intraocular air is diagnostic of disturbance of the orbital wall.[28] Other findings to look for in orbital fractures are entrapment of the inferior rectus, abnormal ocular contour, and fracture of the optic canal.[30] Axial cuts are valuable for assessing facial projection and width in zygomaticomaxillary complex fractures, displacement in nasal fractures, medial canthal tendon position in naso-orbitoethmoid fractures, and orbital contents in the ethmoid sinuses in medial orbital wall fractures.[31]

Preoperative computer planning, intraoperative navigation, and intraoperative CT scans are particularly useful in the treatment of severe midfacial fractures.[3,32]

Treatment overview

Treatment of naso-orbitoethmoid fractures, displaced LeFort fractures, and zygomaticomaxillary fractures typically require treatment with open reduction and internal fixation (ORIF) within 1 week of injury. The decision for orbital fracture repair versus clinical monitoring is based on the presence or absence of globe injury, or damage to the optic nerve or extraocular muscles, the amount of orbital contents in the adjacent paranasal sinus, and the presence or absence of enophthalmos, disturbances of ocular motility, and visual disturbance. Treatment options for nasal fractures include no treatment, early treatment with closed reduction, and late treatment with open reduction.

Mandibular Fractures

Mechanism of injury

Mandibular fractures occur secondary to direct or indirect facial injury, including motor vehicle accidents, falls, sports, and assaults with blunt weapons or guns. Close to half of all patients with maxillofacial injuries have concomitant mandibular fractures.[33]

Clinical signs and symptoms

Findings in patients with mandibular fractures include malocclusion, dentoalveolar fractures, ecchymosis and tenderness of the soft tissue and gingiva adjacent to the fracture, paresthesia in the distribution of the mental nerve, and airway compromise in cases of bilateral and severely comminuted mandibular fractures.

Diagnostic imaging

Historically, plain film series were used to diagnose mandibular fractures and included the following views: Towne (for condylar and subcondylar fractures), bilateral lateral oblique (for condylar, subcondylar, coronoid, ramus, angle, and proximal body fractures), posteroanterior (PA) (for parasymphysis fractures), and sometimes lateral (for posterior borders of the condylar neck, ramus, angle, and inferior mandibular borders).[34]

Some investigators have found the combination of panoramic radiographs and PA plain films to be sufficient for evaluation and treatment of mandibular fractures.[29] However, others recommend CT scanning of all patients with mandibular fractures.[35] CT imaging is necessary for the proper evaluation of lower facial width in cases of secondary reconstruction of maxillofacial trauma.[36] Also, if an initial panoramic radiograph shows a midline mandibular fracture, close clinical examination and CT imaging have been recommended to rule out genial tubercle fracture.[37] Some reports have suggested MRI in the acute setting to diagnose temporomandibular disk morphology and position in certain condylar fractures.[38,39]

We have found intraoperative CT scanning to be particularly useful for the evaluation of mandibular width and splay after ORIF of bilateral mandibular fractures and symphysis fractures (**Fig. 3**). In most cases, there are at least 2 fractures in any fractured mandible, so the surgeon should carefully evaluate for fractures contralateral to the site of impact.[29]

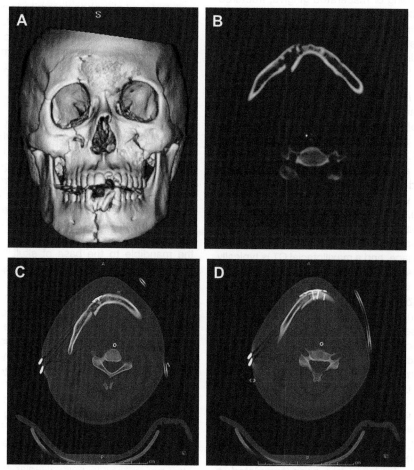

Fig. 3. Outcome assessment for mandibular fracture ORIF using intraoperative CT. (*A*) Preoperative three-dimensional CT scan showing mandible, dentoalveolar, and bilateral LeFort fractures. (*B*) Preoperative CT showing wide mandibular splay. (*C*) Intraoperative CT scan taken after ORIF showing open lingual cortex and insufficient reduction of lingual cortex. Clinically, the patient had good boney reduction, but intraoperative CT scan showed a wide open lingual cortex, thus allowing for immediate correction. (*D*) Intraoperative CT scan taken after ORIF was repeated showing good reduction of the lingual cortex, and thus decreased mandibular splay.

Treatment overview

Treatment options for mandibular fractures vary based on location of the fracture, morphology of the mandible, and severity of injury. They include closed reduction, ORIF, external fixation, and osteocutaneous grafting.

Dentoalveolar Fractures

Mechanism of injury

Dentoalveolar trauma may present in isolation, resulting from lower-velocity blunt facial trauma to the anterior teeth, or in combination with other facial fractures.[40]

Clinical signs and symptoms

Patients with isolated dentoalveolar trauma often present to the dentist or oral and maxillofacial surgeon in an outpatient setting. Clinical signs include bleeding or macerated gingiva, fractured teeth, mobile alveolar segments, and malocclusion. Multiple dentoalveolar trauma classification systems have been described, based both on clinical examination and radiographic findings.[41]

Diagnostic imaging

Diagnosis and treatment planning for these patients can often be accomplished with the use of panoramic and periapical radiographs. Cone-beam CT (CBCT) scanning has been suggested as a useful adjunct in treatment planning for patients with dentoalveolar fractures who would like to proceed with implant placement in the outpatient setting.[42] However, CBCT is not used in the acute hospital setting, because the patient with acute trauma requires head CT to rule out intracranial hemorrhage, and a maxillofacial CT is typically added to the head CT to diagnose facial fractures. In patients with isolated dentoalveolar fractures, CBCT may be combined with dental periapical radiographs in the acute setting to decrease the radiation dose to the patient. Regardless of the imaging technique used, the surgeon should check clinically or radiographically for retained dental fragments in adjacent damaged soft tissues, particularly the lips.

Treatment overview

In the acute setting, most efforts consist of preserving the teeth to maintain as much alveolar bone as possible. After acute management of dentoalveolar injury has been completed, a general dentist should follow the patient to assess for continued tooth viability. Many of these patients require future extractions and implant placement by the oral and maxillofacial surgeon.

Laryngotracheal Injuries

Mechanism of injury

Laryngotracheal injuries are uncommon but can result in significant airway compromise and death if untreated. The most common cause is blunt trauma associated with motor vehicle collisions or sporting injuries, followed by falls and hanging, and less commonly caused by penetrating neck injuries such as gunshot and stab wounds. They are almost always associated with concurrent maxillofacial trauma.[12,43–46]

Clinical signs and symptoms

Clinical signs can vary widely depending on the structures injured, including inspiratory stridor with epiglottic hematoma, dysphagia and aspiration with epiglottic avulsion, severe painful dysphagia with hyoid fracture, hoarseness in glottic injuries with thyroid cartilage fractures, and profound airway compromise in subglottic injuries.[5,9,12,13,25,45–47] Palpable subcutaneous neck emphysema or crepitus may result from a break in the continuity of the airway. These signs along with neck ecchymosis should heighten suspicion for a laryngotracheal injury.[9,12,13,45,46,48,49]

Diagnostic imaging

Once airway stabilization by endotracheal intubation or tracheostomy is complete, the anatomic location of the injury involved should be defined. The location of neck trauma should be defined by its anatomic zone. Zone 1 extends from the level of the clavicles and sternal notch at the thoracic inlet to the cricoid cartilage. Zone 2 extends from the level of the cricoid cartilage to the angle of the mandible. Zone 3 extends from the angle of the mandible to the base of skull.[50] Previously, mandatory endoscopy and angiography for zone 1 and 3 penetrations, and mandatory neck exploration for zone 2 injuries was recommended. CT imaging is the radiographic method of choice, because it allows for anatomic evaluation of the entire laryngotracheal cartilaginous framework. For associated penetrating neck injury or if there is any suspicion of blunt vascular injury CT angiography (CTA) should be performed.[51] Fiber-optic nasopharyngoscopy is often limited by edema, and so, direct laryngoscopy under general anesthesia and rigid esophagoscopy are often necessary for full clinical evaluation of the aerodigestive tract.[47] Given the potential instability of the trachea after trauma, prophylactic tracheostomy may be advised before any endoscopy is performed.

Treatment overview

The treatment spectrum has a wide range: no intervention, advanced airway placement, ORIF, and endolaryngeal stent placement. Injury to the aerodigestive tract may be repaired at the time of endoscopic evaluation or neck exploration.

Traumatic Vascular Injuries

Mechanism of injury
Traumatic vascular injuries are uncommon in maxillofacial traumatic injuries, but must be considered when clinical examination and noninterventional imaging are not diagnostic and clinical suspicion for vascular injury exists. Traumatic vascular injuries of the head and neck typically occur secondary to penetrating neck trauma or high-velocity maxillofacial trauma. In all cases, there is a problem with the vascular wall, ranging from intimal damage, to vessel dissection, to pseudoaneurysm, to complete vessel wall rupture, arteriovenous fistula, or vessel transection.[52]

Clinical signs and symptoms
Traumatic vascular injuries of the head and neck include dissections, aneurysms, arteriovenous malformations, and direct vascular injury from penetrating wounds. These vascular injuries may initially go unrecognized, because clinical signs and symptoms may be delayed hours to weeks after injury, as is the case in traumatic aneurysms without initial rupture. A high index of suspicion for vascular injury is necessary for up to a month after both blunt and penetrating maxillofacial and neck trauma.[53]

The patient with vascular injury to the head and neck may be asymptomatic or may have throbbing pain, face, or neck swelling with or without pulsation, tracheal deviation, spontaneous hemorrhage, epistaxis, or neurologic deficits with signs of stroke. Carotid-cavernous fistulas present with pulsatile exophthalmos, extraocular movement restriction, preseptal edema, and sometimes visual changes.[54]

Diagnostic imaging
Traumatic vascular injury can lead to irreversible neurologic damage or death if not identified and treated early. Occult neurovascular injury, carotid-cavernous fistula, or carotid transection can occur with severe midface and skull base fractures.[14,55]

Many of these patients may start with a noncontrast CT evaluating for facial fractures and intracranial hemorrhage. Noncontrast CT does not allow for specific vascular evaluation, but there are several suspicious findings suggestive of vascular injury, including prevertebral swelling, hematoma along a vessel or a penetration trajectory, infiltration of perivascular fat, or foreign bodies less than 0.5 cm from a vessel wall.[52,56,57]

If these findings are present and there is suspicion for traumatic vascular injury, it is prudent to order further imaging that allows for direct vascular evaluation. Arteriography is the diagnostic modality of choice for evaluation of suspected traumatic vascular injuries, and may be combined with percutaneous or endovascular embolization versus surgical intervention. Noninvasive diagnostic imaging options include MRI, CT, ultrasonography, and Doppler studies, but angiography is typically required before embolization or surgical treatment.[58] CTA has been recommended over digital subtraction angiography for initial evaluation, because of the speed and less invasive nature of CTA. Findings on CTA or MR angiography suggestive of vascular injury include changes in vessel caliber, irregular vessel walls, and filling defects.[52] Three-dimensional reconstruction of the angiographic imaging allows for better visualization of the defects.

Patients who have undergone high-velocity trauma significant enough to cause the injuries discussed earlier are likely to have concomitant cervical spine injuries or intracranial hemorrhage. The radiographic diagnosis and management of these regional injuries are beyond the scope of this article. However, bone window views of the initial CT scan should be evaluated to rule out cervical spine fractures, and serial CT scans should be monitored in the case of suspected or confirmed intracranial hemorrhage.

Treatment overview
Treatment ranges from interventional radiology coil placement or balloon dilation, to open surgical treatment.

IMAGING CONSIDERATIONS IN CHILDREN

The leading cause of death in children aged 1 to 18 years is unintentional injury, largely motor vehicle collisions.[59,60] The leading cause of unintentional injury not leading to death in children is unintentional falls.[61,62] Initial diagnosis of pediatric facial fracture can often be made based on history and physical examination alone, but radiographic imaging for accurate characterization and treatment of fracture is typically necessary.[63,64] Facial trauma in children is of specific interest, because of the growing facial skeleton, the moldability of the facial bones, and the concern for radiation. Detailed knowledge regarding growth of the craniomaxillofacial skeleton is essential in the treatment of these fractures, although it is beyond the scope of this article.[61–67]

Treatment considerations in pediatric versus adult upper and midfacial trauma have many variations because of the effect of these fractures and their treatment on the growing facial skeleton. However, the standard imaging is largely the same: conventional CT scanning. Only specific imaging similarities and differences, not fracture management, are discussed in this section.

Radiation

CT scanning and other forms of radiation in children have raised concern over the past few decades for formation of irradiation cataract and thyroid cancer, as well as multiple other cancers that are less likely to be linked to maxillofacial CT, because of lack of proximity to the facial skeleton.[9,12,13,45,46,48,49] The threshold radiation doses have not yet been determined.[59,60] However, risk estimates have long since suggested that pediatric CT is more precarious than adult CT in terms of lifetime risk of radiation-induced cancer.[68,69] The maxillofacial surgeon should take care to order only CT scans in children when the findings significantly affect the treatment decisions.

Frontal Trauma

The rapid growth of the brain in infancy results in early projection of the cranium and associated trauma. Pediatric skull fractures are more common than midfacial fractures in younger children.[67,70] Direct frontal trauma in children is more likely to result in supraorbital rim and anterior cranial floor or orbital roof fractures because of the lack of pneumatization of the frontal bones.[71,72] As with adults, axial cuts of conventional CT scans are most useful for characterizing anterior versus posterior frontal sinus fractures. Plain films are unreliable.

Orbital Trauma

The pattern of orbital trauma in children parallels the rate of growth of the craniofacial skeleton, as well as the delayed pneumatization of the frontal sinus. Orbital roof fractures are more common in younger children, whereas orbital floor fractures are more likely to occur in children aged 7 years or older, because the orbits are almost fully developed.[72,73]

It is well known that children have a higher rate of trapdoor orbital fractures, resulting in vascular compromise to the inferior rectus, with resulting scarring and shortening of the muscle. These fractures must be diagnosed and treated immediately, because treatment 24 hours after the injury has been linked with a higher rate of diplopia on long-term follow-up.[9,12,13,74,75] Thus, clear imaging of the intraocular muscles is of paramount importance. Conventionally, CT scans have been used for diagnosis of orbital fractures, as discussed earlier. Fractures that seem to approach the orbital canal should be evaluated using 1-mm coronal cuts.[8,11,12,45,46] It has recently been suggested that high-resolution MRI with microscopy coil is superior to conventional CT scanning for the diagnosis of orbital fractures, both because of the decreased radiation and the improved soft tissue portrayal.[9,12,13,43–47]

Nasal Trauma

In patients with isolated nasal trauma and no other suspected injuries, plain films may be used for diagnosis of nasal fractures.[11,76] However, depending on the age of the child and whether or not the nasal bones are fully fused, plain films may prove unhelpful.[77–79] Significant clinical findings such as flattening of the nasal dorsum warrant CT evaluation to rule out occult naso-orbitoethmoid fracture.[67,77]

Clinical examination is still of supreme importance in these patients, because radiographic evidence of nasal fracture is not always present in children with nasal septal hematoma after facial trauma.[79,80] Nasal septal cartilaginous dislocation is an uncommon complication of birth rather than an intrauterine development.[61–65] It can be diagnosed clinically without the need for radiographic verification.[81,82]

Mandibular Trauma

Historically, plain films were used, necessitating multiple views, as discussed earlier. However, it may prove difficult for children who have just been traumatized to cooperate for these films. If only 1 film can be obtained, the orthopantomogram is the single radiograph that provides the most information.[64,83] However, it has been suggested that the sensitivity and specificity of panoramic radiographs is inferior to CT scans when evaluating specifically for condylar fractures in children.[84–86] Dental radiographs often prove useful for evaluating teeth or tooth buds in the line of fracture.[66,67]

Literature regarding mandibular fractures in neonates and infants is lacking. The cause of neonatal mandibular fractures is usually birth trauma. No standard of care for imaging these fractures has been set, although both CT and plain films, including occlusal, periapical, and extraoral lateral oblique plain films, have been used for diagnosis.[87–89] Some sort of imaging is advisable if mandibular fracture is suspected, because conservative management of these fractures is not always the best option, and minimally displaced neonatal mandibular fractures can often be missed on clinical examination.[90]

ROLE OF POSTOPERATIVE IMAGING
Postoperative Radiography in Other Settings

In an effort to minimize unnecessary radiation and cost, investigators in other clinical domains have assessed the value of routine postprocedure radiography. Investigators have looked at the usefulness of routine postoperative radiography after feeding tube placement, chest tube removal, central line placement, and foreign body ingestion.[68,69,71–73,91,92] In all cases except foreign body ingestion, routine postoperative radiographs were found to be unnecessary. In cases in which complications requiring intervention were found postoperatively, clinical suspicion existed irrespective of the radiographs. Postoperative radiography should be reserved for cases in which the surgeon suspects a complication during the operation, or postoperative clinical findings are consistent with a complication.

Health Care Costs

Given the increased attention to multiple inefficiencies in the US health care system over the past decade, providers are becoming more cognizant of unnecessary spending and attempting to use health care resources more wisely. Several specialties have come to the conclusion that routine postoperative radiographs are more often habitual than clinically necessary. Routine chest radiographs evaluating for pneumothorax after percutaneous dilational tracheostomy and thoracostomy have been shown to cost more than $13,000 and $22,000, respectively. Investigators have come to the conclusion that the radiographic findings resulted in no significant changes in patient management, and chest radiographs should be taken only after particularly difficult procedures, or when there are worrisome clinical signs and symptoms.[93–95]

Radiation Exposure

Although modern radiography equipment has decreased total radiation dose, minor risk of adverse effects still exists, and the goal should be to lower this risk as much as possible and perform the necessary imaging to allow for proper diagnosis.

The largest case-control study to date examining the correlation between dental ionizing radiation and intracranial meningioma was recently published. This population-based case-control study of 1433 patients with intracranial meningiomas diagnosed between 2005 and 2011 found both statistically and clinically significantly increased risk of meningiomas with bitewing and panoramic radiographs. Overall, patients with meningioma were twice as likely to have received bitewing radiographs than controls (odds ratio, 1.4–2.9). An almost 5-fold increased risk was observed in patients who had at least 1 panoramic radiograph as a child when younger than 10 years. No association was found between full mouth radiographs and intracranial meningiomas. No association was found between tumor location supratentorial versus infratentorial and dental radiographs of any category.[81]

Dental radiographs, without specification of full mouth series versus panoramic radiographs, have been claimed as risk factors for intracranial meningiomas, thyroid cancer, and parotid tumors.[83,84,86] Another recent but smaller case-control study from the United Kingdom, matching 313 patients with thyroid cancer to similar controls, found that dental radiographs (no distinction was made between panorex and full mouth series) were significantly associated with an increased risk of thyroid cancer, with a dose-response pattern. In multiple other studies, dental radiographs full mouth series, particularly those taken before 1960, were most highly indicated as risk factors. Investigators did not find a direct association between panoramic radiographs and the tumors studied.

Grange[96] reported effective dose measured in milliSieverts (mSv), with the average background radiation in the United Kingdom being 2.2 mSv per year. With this scale, various radiographs may be correlated to an equivalent period of natural background radiation: 0.002 days (a few hours) for a single bitewing/periapical film, less than 1.5 days for a panoramic radiograph, and 3 days for a PA chest radiograph. Radiation protection is always aimed at reducing risks of harm by decreasing doses received to as low as reasonably practicable. Ludlow and colleagues[97] calculated radiation dosimetry on an average of 5 digital panoramic radiographic units and found that the average ionizing radiation dose from 1 panoramic radiograph was equivalent to 2 days of background radiation, correlating to 16 microSieverts (μSv) and 32 μSv, respectively.

The guidelines in the *Vital Guide to Radiography and Radiation Protection*[96] state that the practitioner ordering the radiograph must anticipate that information in the image significantly affects their treatment decisions. The most recent recommendations from the American Dental Association on the use of dental radiographs were published in the *Journal of the American Dental Association* in 2006.[98] Although no specific recommendations are stated regarding postwire removal radiographs, they do recommend against taking routine radiographs to search for occult disease in the absence of clinical suspicion. The US Food and Drug Administration recommendations for prescribing dental radiographs were most recently revised in 2004.[99] These guidelines state that clinical suspicion should be the guiding factor in radiograph prescription, and they list evidence of foreign objects as an indication for radiographic examination.

Postoperative Radiography in Facial Fracture Management

Multiple investigators have found routine radiography after simple maxillofacial trauma cases to be less than useful. We agree with this conclusion and order posttreatment radiography only when we suspect the need for further operative intervention to correct the facial deformity. We use intraoperative CT in most of these cases, because it allows for immediate correction.

Jain and Alexander[43] performed a prospective, multicenter study evaluating the need for postoperative radiographs after maxillofacial fracture fixation in 431 patients. Although one of the primary arguments for routine postoperative radiography in trauma patients is the ability to identify fractures that need reoperation before the patients' discharge, this study detected no such fractures, and any decisions made to reoperate were purely based on clinical findings. The home institution in this study also noted that postoperative radiographs led to a delay of 2 to 3 days in patient discharge.

Bali and Lopes[76] investigated the effectiveness of postoperative radiography in 278 facial fractures in 257 patients, about half retrospectively and half prospectively.[11] There were 3 cases in which a patient required reoperation, and each case was based on a clinical decision rather than a radiographic finding: 2 fractured mandibles with postoperative occlusal discrepancy, and a fractured zygoma that was initially treated closed, but clinically determined to need reoperation with ORIF. These investigators even noted that 5% of postoperative radiographs taken during the prospective portion of their study showed an unfavorable reduction, which was disregarded because of a satisfactory clinical outcome.

Durham[77] and Childress and Newlands[79] looked at the usefulness of postoperative radiography in patients treated for mandibular fractures: a prospective study of 100 patients, and a retrospective study of 289 patients, respectively.[78] Durham found the sensitivity of postoperative radiographs in determining postoperative complications to be just 20%, "well below what [they] had hoped for," an equally poor specificity of 5%, and a positive predictive value (PPV) of just 20%. Clinical evidence of malocclusion was more predictive of the need for reoperation, with sensitivity 42%, specificity 2%, and PPV 60%. Both studies concluded that postoperative radiographs add little information to physical examination and history in terms of identification of complications. The investigators suggested reserving postoperative radiographic evaluation for patients with gross malocclusion,[67,77] and those with complaints or other physical findings suggestive of complications.[79,80] Ogden and colleagues[100] came to the same conclusion in regards to management of zygomatic complex fractures. In their review of 183 simple fractures treated via a Gillies approach, there was only 1 indeterminate case, in which the postoperative radiograph may have aided in the decision to reoperate. Based on this finding, the investigators challenged the accepted protocol of ordering postoperative radiographs without specific clinical indicators.

Numerous studies and our experience have concluded that clinical examination and patient history are more effective and efficient means of evaluating potential need for retreatment after facial fracture management than routine postoperative radiography.

SUMMARY

Optimal diagnostic imaging is a critical component of successful management of complex posttraumatic craniomaxillofacial deformity. Many of these injuries, although not necessary life threatening, are irreversibly life altering. Most of the time, the best outcome is provided in the primary setting, and therefore every effort must be made to optimize treatment outcome during the initial operative treatment. Optimizing treatment requires judicious use of CT imaging, tempered by the limitations and risks associated with repeated radiation exposure. Until optimal radiation thresholds are established, the surgeon must use their best judgment, in consultation with an informed patient, to obtain enough preoperative, intraoperative, and postoperative data with which to optimally manage each patient.

REFERENCES

1. Bui TG, Bell RB, Dierks EJ. Technological advances in the treatment of facial trauma. Atlas Oral Maxillofac Surg Clin North Am 2012;20: 81–94. Available at. http://eutils.ncbi.nlm.nih.gov/entrez/eutils/elink.fcgi?dbfrom=pubmed&id=22365431&retmode=ref&cmd=prlinks. Accessed May 12, 2013.

2. Markiewicz MR, Gelesko S, Bell RB. Zygoma reconstruction. Oral Maxillofac Surg Clin North Am 2013;25:167–201.

3. Bell RB, Markiewicz MR. Computer-assisted planning, stereolithographic modeling, and intraoperative navigation for complex orbital reconstruction: a descriptive study in a preliminary cohort. J Oral Maxillofac Surg 2009;67:2559–70.

4. Johnson F, Semaan MT, Megerian CA. Temporal bone fracture: evaluation and management in the modern era. Otolaryngol Clin North Am 2008;41: 597–618.

5. Zapalac JS, Marple BF, Schwade ND. Skull base cerebrospinal fluid fistulas: a comprehensive diagnostic algorithm. Otolaryngol Head Neck Surg 2002;126:669–76.

6. Brandt KE, Burruss GL, Hickerson WL, et al. The management of mid-face fractures with intracranial injury. J Trauma 1991;31:15–9.

7. Holmgren EP, Dierks EJ, Homer LD, et al. Facial computed tomography use in trauma patients who require a head computed tomogram. J Oral Maxillofac Surg 2004;62:913–8.

8. Hodge D, Tecklenburg F, Fleisher G. Coin ingestion: does every child need a radiograph? Ann Emerg Med 1985;14:443–6.

9. Michel M, Jacob S, Roger G, et al. Eye lens radiation exposure and repeated head CT scans: a problem to keep in mind. Eur J Radiol 2012;81: 1896–900.

10. Lambert DM, Mirvis SE, Shanmuganathan K, et al. Computed tomography exclusion of osseous paranasal sinus injury in blunt trauma patients: the "clear sinus" sign. J Oral Maxillofac Surg 1997; 55:1207–10.

11. Morris CD, Kushner GM, Tiwana PS. Facial skeletal trauma in the growing patient. Oral Maxillofac Surg Clin North Am 2012;24:351–64.

12. Lund E, Halaburt H. Irradiation dose to the lens of the eye during CT of the head. Neuroradiology 1982;22:181–4.

13. Davidson HC. Imaging of the temporal bone. Neuroimaging Clin N Am 2004;14:721–60.

14. Yang WG, Chen CT, de Villa GH, et al. Blunt internal carotid artery injury associated with facial fractures. Plast Reconstr Surg 2003;111:789–96.

15. Stanwix MG, Nam AJ, Manson PN, et al. Critical computed tomographic diagnostic criteria for frontal sinus fractures. J Oral Maxillofac Surg 2010;68: 2714–22.

16. Bell RB, Chen J. Frontobasilar fractures: contemporary management. Atlas Oral Maxillofac Surg Clin North Am 2010;18:181–96.

17. Raveh J, Laedrach K, Vuillemin T, et al. Management of combined frontonaso-orbital/skull base fractures and telecanthus in 355 cases. Arch Otolaryngol Head Neck Surg 1992;118:605–14.

18. Erbele ID, Sorensen MP, Rivera A. Otologic and temporal bone injuries, triage, and management. Atlas Oral Maxillofac Surg Clin North Am 2013;21: 117–25.

19. Swartz JD, Harnsberger R, Mukherji SK. The temporal bone. Radiol Clin North Am 1998;36:819–53.

20. Brodie HA, Thompson TC. Management of complications from 820 temporal bone fractures. Am J Otol 1997;18:188–97.

21. Schuknecht B, Graetz K. Radiologic assessment of maxillofacial, mandibular, and skull base trauma. Eur Radiol 2005;15:560–8.

22. Ghorayeb BY, Yeakley JW. Temporal bone fractures: longitudinal or oblique? The case for oblique temporal bone fractures. Laryngoscope 1992;102: 129–34.

23. Dahiya R, Keller JD, Litofsky NS, et al. Temporal bone fractures: otic capsule sparing versus otic capsule violating clinical and radiographic considerations. J Trauma 1999;47:1079–83.

24. Ishman SL, Friedland DR. Temporal bone fractures: traditional classification and clinical relevance. Laryngoscope 2004;114:1734–41.

25. Stone JA, Castillo M, Neelon B, et al. Evaluation of CSF leaks: high-resolution CT compared with contrast-enhanced CT and radionuclide cisternography. AJNR Am J Neuroradiol 1999;20:706–12.

26. Lund VJ, Savy L, Lloyd G, et al. Optimum imaging and diagnosis of cerebrospinal fluid rhinorrhoea. J Laryngol Otol 2000;114:988–92.

27. Bell RB, Dierks EJ, Homer L, et al. Management of cerebrospinal fluid leak associated with craniomaxillofacial trauma. J Oral Maxillofac Surg 2004;62: 676–84.

28. Blice JB. Ocular injuries, triage, and management in maxillofacial trauma. Atlas Oral Maxillofac Surg Clin North Am 2013;21:97–103.

29. Ellis E III, Scott K. Assessment of patients with facial fractures. Emerg Med Clin North Am 2000; 18:411–48.

30. Urolagin SB, Kotrashetti SM, Kale TP, et al. Traumatic optic neuropathy after maxillofacial trauma: a review of 8 cases. J Oral Maxillofac Surg 2012; 70:1123–30.

31. Avery LA, Susarla SM, Novelline RA. Multidetector and three-dimensional CT evaluation of the patient with maxillofacial injury. Radiol Clin North Am 2011; 49:183–203.

32. Wilde F, Lorenz K, Ebner AK, et al. Intraoperative imaging with a 3D C-Arm system after zygomatico-orbital complex fracture reduction. J Oral Maxillofac Surg 2012;12:1–17.

33. Ellis E, Moos KF, el-Attar A. Ten years of mandibular fractures: an analysis of 2,137 cases. Oral Surg Oral Med Oral Pathol 1985;59:120–9.

34. Hutson RK, Christian BA. Diagnostic Imaging of Facial Fractures. In: Marciani RD, Carlson ER,

Braun TW, editors. Oral and maxillofacial surgery. 2nd edition. St Louis, MO: Saunders Elsevier; 2009. p. 91–102.

35. Czerwinski M, Parker WL, Williams HB. Algorithm for head computed tomography imaging in patients with mandible fractures. J Oral Maxillofac Surg 2008;66:2093–7.

36. Laine P, Kontio R, Salo A, et al. Secondary correction of malocclusion after treatment of maxillofacial trauma. J Oral Maxillofac Surg 2004;62:1312–9.

37. Ryan JM, Ross D, Obeid G. Genial tubercle fracture: a case report and review of the literature. J Oral Maxillofac Surg 2010;68:2338–41.

38. Gerhard S, Ennemoser T, Rudisch A, et al. Condylar injury: magnetic resonance imaging findings of temporomandibular joint soft-tissue changes. Int J Oral Maxillofac Surg 2007;36:214–8.

39. Emshoff R, Rudisch A, Ennemoser T, et al. Magnetic resonance imaging findings of temporomandibular joint soft tissue changes in type V and VI condylar injuries. J Oral Maxillofac Surg 2007;65:1550–4.

40. Marão HF, Panzarini SR, Manrrique GR, et al. Importance of clinical examination in dentoalveolar trauma. J Craniofac Surg 2012;23:e404.

41. Feliciano KM, de França Caldas A Jr. A systematic review of the diagnostic classifications of traumatic dental injuries. Dent Traumatol 2006;22:71–6.

42. Palomo L, Palomo JM. Cone beam CT for diagnosis and treatment planning in trauma cases. Dent Clin North Am 2009;53:717–27.

43. Jain MK, Alexander M. The need of postoperative radiographs in maxillofacial fractures–a prospective multicentric study. Br J Oral Maxillofac Surg 2009;47:525–9.

44. Kolk A, Stimmer H, Klopfer M, et al. High resolution magnetic resonance imaging with an orbital coil as an alternative to computed tomography scan as the primary imaging modality of pediatric orbital fractures. J Oral Maxillofac Surg 2009;67:348–56.

45. Ron E, Lubin JH, Shore RE, et al. Thyroid cancer after exposure to external radiation: a pooled analysis of seven studies. Radiat Res 1995;141:259–77.

46. Verscheuren D, Bell RB, Bagheri SC, et al. Management of laryngo-tracheal injuries associated with craniomaxillofacial trauma. J Oral Maxillofac Surg 2006;64:203–14.

47. Bell RB, Verscheuren DS, Dierks EJ. Management of laryngeal trauma. Oral Maxillofac Surg Clin North Am 2008;20:415–30.

48. Ainsbury EA, Bouffler SD, Dörr W, et al. Radiation cataractogenesis: a review of recent studies. Radiat Res 2009;172:1–9.

49. Goudy SL, Miller FB, Bumpous JM. Neck crepitance: evaluation and management of suspected upper aerodigestive tract injury. Laryngoscope 2002;112:791–5.

50. Bell RB, Osborne T, Dierks EJ, et al. Management of penetrating neck injuries: a new paradigm for civilian trauma. J Oral Maxillofac Surg 2007;65:691–705.

51. Shiroff AM, Gale SC, Martin ND, et al. Penetrating neck trauma: a review of management strategies and discussion of the "No Zone" approach. Am Surg 2013;79:23–9.

52. Stallmeyer MJ, Morales RE, Flanders AE. Imaging of traumatic neurovascular injury. Radiol Clin North Am 2006;44:13–39.

53. Prêtre R, Reverdin A, Kalonji T, et al. Blunt carotid artery injury: difficult therapeutic approaches for an underrecognized entity. Surgery 1994;115:375–81.

54. Teitelbaum GP, Bernstein K, Choi S, et al. Endovascular coil occlusion of a traumatic basilar-cavernous fistula: technical report. Neurosurgery 1998;42:1394–7 [discussion: 1397–8].

55. Kerwin AJ, Bynoe RP, Murray J, et al. Liberalized screening for blunt carotid and vertebral artery injuries is justified. J Trauma 2001;51:308–14.

56. Múnera F, Cohn S, Rivas LA. Penetrating injuries of the neck: use of helical computed tomographic angiography. J Trauma 2005;58:413–8.

57. Sclafani AP, Sclafani SJ. Angiography and transcatheter arterial embolization of vascular injuries of the face and neck. Laryngoscope 1996;106:168–73.

58. Cunningham L, Van Sickels JE, Brandt T. Angiographic evaluation of the head and neck. Atlas Oral Maxillofac Surg Clin North Am 2003;11:73–86.

59. Centers for Disease Control, Prevention, National Center for Injury Prevention. 10 leading causes of death by age group, United States–2010. National Center for Health Statistics; 1–1, 2012. Available at: http://www.cdc.gov/injury/wisqars/pdf/10LCID_All_Deaths_By_Age_Group_2010-a.pdf. Accessed June 23, 2013.

60. Centers for Disease Control, Prevention, National Center for Injury Prevention and Control. 10 leading causes of injury deaths by age group highlighting unintentional injury deaths, United States–2010. National Center for Health Statistics; 1–1, 2012. Available at: http://www.cdc.gov/injury/wisqars/pdf/10LCID_Unintentional_Deaths_2010-a.pdf. Accessed June 23, 2013.

61. Uhing MR. Management of birth injuries. Pediatr Clin North Am 2004;51:1169–86.

62. Centers for Disease Control and Prevention, National Center for Injury Prevention and Control. National estimates for leading causes of deaths in the US 2009 and 2010. National Center for Health Statistics; 1–1, 2012. Available at: http://www.cdc.gov/Injury/wisqars/pdf/National_Estim_10_Leading_Causes_Nonfatal_Injuries_Tx_Hospital-ED_US2010-a.pdf. Accessed June 23, 2013.

63. Uhing MR. Management of birth injuries. Clin Perinatol 2005;l32:19–38.

64. Chung WL, Papadopoulos H, Costello BJ. Pediatric craniomaxillofacial trauma. Selected Readings in Oral and Maxillofacial Surgery 2012;13:1–28.

65. Costello BJ, Rivera RD, Shand J, et al. Growth and development considerations for craniomaxillofacial surgery. Oral Maxillofac Surg Clin North Am 2012; 24:377–96.

66. Suei Y, Mallick PC, Nagasaki T, et al. Radiographic evaluation of the fate of developing tooth buds on the fracture line of mandibular fractures. J Oral Maxillofac Surg 2006;64:94–9.

67. Koltai PJ, Rabkin D. Management of facial trauma in children. Pediatr Clin North Am 1996;43:1253–75.

68. Whitehouse MR, Patel A, Morgan JA. The necessity of routine post-thoracostomy tube chest radiographs in post-operative thoracic surgery patients. Surgeon 2009;7:79–81.

69. Brenner D, Elliston C, Hall E, et al. Estimated risks of radiation-induced fatal cancer from pediatric CT. AJR Am J Roentgenol 2001;176:289–96.

70. Pacharn P, Heller DN, Kammen BF, et al. Are chest radiographs routinely necessary following thoracostomy tube removal? Pediatr Radiol 2002;32:138–42.

71. Genther DJ, Thorne MC. Utility of routine postoperative chest radiography in pediatric tracheostomy. Int J Pediatr Otorhinolaryngol 2010;l74:1397–400.

72. Cobb AR, Jeelani NO, Ayliffe PR. Orbital fractures in children. Br J Oral Maxillofac Surg 2013;51:41–6.

73. Farrell J, Walshe J, Gellens M, et al. Complications associated with insertion of jugular venous catheters for hemodialysis: the value of postprocedural radiograph. Am J Kidney Dis 1997;30:690–2.

74. Donaldson D. Chest radiographs after dilatational percutaneous tracheotomy: are they necessary? Otolaryngol Head Neck Surg 2000;123:236–9.

75. Gerbino G, Roccia F, Bianchi FA, et al. Surgical management of orbital trapdoor fracture in a pediatric population. J Oral Maxillofac Surg 2010;68:1310–6.

76. Bali N, Lopes V. An audit of the effectiveness of postoperative radiographs–do they make a difference? Br J Oral Maxillofac Surg 2004;42:331–4.

77. Durham J. Postoperative radiographs after open reduction and internal fixation of the mandible: are they useful? Br J Oral Maxillofac Surg 2006; 44:279–82.

78. Stucker FJ, Bryarly RC, Shockley WW. Management of nasal trauma in children. Arch Otolaryngol 1984;110:190–2.

79. Childress CS, Newlands SD. Utilization of panoramic radiographs to evaluate short-term complications of mandibular fracture repair. Laryngoscope 1999;109:1269–72.

80. Sayin I, Yazici ZM, Bozkurt E, et al. Nasal septal hematoma and abscess in children. J Craniofac Surg 2011;22:e17–9.

81. Claus EB, Calvocoressi L, Bondy ML, et al. Dental x-rays and risk of meningioma. Cancer 2012; 118(18):4530–7.

82. Podoshin L, Gertner R, Fradis M, et al. Incidence and treatment of deviation of nasal septum in newborns. Ear Nose Throat J 1991;70:485–7.

83. Memon A, Godward S, Williams D, et al. Dental x-rays and the risk of thyroid cancer: a case-control study. Acta Oncol 2010;49:447–53.

84. Preston-Martin S, Henderson BE, Bernstein L. Medical and dental x rays as risk factors for recently diagnosed tumors of the head. Natl Cancer Inst Monogr 1985;69:175–9.

85. Chacon GE, Dawson KH, Myall RW, et al. A comparative study of 2 imaging techniques for the diagnosis of condylar fractures in children. J Oral Maxillofac Surg 2003;61(6):668–72.

86. Longstreth WT, Phillips LE, Drangsholt M, et al. Dental X-rays and the risk of intracranial meningioma: a population-based case-control study. Cancer 2004;100:1026–34.

87. Vasconcelos BC, Lago CA, Nogueira RV, et al. Mandibular fracture in a premature infant: a case report and review of the literature. J Oral Maxillofac Surg 2009;67:218–22.

88. Bhatt N, Khachi GJ, Yu JC. Resorbable suture fixation of neonatal mandibular fractures: a novel technique. Plast Reconstr Surg 2010;126:258e–60e.

89. Lustmann J, Milhem I. Mandibular fractures in infants: review of the literature and report of seven cases. J Oral Maxillofac Surg 1994;52:240–5 [discussion: 245–6].

90. Posnick JC. Discussion: mandibular fractures in infants: review of the literature and report of seven cases. J Oral Maxillofac Surg 1994;52: 245–6.

91. Harrison AM, Clay B, Grant MJ, et al. Nonradiographic assessment of enteral feeding tube position. Crit Care Med 1997;25:2055–9.

92. McCormick JT, O'Mara MS, Papasavas PK, et al. The use of routine chest X-ray films after chest tube removal in postoperative cardiac patients. Ann Thorac Surg 2002;74:2161–4.

93. Tarnoff M, Moncure M, Jones F, et al. The value of routine posttracheostomy chest radiography. Chest 1998;113:1647–9.

94. Donaldson D, Emami A, Wax M. Chest radiographs after percutaneous dilational tracheostomy: are they necessary? Otolaryngol Head Neck Surg 1999;162:236–9.

95. Kumar J, Grant C, Hughes M, et al. Role of routine chest radiography after percutaneous dilatational tracheostomy. Br J Anaesth 2008;100:663–6. Available at: http://bja.oxfordjournals.org/cgi/reprint/100/5/663. Accessed January 7, 2012.

96. Grange S. Vital guide to radiography and radiation protection. Vital 2009;7:43–6.

97. Ludlow JB, Davies-Ludlow LE, Brooks SL. Dosimetry of two extraoral direct digital imaging devices: NewTom cone beam CT and Orthophos Plus DS panoramic unit. Dentomaxillofac Radiol 2003;32: 229–34.

98. American Dental Association Council on Scientific Affairs. The use of dental radiographs: update and recommendations. J Am Dent Assoc 2006;137:1304–12.

99. American Dental Association: Council on Dental Benefit Programs & Council on Scientific Affairs. Guidelines for the Selection of Patients for Dental Radiographic Examinations 2004;1–23.

100. Ogden G, Cowpe J, Adi M. Are post-operative radiographs necessary in the management of simple fractures of the zygomatic complex? Br J Oral Maxillofac Surg 1987;26:292–6.

Helping Anesthesiologists Understand Facial Fractures

Chad G. Robertson, DDS, MD, MSc, FRCD(C)*,
Jean Charles Doucet, DDS, MD, MSc, FRCD(C)

KEYWORDS

- Facial injuries • Airway management • Anesthesiology • Laryngoscopy • Intubation

KEY POINTS

- Patients with facial fractures often present specific anesthesia-related challenges.
- Limited preoperative mandibular opening alone should not be considered a predictor of difficult intubation.
- Reestablishing proper dental occlusion is required for the treatment of fractures involving the maxilla or mandible.
- Unless contraindicated, nasotracheal intubation is usually the option of choice for the intraoperative airway management of patients with maxillofacial trauma.
- When nasotracheal intubation is contraindicated, submental intubation and retromolar intubation should be considered as alternatives to a tracheostomy.

Injuries to the oral and maxillofacial region are commonly encountered, and the appropriate management of patients with these injuries frequently requires the expertise of an anesthesiologist. Injuries to this region may involve any combination of soft tissue, bone, and teeth. Injuries to these structures often produce anesthesia-related challenges, which must be overcome to achieve optimal outcomes. This article addresses the common challenges faced by anesthesiologists specific to patients with facial fractures.

HOW SEVERE IS THE TRAUMA?

Facial fractures may be the result of motor vehicle collisions, industrial/workplace accidents, interpersonal violence, sporting activity, and falls. The mechanism of injury is an important factor in determining the scope and severity of injury. Although most facial fractures are the result of isolated blunt-force trauma to the face and are rarely life threatening, they may be associated with life-threatening injuries to the head, cervical spine, chest, abdomen, pelvis, and/or extremities. Trauma patients must be assessed and managed according to the principles of Advanced Trauma Life Support (ATLS). The primary survey in ATLS involves the following:

A: Airway with cervical spine protection
B: Breathing and ventilation
C: Circulation and hemorrhage control
D: Disability or neurologic status
E: Exposure and environment with temperature control

Within the ATLS protocol, resuscitation and evaluation are carried out concurrently. The establishment and maintenance of an airway and restoration of ventilation are clearly of prime importance in the resuscitation of trauma patients. With facial

Financial Disclosures and Conflicts of Interest: Nil.
Department of Oral and Maxillofacial Sciences, Dalhousie University, 5981 University Avenue, PO Box 15000, Halifax, Nova Scotia B3H 4R2, Canada
* Corresponding author.
E-mail address: cgrobert@dal.ca

Oral Maxillofacial Surg Clin N Am 25 (2013) 561–572
http://dx.doi.org/10.1016/j.coms.2013.07.005

trauma, it is important to perform a quick visual inspection of the oral cavity for tooth and bone fragments, large blood clots, and foreign bodies before bag-mask-ventilation or insertion of transoral airway devices.

The incidence of cervical spine (c-spine) injury in association with facial fractures has been reported to be 3% to 7%.[1–3] This incidence, along with the potential catastrophic consequences of undiagnosed c-spine injury, requires that patients with facial fractures must be considered to have a c-spine injury until this has been ruled out, which is done by clinical and radiographic assessment. The maintenance of in-line cervical immobilization is necessary until the c-spine is cleared. In alert and stable trauma patients, the Canadian C-spine rule (**Fig. 1**) can be applied to assist in determining the need for cervical spine imaging.[4–7] The implementation of this rule can reduce health care costs, radiation exposure to patients, and emergency department wait times with limited risk to patients.

In patients with acute facial trauma, bag-valve-ventilation and laryngoscopy can be difficult as the result of the following:

- C-spine precautions limiting the ability to position the head and neck optimally
- Bleeding
- Inability to maintain a seal with an unstable mandible and/or maxilla
- Soft tissue edema
- Nasal obstruction
- Foreign bodies

These factors may also compromise the use of the following alternative devices:

- Transillumination with lighted stylet
- Laryngeal mask airway
- Bullard laryngoscope (Gyrus ACMI, Southborough, MA, USA)
- GlideScope (Verathon Medical, Burnaby, BC, Canada)
- Bronchoscope

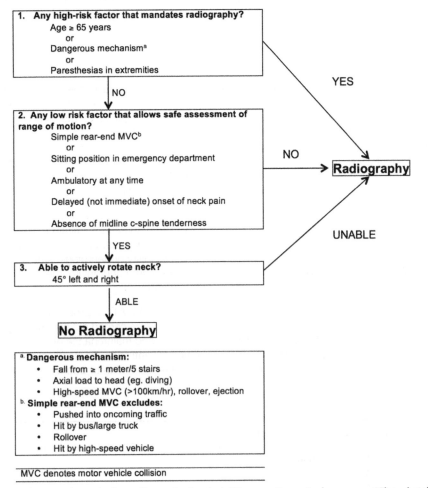

Fig. 1. The Canadian c-spine rule for radiography in alert (Glasgow Coma Scale score = 15) and stable trauma patients when c-spine injury is a concern.

Thus, additional alternatives should be available, such as the Combitube (Tyco Healthcare Group LP, Gosport, UK), King LT-D (King Systems Corp, Noblesville, IN, USA), and personnel to perform a surgical airway.

Once the primary survey is complete, the resuscitation initiated, and the airway, breathing, and circulation are reassessed, the secondary survey is commenced. This head-to-toe assessment includes a physical examination, special procedures, radiologic evaluation, and laboratory investigations. Repeated reassessment of trauma patients is imperative because the patients' status may change because of the delayed development of clinically apparent sequelae of previously unrecognized injuries or the worsening of known conditions.

In addition to c-spine injuries, patients with facial fractures are also at risk for brain injury. The incidence of brain injury in association with facial fractures has been reported to be in the range of 67%.[3,8] The Canadian CT head rule (**Box 1**) is a validated clinical decision rule, which has the sensitivity to capture patients with minor head injury who require head computed tomography (CT) scans and the potential to minimize the use of CT scans without jeopardizing patient care.[9–11] With particular relevance to anesthesiology,

---

Box 1
Canadian CT head rule

CT head rule is only required for patients with minor head injuries with any one of the following:

High risk (for neurologic intervention)

    Glasgow Coma Scale (GCS) score of less than 15 at 2 hours after injury

    Suspected open or depressed skull fracture

    Any sign of basal skull fracture (hemotympanum, raccoon eyes, cerebrospinal fluid otorrhea/rhinorrhea, Battle sign)

    Vomiting 2 or more episodes

    Aged 65 years or older

Medium risk (for brain injury on computed tomography)

    Amnesia before impact more than 30 minutes

    Dangerous mechanism (pedestrian struck by motor vehicle, occupant ejected from motor vehicle, fall from height greater than 3 feet or 5 stairs)

Minor head injury

    Defined as witnessed loss of consciousness, definite amnesia, or witnessed disorientation in patients with a GCS score of 13 to 15

---

appropriate fluid resuscitation, oxygenation, ventilation, and stable intracranial dynamics with avoidance of intracranial hypertension are important in minimizing secondary brain injury and mortality in patients with head injuries.

It is during the secondary survey that the extent of the oral and maxillofacial injuries is determined. Most of these injuries are not life threatening. It is not until patients have been resuscitated, stabilized, and the life-threatening injuries addressed that the definitive management of facial fractures is typically undertaken. The management of facial fractures will often necessitate a general anesthetic with tracheal intubation to facilitate the appropriate treatment.

CAN PATIENTS WITH FACIAL FRACTURES BE SAFELY INTUBATED?

Because most patients with facial fractures do not require resuscitative efforts or urgent intubation on presentation, it is when patients are being prepared for the operating room for definitive fracture management that the anesthesiologist most often becomes directly involved in the patients' care. Under these circumstances, there is generally time to evaluate the patients' airway for anticipated difficulty. The importance of preoperative airway assessment cannot be underestimated. Failure to identify a difficult airway may result in a lack of preparedness and has the potential to create an emergent airway situation because of an inability to intubate and ventilate patients, which clearly has potentially disastrous consequences.

In addition to the factors previously listed, which may result in difficult bag-mask-ventilation in patients with acute facial trauma, one must also assess the general anatomic features that are predictive of a difficult airway. These features include obese, elderly, and edentulous patients, as well as patients with facial hair. These factors may be present in patients with facial trauma just as they are in any population undergoing general anesthesia.

The LEMON assessment is a method of quickly identifying clinical anatomic factors that predispose to difficult laryngoscopy and intubation.[12] The components of this assessment tool are the following:

    Look externally: Assess the physical features associated with difficult laryngoscopy and intubation, such as a retropositioned mandible and short neck.

    Evaluate 3-3-2: The first *3* represents an interincisal opening of at least 3 of one's own finger breadths. The second *3* represents a thyromental distance of 3 finger breadths. The 2 represents 2 finger breadths between the superior notch of the thyroid cartilage to the superior aspect of the hyoid bone. Measurements less than these are predictive of difficult laryngoscopy and intubation.

Mallampati class: This classification system uses 4 categories to assess the transoral visibility of the uvula and oropharynx when patients are asked to open their mouth wide and protrude their tongue. Glottic visualization on laryngoscopy is less likely to be achieved in class III and IV patients than in class I and II patients.[13,14]

Obstruction: Signs of upper airway obstruction include muffled voice, difficulty swallowing, and stridor. Obstruction of the upper airway is considered an indicator of a difficult airway.

Neck mobility: Neck flexion and head extension is considered the optimal position of the head and neck for laryngoscopy and intubation. Patients with limited neck mobility or with c-spine immobilization should be considered to have a difficult airway.

A limited mandibular opening is often used as a predictor of difficult intubation and is incorporated in the Evaluate portion of the LEMON assessment. In addition, a limited mandibular opening will have a negative influence on the Mallampati score. A recent study at Dalhousie University prospectively assessed the preoperative predictors of difficult intubation in patients with isolated mandibular fractures undergoing treatment of their fractures under general anesthesia.[15] Ninety-four patients with isolated mandibular fractures were evaluated using the LEMON evaluation preoperatively. All patients also had glottic views on direct laryngoscopy classified according to the Cormack and Lehane Classification[16] following induction. Grade 1 and 2 laryngeal views were considered easy intubations and grade 3 and 4 views were considered difficult intubations. No association was found between difficult intubation and the LEMON evaluation. A total of 95.7% of patients were predicted to have difficult intubations based on an inability to open their mouth at least 3 finger breadths. Only 3 of these 91 patients actually had grade 3 or 4 views on direct laryngoscopy. In addition, patients were found to have a mean preoperative maximum interincisal opening of 23.4 mm and a mean interincisal opening following induction of 47.3 mm. Patients with mandibular fractures are likely to have limited voluntary mandibular opening because of pain, and this alone should not be considered predictive of a difficult airway.

Although the Dalhousie study demonstrated that patients with mandibular fractures generally do not have limited mandibular opening following induction, there are some conditions under which this may not be the case.

1. Patients who have delayed treatment may develop infection in fascial spaces involving the muscles of mastication. Under these circumstances, there may not be any additional mandibular opening following induction.
2. Zygomaticomaxillary complex fractures, which are displaced posteriorly, can interfere with the mandibular opening by impinging on the coronoid process of the mandible, thus limiting translation of the mandibular condyle until the zygomaticomaxillary complex is reduced.
3. Patients in which the mandibular condyle has been displaced into the middle cranial fossa may experience limited mandibular opening until the condyle is distracted from the middle cranial fossa.
4. Foreign bodies in the temporomandibular joint, which inhibit translation of the mandibular condyle may experience limited mandibular opening.
5. Patients with a history of head and neck radiation therapy may have long-term limited mandibular opening.
6. Patients with a preexisting history of temporomandibular joint disease or ankylosis may have limited mandibular opening.

Following the airway assessment, the anesthesiologist must make a determination regarding whether to proceed directly to induction, paralysis, and intubation or whether the airway is sufficiently difficult to warrant the use of the difficult airway algorithm[17] or an awake intubation.

HOW SHOULD I INTUBATE PATIENTS?
Will the Surgeon Need to Establish Occlusion?

Reestablishing proper dental occlusion is one of the main objectives in the reconstruction of maxillofacial trauma. The surgeon uses the occlusion as a guide to ensure adequate fracture reduction. Typically, the occlusion is reestablished using maxillomandibular fixation (MMF) using either Erich arch bars or intermaxillary fixation screws.

Table 1 lists the common indications for MMF in maxillofacial trauma. As a general rule, MMF is required for the reduction of all mandibular and maxillary fractures. However, establishing occlusion is usually not required in the treatment of isolated zygomatic, orbital, nasal, or frontal bone fractures.

Table 1 Need to establish occlusion?	
Yes	**No**
Mandibular fractures	Zygomatic complex fractures
Symphyseal	Zygomatic arch fractures
Parasymphyseal	Orbital fractures
Body	Nasal bone fractures
Angle	Isolated naso-orbito-ethmoidal fractures
Ramus	Frontal bone fractures
Subcondylar	
Condylar	
Maxillary fractures	
Lefort I, II, and III	
Dentoalveolar fractures	
Panfacial fractures	

After evaluating the patient factors and applying these general rules, the anesthesiologist and surgeon can determine the most appropriate approach to intubate patients. **Table 2** summarizes the indications, contraindications, and complications of the common techniques of airway access in patients with maxillofacial trauma.

Orotracheal Intubation

In patients with maxillofacial trauma, orotracheal intubation has been proven to be a fast and reliable method of securing a definitive airway.[18,19] Unfortunately, orotracheal intubation is usually not the method of choice because it will most often interfere with surgical access. An endotracheal tube inserted orally will obviously impede on the proper restoration of the patients' occlusion when intraoperative MMF is required. Certain types of maxillofacial trauma also have the potential to limit the mouth opening after induction creating a difficult laryngoscopy. These types of trauma could include certain types of condylar fractures or a zygomatic arch fracture impeding on the coronoid process. **Table 2** summarizes the indications, contraindications, and complications associated with the orotracheal intubation.

Direct laryngoscopy

Endotracheal intubation is most commonly achieved via direct laryngoscopy. Visualization of the glottis is achieved using a curved Macintosh blade or a straight Miller blade. The insertion of the tip of the curved Macintosh blade in the vallecula and the elevation of the base of the tongue will create traction on the epiglottis and expose the larynx (**Fig. 2**). A straight Miller blade can also be inserted posterior to the epiglottis to expose the larynx.

In a trauma setting, most of the intubations using direct laryngoscopy are successful. Most of the trauma centers report a failed intubation rate of 1% to 2%.[20–22] Direct laryngoscopy has also been reported to be the fastest technique. Lee and colleagues,[19] in 2009, reviewed the intraoperative airway management of patients with facial fractures and reported on the total procedure time defined as "from induction to successful intubation, tube fixation, and turn on the ventilator." They reported an average time of 4 minutes 33 seconds with orotracheal intubation by direct laryngoscopy and 5 minutes with nasotracheal intubation by direct laryngoscopy compared with an average time of 6 minutes 1 second with fiberoptic nasotracheal intubation and 12 minutes 25 seconds with tracheostomy.[19]

Nonvisual intubation techniques

Maxillofacial trauma is a common predictor of difficult laryngoscopy[20]; this is especially true if foreign materials (blood, emesis, debris, edema, and so forth) compromise direct visualization. A review of the emergency management of maxillofacial injuries with severe oronasal hemorrhage reported a success rate of endotracheal intubation of only 80%.[23] This visualization issue led to the development of nonvisual intubation techniques, which have been proven to be effective, safe, and of low cost.[24] These techniques include intubating stylets, light wands, and retrograde intubation.

Intubating stylets Intubating stylets, often referred as *gum elastic bougie* have been introduced as adjuncts to endotracheal intubation in cases of difficult laryngoscopy. Macintosh[25] first introduced this type of device in 1949, and many other intubating guides have been developed since.[26,27] These devices consist of a long, thin, and fairly stiff wand that can be passed through the laryngeal inlet to serve as a guide for the placement of an endotracheal tube (**Fig. 3**). Its use is widespread, and it is often the initial device recommended in cases of difficult laryngoscopy.[28]

Light wands Light wands are lighted stylets that use the principle of transillumination of the soft tissues of the anterior neck to guide an endotracheal or nasotracheal tube into the trachea. This device has been proven to be effective in cases of difficult laryngoscopy, with Hung and colleagues[29] reporting a success rate of 99% after intubating 265 patients with a difficult airway. Unfortunately, because this technique is blind and relies on transillumination, it is relatively

Table 2
Airway access in maxillofacial injury

	Indications	Contraindications	Complications

Orotracheal	Emergency airway
	Intraoperative MMF not
	  required
	Nasal pyramid fractures
	  (Lefort II and III, NOE,
	  nasal bone)
	Skull base fractures
		Limited mouth opening
		Intraoperative MMF
		  required
		Laryngeal trauma
			Hemorrhage
			Infection
			Airway injury
			Dental injury

Nasotracheal	Intraoperative MMF
	  required (except for
	  nasal pyramid fractures)
	Limited mouth opening
		Emergency airway
		Course of tube uncertain
		  (nasal pyramid fractures,
		  base of skull fractures)
		Traumatic brain injury
		  (possible increase in ICP)
		Coagulopathy
		Laryngeal trauma
			Epistaxis
			Otitis media
			Sinusitis
			False passage
			Dental injury

Submental	Nasotracheal intubation
	  contraindicated and
	  intraoperative MMF
	  required
		Limited mouth opening
		Local injury
		Coagulopathy
		Prolonged intubation
		  required (>7 d)
		Laryngeal trauma
			Hemorrhage
			Accidental extubation
			Tube damage
			Local infection/scar/fistula/
			  mucocele

Retromolar	Nasotracheal intubation
	  contraindicated and
	  intraoperative MMF
	  required
		Limited retromolar space
		Limited mouth opening
		Laryngeal trauma
			Accidental extubation
			Risk of inadequate
			  occlusion
			Long buccal nerve palsy

Tracheostomy	Surgical airway required Prolonged postoperative ventilation Laryngeal trauma	Coagulopathy Expanding hematoma	Hemorrhage Infection Subcutaneous emphysema Esophageal injury False passage Pneumothorax Aspiration pneumonia Tracheal stenosis Tracheoesophageal fistula Vocal cord paralysis

Abbreviations: ICP, intracranial pressure; NOE, naso-orbital-ethmoidal.

Data from Griesdale DE, Liu D, McKinney J, et al. Glidescope® video-laryngoscopy versus direct laryngoscopy for endotracheal intubation: a systematic review and meta-analysis. Can J Anaesth 2012;59:41–52; and Arrowsmith JE, Robertshaw HJ, Boyd JD. Nasotracheal intubation in the presence of frontobasal skull fracture. Can J Anaesth 1998;45:71–5.

contraindicated in cases of severe upper airway and neck trauma. Despite this, a recent case report described its successful use in a patient with significant lacerations in the upper chest and submandibular area.[30]

Retrograde intubation Retrograde intubation has been recommended as an alternative method of intubation for patients who can be ventilated but not intubated using conventional techniques.[31] The technique basically consists of a cricothyroid membrane puncture followed by the insertion of a catheter or guidewire that is advanced and retrieved in the oropharynx. After retrieval, an endotracheal tube is advanced over the guide into the trachea. This method of intubation is not often used because of its technique sensitivity and limited success rate.[32]

Visual intubation techniques
Fiberoptic-assisted visual intubation techniques have been developed for the management of the anticipated difficult airway. These devices are now part of the essential strategies used in the difficult airway algorithm.[31] Commonly used fiberoptic-guided intubation tools include the flexible bronchoscope and the video laryngoscope.

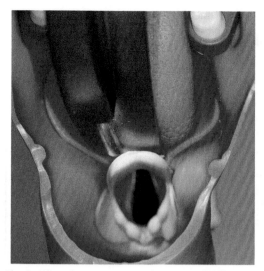

Fig. 2. Direct laryngoscopy with Macintosh blade.

emergency airway management of trauma patients, including cases of penetrating neck trauma,[34–36] massive oropharyngeal bleeding,[37] and unstable bilateral mandibular fractures.[38]

Video laryngoscopic intubation Rigid video-laryngoscope devices combine a laryngoscope-type blade with a video camera to permit non–line-of-sight viewing of the glottis. The use of these devices is similar to direct laryngoscopy, making them fairly easy to use, even for inexperienced operators.[39] A recent meta-analysis showed that the GlideScope video laryngoscope (Verathon Medical, Bothell, WA) is associated with improved glottic visualization, especially in patients with difficult airways.[40] Video laryngoscopy has also been shown to facilitate a better laryngeal view in the trauma setting where manual-in-line stabilization is used to prevent c-spine injury.[41]

Nasotracheal Intubation

Unless contraindicated, nasotracheal intubation is usually the option of choice for the intraoperative airway management of patients with maxillofacial trauma. This technique provides numerous advantages to the trauma surgeon, including improved visibility and the possibility of intraoperative MMF. It can be performed on awake patients or on patients under general anesthesia via direct laryngoscopy, via fiberoptic guidance, or even via a blind nasal intubation technique (**Fig. 5**). It

Flexible bronchoscopic intubation The flexible bronchoscope is widely accepted as an invaluable tool for the management of difficult airways.[33] It can be used in the setting of a general anesthesia or an awake intubation. Using an oral or nasal route, the tip of the bronchoscope can be advanced through the glottis and trachea using direct visualization (**Fig. 4**). An endotracheal tube can then be advanced over the bronchoscope into the trachea. Although more time consuming, bronchoscopic intubation has been successfully used in the

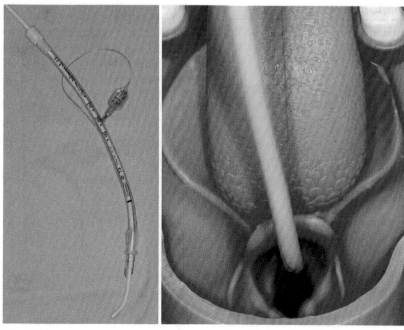

Fig. 3. Intubating stylet.

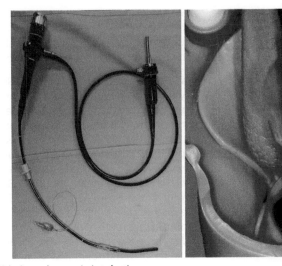

Fig. 4. Flexible bronchoscopic intubation.

is also the route of choice in patients with a significantly limited mouth opening.

Table 2 lists the common indications, contraindications, and complications associated with nasotracheal intubation. The nasal route is contraindicated in cases of basal skull fracture because of a possible intracranial placement. This evidence is based only on 2 case reports[42,43] and is somewhat a subject of debate.[44] Successful fiberoptic nasotracheal intubation has also been described in case reports of patients with suspected basal skull fractures.[45–47]

Submental Intubation

The submental intubation technique is the option of choice for patients with maxillofacial trauma in whom nasotracheal intubation is contraindicated; intraoperative MMF will be required, and prolonged postoperative ventilation is unlikely. **Table 2** summarizes the indications, contraindications, and complications associated with the submental intubation.

The technique basically consists of the conversion of an orotracheal route into a submental-tracheal route and can be summarized as follows. Orotracheal intubation is initially achieved using an armored endotracheal tube with a detachable connector (**Fig. 6**). The skin is then prepared using povidone iodine and then infiltrated with a local anesthetic with epinephrine. A 2-cm skin incision is then performed in the submental area, adjacent to the midline, and parallel to the inferior border of the mandible. A second incision is also performed at the level of the lingual mucogingival junction in the area where the endotracheal tube is desired to exit. Both incisions are then connected (from outside to inside) using a curved artery forceps

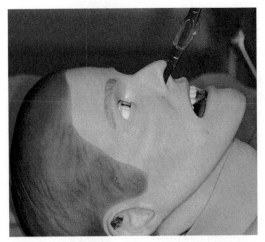

Fig. 5. Nasotracheal intubation via fiberoptic guidance.

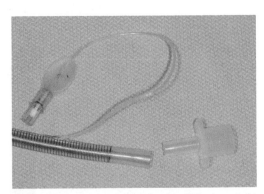

Fig. 6. Armored endotracheal tube with detachable connector.

and blunt dissection through the subcutaneous fat, platysma, deep cervical fascia, and mylohyoid muscle. While leaving the curved artery forceps in place, the tube is then disconnected from the breathing circuit, and the connector is detached. The deflated cuff and endotracheal tube are then pulled through the submandibular incision using the curved artery forceps. The connector is then replaced, the breathing circuit reconnected, and the cuff reinflated. The tube is then secured to the skin using a strong silk suture (**Fig. 7**). At the end of the procedure, the tube is pulled back into an orotracheal route and the skin incision is closed.

In 1986, Hernandez[48] first described this technique to avoid a tracheostomy in a patient with maxillofacial trauma. The method has since gained wide acceptance. Jundt and colleagues,[49] in 2012, recently published a literature review of 842 patients who underwent submental intubation. The technique was successful in 100% of cases.[49] The average procedural time was 9.9 minutes, with ranges varying from less than 4 minutes to 30 minutes.[49] No major complications were reported, and minor complications occurred in 7% of patients.[49] Accidental extubations only occurred in the pediatric population on 2 occasions.[49] The most frequent complications reported were superficial skin infections (N = 23), damage to the tube apparatus (N = 10), and fistula formation (N = 10).[49] Other reported complications included right mainstem bronchus intubation or obstruction (N = 5), hypertrophic scarring (N = 3), excessive bronchial flexion (N = 2), venous bleeding (N = 2), transient lingual nerve paresthesia (N = 1), mucocele (N = 1), and dislodgement of the throat pack sticker in the submental wound (N = 1).[49]

Therefore, submental intubation is a safe and reliable technique that should be considered as an alternative to a tracheostomy in selected patients with maxillofacial trauma.

Retromolar Intubation

The retromolar intubation can be viewed as an alternative to the submental intubation. Therefore, it is indicated when nasotracheal intubation is contraindicated, intraoperative MMF is required, and prolonged postoperative ventilation is unlikely. **Table 2** lists the indications, contraindications, and complications associated with the retromolar intubation.

The technique can be described as follows. After conventional orotracheal intubation using an armored tube, the surgeon repositions the tube in the retromolar space (or missing tooth space) (**Fig. 8**). The tube is then secured in place using a silk suture or a ligature wire around a molar tooth. The patient can then be placed in MMF while the anesthesiologist monitors peak airway pressures and oxygen saturation. At the end of the procedure, the tube can be repositioned to the midline. A semilunar osteotomy of the anterior ramus (with extraction of the mandibular third molar if present) has also been described and could be used in cases when the retromolar space is limited.[50]

The retromolar intubation provides the advantages of being easy to perform, time efficient, and noninvasive. The major disadvantage is that the tube can possibly interfere with the surgical field. The possibility of a long buccal nerve palsy

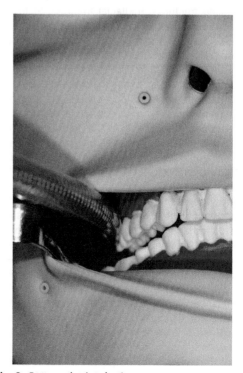

Fig. 8. Retromolar intubation.

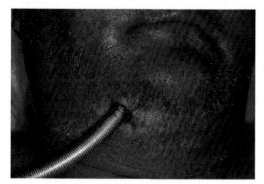

Fig. 7. Secured submental intubation.

has also been reported.[51] Its use was usually recommended in the pediatric population before 15 years of age because of the increased retromolar space (before the eruption of the third molars).[52,53] It has also been successfully used in the adult population.[19,50,51,54] Lee and colleagues,[19] in 2009, reported the use of retromolar intubation in 91 cases of midface fractures. The occlusion and nasal reconstruction of most patients was deemed satisfactory, with only 2 patients requiring a secondary correction of a residual nasal deformity.[19]

Tracheostomy

The decision behind electing to intubate patients via a tracheostomy depends on multiple factors, including the patients' comorbidities; the surgeon's experience; and, most importantly, the cause and extent of the injury.[55] Generally, a surgical airway is indicated when orotracheal and nasotracheal intubations are not possible or when prolonged postoperative ventilation will be required.[55–57] Common injuries requiring a tracheostomy include laryngotracheal injuries, gunshot wounds, and severe panfacial fractures.[55,56] Holmgren and colleagues,[55] in 2007, retrospectively reviewed 1079 patients who sustained facial fractures over a 10-year period. Of these patients, 11.6% received a tracheostomy at the time of the fracture repair.[55] Common facial injures requiring a tracheostomy included multiple mandible fractures, midfacial fractures at the Le Fort III level, panfacial fractures, and larynx fractures.[55] **Table 2** summarizes the indications, contraindications, and complications associated with a tracheostomy.

Before electing to perform a tracheostomy, it is important to consider its associated morbidity. The initial reviews have reported a complication rate ranging from 6.7% to 48.0%, with a 1.6% mortality rate.[58,59] Recent studies have reported lower complication rates varying from 2.7% to 14.1%, with an overall mortality rate of only 0.85%.[60,61] The perioperative complications include hemorrhage, pneumothorax, aspiration, esophageal injury, accidental decannulation/false passage, and subcutaneous emphysema. The postoperative complications include mucous plugging, tracheitis/infection, bleeding, tracheal stenosis, tracheomalacia, tracheocutaneous or tracheoesophageal fistulas, and vocal cord paralysis.[55,61,62]

Patients with maxillofacial trauma requiring a tracheostomy usually have a more complex hospital course.[55] This point was shown by Holmgren and colleagues[55] who reviewed 125 patients with facial fractures who required a tracheostomy compared with 224 patients with facial fractures who did not require a tracheostomy. Their initial Glasgow Coma Score was lower (6.8 with tracheostomy and 12.4 without), whereas their facial injury severity score was higher (6.22 with tracheostomy and 3.16 without).[55] Patients with a tracheostomy had both a longer intensive-care-unit stay (7.21 days with tracheostomy and 1.33 days without) and hospital length of stay (19.71 days with tracheostomy and 6.82 days without).[55] The incidence of death was also higher (7.2% with tracheostomy and 0% without).[55] All of these differences were statistically significant (all $P<.000001$).[55]

SUMMARY

Facial fractures are commonly encountered injuries that frequently require intervention. Although they are commonly isolated injuries, they may be associated with more extensive systemic trauma, including c-spine and head injuries. Implementation of ATLS principles is important in the resuscitation and stabilization of such patients. Some commonly used airway assessment tools may not offer any predictive value in patients with facial fractures, particularly because of the limited voluntary mandibular opening resulting from pain associated with mandibular fractures. The nature of the facial fractures, the treatment required to manage them, the concomitant injuries, and the airway challenges patients present with must be taken into account in determining the most appropriate method of intubation for individual patients. This determination requires close communication between the anesthesiologist and the surgeon managing the facial fractures.

REFERENCES

1. Hackl W, Hausberger K, Sailer R, et al. Prevalence of cervical spine injuries in patients with facial trauma. Oral Surg Oral Med Oral Pathol Oral Radiol Endod 2001;92:370–6.
2. Elahi MM, Brar MS, Ahmed N, et al. Cervical spine injury in association with craniomaxillofacial fractures. Plast Reconstr Surg 2008;121:201–8.
3. Mulligan RP, Friedman JA, Mahabir RC. A nationwide review of the associations among cervical spine injuries, head injuries, and facial fractures. J Trauma 2010;68:587–92.
4. Stiell IG, Wells GA, Vandemheen KL, et al. The Canadian C-spine rule for radiography in alert and stable trauma patients. JAMA 2001;286:1841–8.
5. Stiell IG, Clement CM, McKnight RD, et al. The Canadian C-spine rule versus the NEXUS low-risk criteria in patients with trauma. N Engl J Med 2003;349:2510–8.

6. Stiell IG, Clement CM, Grimshaw J, et al. Implementation of the Canadian C-spine rule: prospective 12 centre cluster randomised trial. BMJ 2009; 339:b4146.

7. Michaleff ZA, Maher CG, Verhagen AP, et al. Accuracy of the Canadian C-spine rule and NEXUS to screen for clinically important cervical spine injury in patients following blunt trauma: a systematic review. CMAJ 2012;184:E867–76.

8. Grant AL, Ranger A, Young GB, et al. Incidence of major and minor brain injuries in facial fractures. J Craniofac Surg 2012;23:1324–8.

9. Stiell IG, Wells GA, Vandemheen K, et al. The Canadian CT head rule for patients with minor head injury. Lancet 2001;357:1391–6.

10. Smits M, Dippel DW, de Haan GG, et al. External validation of the Canadian CT head rule and the New Orleans criteria for CT scanning in patients with minor head injury. JAMA 2005;294:1519–25.

11. Korley FK, Morton MJ, Hill PM, et al. Agreement between routine emergency department care and clinical decision support recommended care in patients evaluated for mild traumatic brain injury. Acad Emerg Med 2013;20:463–9.

12. Murphy M, Doyle D. Evaluation of the airway. In: Hung O, Murphy MF, editors. Management of the difficult and failed airway. 2nd edition. New York: McGraw-Hill; 2012. p. 3–14.

13. Mallampati SR. Clinical sign to predict difficult tracheal intubation (hypothesis). Can Anaesth Soc J 1983;30:316–7.

14. Mallampati SR, Gatt SP, Gugino LD, et al. A clinical sign to predict difficult tracheal intubation: a prospective study. Can Anaesth Soc J 1985;32:429–34.

15. Cobb J, Robertson C, Precious D. Effect of isolated mandible fracture on direct laryngoscopy and intubation difficulty. In: Programs and abstracts of the 91st AAOMS Annual Meeting and Scientific Sessions. Toronto: 2009. J Oral Maxillofac Surg 2009; 67(Suppl 2):34.

16. Cormack RS, Lehane J. Difficult tracheal intubation in obstetrics. Anaesthesia 1984;39:1105–11.

17. Murphy M, Crosby E. The algorithms. In: Hung O, Murphy MF, editors. Management of the difficult and failed airway. 2nd edition. New York: McGraw-Hill; 2012. p. 15–29.

18. Clinton J, Ruiz E. Emergency airway management: methods to meet the challenge. Top Emerg Med 1988;10:31–41.

19. Lee SS, Huang SH, Wu SH, et al. A review of intraoperative airway management for midface facial bone fracture patients. Ann Plast Surg 2009;63: 162–6.

20. Stephens CT, Kahntroff S, Dutton RP. The success of emergency endotracheal intubation in trauma patients: a 10-year experience at a major adult trauma referral center. Anesth Analg 2009;109: 866–72.

21. Dunham CM, Barraco RD, Clark DE, et al. Guidelines for emergency tracheal intubation immediately after traumatic injury. J Trauma 2003;55: 162–79.

22. Sise MJ, Shackford SR, Sise CB, et al. Early intubation in the management of trauma patients: indications and outcomes in 1,000 consecutive patients. J Trauma 2009;66:32–9.

23. Cogbill TH, Cothren CC, Ahearn MK, et al. Management of maxillofacial injuries with severe oronasal hemorrhage: a multicenter perspective. J Trauma 2008;65:994–9.

24. Christodoulou C, Hung O. Nonvisual intubation techniques. In: Hung O, Murphy MF, editors. Management of the difficult and failed airway. 2nd edition. New York: McGraw-Hill; 2012. p. 186–200.

25. Macintosh R. An aid to oral intubation [letter]. BMJ 1979;1:28.

26. Venn P. The gum elastic bougie. Anaesthesia 1993; 48:274–5.

27. Hodzovic I, Latto IP, Wilkes AR, et al. Evaluation of Frova, single-use intubation introducer, in a manikin. Comparison with Eschmann multiple-use introducer and Portex single-use introducer. Anaesthesia 2004;59:811–6.

28. Henderson JJ, Popat MT, Latto IP, et al. Difficult Airway Society guidelines for management of the unanticipated difficult intubation. Anaesthesia 2004;59:675–94.

29. Hung OR, Pytka S, Morris I, et al. Lightwand intubation: II–clinical trial of a new lightwand for tracheal intubation in patients with difficult airways. Can J Anaesth 1995;42:826–30.

30. Jain S, Bhadani U. Lightwand: a useful aid in faciomaxillary trauma. J Anesth 2011;25:291–3.

31. American Society of Anesthesiologists Task Force on Management of the Difficult Airway. Practice guidelines for management of the difficult airway: an updated report by the American Society of Anesthesiologists Task Force on Management of the Difficult Airway. Anesthesiology 2003;98: 1269–77.

32. Lenfant F, Benkhadra M, Trouilloud P, et al. Comparison of two techniques for retrograde tracheal intubation in human fresh cadavers. Anesthesiology 2006;104:48–51.

33. Rosenblatt WH, Wagner PJ, Ovassapian A, et al. Practice patterns in managing the difficult airway by anesthesiologists in the United States. Anesth Analg 1998;87:153–7.

34. Shearer VE, Giesecke AH. Airway management for patients with penetrating neck trauma: a retrospective study. Anesth Analg 1993;77: 1135–8.

35. Mandavia DP, Qualls S, Rokos I. Emergency airway management in penetrating neck injury. Ann Emerg Med 2000;35:221–5.

36. Desjardins G, Varon AJ. Airway management for penetrating neck injuries: the Miami experience. Resuscitation 2001;48:71–5.

37. Preis CA, Hartmann T, Zimpfer M. Laryngeal mask airway facilitates awake fiberoptic intubation in a patient with severe oropharyngeal bleeding. Anesth Analg 1998;87:728–9.

38. Neal MR, Groves J, Gell IR. Awake fibreoptic intubation in the semi-prone position following facial trauma. Anaesthesia 1996;51:1053–4.

39. Nouruzi-Sedeh P, Schumann M, Groeben H. Laryngoscopy via Macintosh blade versus GlideScope: success rate and time for endotracheal intubation in untrained medical personnel. Anesthesiology 2009;110:32–7.

40. Griesdale DE, Liu D, McKinney J, et al. Glidescope® video-laryngoscopy versus direct laryngoscopy for endotracheal intubation: a systematic review and meta-analysis. Can J Anaesth 2012;59:41–52.

41. Aziz M. Use of video-assisted intubation devices in the management of patients with trauma. Anesthesiol Clin 2013;31:157–66.

42. Muzzi DA, Losasso TJ, Cucchiara RF. Complication from a nasopharyngeal airway in a patient with a basilar skull fracture. Anesthesiology 1991;74:366–8.

43. Schade K, Borzotta A, Michaels A. Intracranial malposition of nasopharyngeal airway. J Trauma 2000;49:967–8.

44. Roberts K, Whalley H, Bleetman A. The nasopharyngeal airway: dispelling myths and establishing the facts. Emerg Med J 2005;22:394–6.

45. Arrowsmith JE, Robertshaw HJ, Boyd JD. Nasotracheal intubation in the presence of frontobasal skull fracture. Can J Anaesth 1998;45:71–5.

46. Huang JJ, Wu J, Brandt K. Airway management of a patient with facial trauma. J Clin Anesth 2002;14:302–4.

47. Lee BB. Nasotracheal intubation in a patient with maxillo-facial and basal skull fractures. Anaesthesia 2004;59:299–300.

48. Hernández Altemir F. The submental route for endotracheal intubation. A new technique. J Maxillofac Surg 1986;14:64–5.

49. Jundt JS, Cattano D, Hagberg CA, et al. Submental intubation: a literature review. Int J Oral Maxillofac Surg 2012;41:46–54.

50. Martinez-Lage JL, Eslava JM, Cebrecos AI, et al. Retromolar intubation. J Oral Maxillofac Surg 1998;56:302–5.

51. Dutta A, Kumar V, Saha SS, et al. Retromolar tracheal tube positioning for patients undergoing faciomaxillary surgery. Can J Anaesth 2005;52:341.

52. Arora S, Rattan V, Bhardwaj N. An evaluation of the retromolar space for oral tracheal tube placement for maxillofacial surgery in children. Anesth Analg 2006;103:1122–5.

53. Habib A, Zanaty OM. Use of retromolar intubation in paediatric maxillofacial trauma. Br J Anaesth 2012;109:650–1.

54. Malhotra N. Retromolar intubation–a simple alternative to submental intubation. Anaesthesia 2006;61:515–6.

55. Holmgren EP, Bagheri S, Bell RB, et al. Utilization of tracheostomy in craniomaxillofacial trauma at a level-1 trauma center. J Oral Maxillofac Surg 2007;65:2005–10.

56. Mohan R, Iyer R, Thaller S. Airway management in patients with facial trauma. J Craniofac Surg 2009;20:21–3.

57. Das S, Das TP, Ghosh PS. Submental intubation: a journey over the last 25 years. J Anaesthesiol Clin Pharmacol 2012;28:291–303.

58. Chew JY, Cantrell RW. Tracheostomy. Complications and their management. Arch Otolaryngol 1972;96:538–45.

59. Taicher S, Givol N, Peleg M, et al. Changing indications for tracheostomy in maxillofacial trauma. J Oral Maxillofac Surg 1996;54:292–5.

60. Haspel AC, Coviello VF, Stevens M. Retrospective study of tracheostomy indications and perioperative complications on oral and maxillofacial surgery service. J Oral Maxillofac Surg 2012;70:890–5.

61. Halum SL, Ting JY, Plowman EK, et al. A multi-institutional analysis of tracheotomy complications. Laryngoscope 2012;122:38–45.

62. Scully J, Matheson J, Ramming S, et al. Emergency airway management in the traumatized patient. In: Fonseca RJ, Walker RV, Betts NJ, editors. Oral and maxillofacial trauma. 3rd edition. St Louis (MO): Elsevier; 2005. p. 135–74.

Management of Fractures of the Condyle, Condylar Neck, and Coronoid Process

Reha Kisnisci, DDS, PhD

KEYWORDS

- Condylar fracture • Condylar neck fracture • Management • Coronoid fracture

KEY POINTS

- There have been significant developments in craniomaxillofacial trauma care and the management of mandibular condylar injuries in the last several decades.
- The treatment of condylar fractures has been carried out by either functional methods and appliances or by maxillomandibular immobilization techniques.
- Several surgical techniques and innovative concepts have been introduced in order to minimize perioperative challenges.
- An appreciation of the impact on facilitated functional recovery after anatomic reconstruction and functional stabilization has gained popularity.
- There is an increased tendency for surgeons to perform open reduction of the displaced condylar fracture.

INTRODUCTION

Over recent decades, significant headway in craniomaxillofacial trauma care has been achieved. Although perhaps not to the same extent, advancements in the management of mandibular condylar injuries have nevertheless proved to be no exception. Essentially, condylar fractures have been treated by closed means either by functional methods and appliances or by maxillomandibular immobilization techniques for a lengthy period, almost without operative interventions apart from a few reported attempts in the early years of the last century.[1] Subsequently, controversy has evolved with regard to treatment by closed reduction, in which an anatomic alignment was not expected, versus open reduction.[2–4] Several surgical techniques and innovative concepts are introduced in order to minimize perioperative challenges, which are often considered the cause of postoperative complications. In addition, an appreciation of the marked impact on facilitated functional recovery after proper anatomic reconstruction and functional stabilization has gained widespread popularity. Thus, there is an increased tendency for surgeons to perform open reduction of the displaced condylar fracture.[3,5–9]

RECENT ADVANCEMENTS

Recently, there have been an increased number of enhanced study designs, with randomized prospective reports, comparative clinical analysis, and novel techniques reporting not only clinically relevant interpretations to be applied in daily clinical practice but also broadened management strategies.[7,9–16] Significant improvements in diagnostic modalities, adequate surgical access, and operative concepts for complex and difficult

Disclosures: The author has nothing to disclose.
Department of Oral and Maxillofacial Surgery, School of Dentistry, Ankara University, Mesa Koru Sitesi Orkide Blok No:52, Ankara 06530, Turkey
E-mail address: kisnisci@gmail.com

Oral Maxillofacial Surg Clin N Am 25 (2013) 573–590
http://dx.doi.org/10.1016/j.coms.2013.07.003
1042-3699/13/$ – see front matter © 2013 Elsevier Inc. All rights reserved

fractures have been achieved. Accordingly, operative indications have expanded to include some conditions previously believed to be inoperable (**Box 1**).

Condylar fractures in children are commonly managed by closed techniques; however, technical improvements have enabled a change in managing such cases.[15] Similarly, high condylar or intracapsular fractures were among the most challenging cases; for many years, they were not considered for operative treatment and were reserved only for conservative modalities. Contrary to other human joints, involvement of capsular and diskoligamentous soft tissues of

the temporomandibular joint (TMJ) restricted operative indications of condylar fractures in the past. Some recent studies have advocated direct operative management of these structures, because if left disrupted, they might be considered as nefarious factors capable of influencing long-term functional outcomes. Condylar soft tissues and diskoligamentous involvement may require careful assessment and open reduction to avoid functional disturbances.

Taken together, newer medical technologies and devices, techniques, and enhanced operative expertise added to the fact that anatomic alignment of condylar fractures by closed means is rarely achievable, have all encouraged surgeons to perform open, reconstructive, anatomic reduction and internal fixation.

Box 1
Recent advancements in the management of condylar injuries

Enhanced imaging modalities/interpretations

- Detection of soft tissue injuries (ie, diskoligamentous attachments)

- Detection of fracture line in relation to capsule

- Assessment of precise location, angulation, comminution, characteristics, and positioning of fracture

- Minimize postoperative misinterpretation

- Assessment of hardware placement, alignment, and interferences

Surgical anatomic studies/revisited techniques/innovative and modified surgical approaches

Importance/understanding of anatomic reduction

Identifying key areas for proper anatomic reduction and internal fixation

- Improved open or assisted reduction techniques

- Improved open or assisted internal fixation techniques

Intracapsular fracture management

Sustainable concomitant bone defect reconstruction

Operative management possibilities in children

Soft tissue injury management (when and if needed)

Improvements/wide selection of fixation materials

Increased availability for early functional recovery

Early and effective postoperative physical therapy

CHALLENGES

Basic operative indications and principles after injuries of the joints of the locomotor system were established some time ago, but the operative management of mandibular condyle fractures was slow to adopt these principles because of the propensity for surgeons to use closed modalities without emphasis on immediate anatomic reduction. In contrast, the management of fractures at other sites in the mandible adapted fundamental orthopedic fracture treatment principles early on, and indications of operative managements became less restricted than condylar fractures. The specific surgical fundamentals for the mandible included proper anatomic reduction, functionally stable fixation, followed by subsequent musculoskeletal physical therapy in order to accelerate recovery to premorbid status. In orthopedic practice, closed reduction might be chosen to be performed under the guidance of imaging in selected indications followed by immobilization for maintaining repositioned bony segments, whereas immediate anatomic reduction was rarely accomplished in condylar fractures and relied only on postoperative occlusal stabilization or guidance treatments to exploit growth potential. Generally, open reduction techniques yield better results for accelerated recovery and decreased incidence of long-term functional problems. Surgeons hesitantly opted for operative condylar fracture treatments mainly because of troublesome surgical exposure, particularly by the immediacy of facial nerve branches. Unavoidable scars caused by cutaneous incision, risks of facial palsy, and difficulty of incorporating technological innovations, with long-term learning curves and extended operating time, account for some of the drawbacks related to operative interventions.

Condylar fractures appeal to researchers who are planning projects to illuminate obscurities, compare treatment approaches, investigate outcome measures, and seek options for accelerated recovery to minimize functional and physiologic challenges or complications. However, multiple hindrances exist to conducting prospective and randomized clinical projects to obtain convincing management schemes for condylar fractures. Case selection bias, divergent approaches of care, ethics, assessment of outcomes, and exclusion variables may limit clinical trials.[17]

Another reason for not abandoning closed management to justify surgical modalities, despite several developments, is the possibly unavoidable operative complications. In addition, reduction and alignment of fractured bones relying on dental occlusion is not as sound and reliable as dentate parts of the mandible with the fracture lines crossing or engaging teeth. On the other hand, closed techniques without direct reduction maneuvers and functionally stable fixation may result in serious problems, including facial disfigurement, oral dysfunction, obstructive sleep apnea, and craniomandibular ankylosis.

Some cases may be compounded by concomitant fracture of the contralateral condyle. Bilateral fractures are sometimes regarded as a duplicate of single condylar fracture, in which protocols identical to those for unilateral fractures may apply. Sometimes, bilateral fractures are judged and considered to be different fractures, each of which requires independent treatment. An example is to treat each of the mildly displaced bilateral fractures by closed means, considering the mandible to be as reliable as it would be in a unilateral condylar fracture. However, with bilateral injuries, the mandible is different in unilateral fractures, both biomechanically and functionally, which may lead to misinterpretation of the outcomes if evaluated by the mean values of unilateral condyle fracture outcome measures. Therefore, selection and treatment criteria of the outcomes should be considered with caution, particularly if bilateral fractures are considered simply as 2 unilateral fractures. Each circumstance requires different criteria on which to make comparisons.

GOALS AND FUNCTIONAL IMPORTANCE OF MANAGEMENT

The main goals of management of mandibular condyle injuries are to restore premorbid dental occlusion, obtain painless normal range of movements, and to correct and avoid functional, esthetic, and developmental complications. The TMJ plays a significant role as a part of the entire craniofacial structure. Its distinct entity enables it to assume physical loads between the mandible and cranium. Forces of exceeding magnitudes over time or sudden impacts may affect the integrity of the TMJ, leading to various disorders and a spectrum of injuries of the soft or hard tissues.

The TMJ is unique in that it transfers forces through a simple class III lever, but with a complex system of vectors.[18] The constituent parts derive mainly internally from the temporalis and masseter muscles and externally from biting and chewing points. Biting and chewing functions also have varying force levels depending on location, side, and state of edentulism. The forces are predominantly compressive forces on the balancing side. For the same reasons as those for unilateral injuries, bilateral fractures of the mandibular condyles influence mobility, mastication, and bite force on both sides as a result of the injury.

The TMJ is a supportive system in mandibular movements, although disorders and trauma may be compensated by simple hinge movements. However, limited translation movements may be expected in most of the injured or deranged joints. It is commonly accepted that the contralateral joint assumes more forces when molar biting takes place in normal circumstances.[19] In the event of unilateral mandibular condyle fracture, contralateral muscles take on additional loads in order to ease and lower the load on injured condyle. Reduction of load on the injured condyle biting on the contralateral side may be achieved particularly by taking more loads by the masseter muscle.

Once the mandibular condyle fracture is surgically reduced, followed by internal fixation, then stabilizing muscle functions or a need for neuromuscular protection decreases.[20] In addition, even if patients refrain from biting on the fractured condyle side, load is mostly generated at the uninjured side, although much reduced compared with the normal cycle of muscle activities. In this manner, cases with unilateral mandibular condyle fractures reveal a protective mechanism by which, after injury, patients return from subnormal to almost normal function through adaptive responses of the musculature. The lateral pterygoid muscle is disabled from normal function on the side of mandibular condyle fractures.[21] This situation affects the type of mandibular mobility and not only limits the vertical range of movement but also prevents the TMJ from executing translation, resulting in deviation toward the fractured side. Some investigators have reported that this deviation may persist when fractures of mandibular condyle are managed by closed treatment.[22] On the other hand, patients who have undergone open reduction and internal fixation show a compensatory functional load, in which increased equilibrium between biting and balancing sides occurs.[20]

PHYSIOLOGIC CONSIDERATIONS

Modern interpretation and understanding of the temporomandibular articulation embraces the treatment of injuries to the area, by taking into account the appropriate properties of condyle. The TMJ, and hence the condyle, is modulated through functional activities. Many researchers have presented evidence to support the hypothesis that the condyle is a load-bearing joint even when transmitting physiologic and functional forces. Others believe that TMJ is unique in being capped with fibrocartilage (to withstand forces resulting from its translating movement along the slope of the glenoid fossa) instead of hyaline cartilage, as is the case in other joints. Many researchers believe that there is increased strain at both condyles, albeit more on the balancing side than on the working side, but nevertheless, they are agreed that there is load during function.

The ignored adaptive role of function at the condylar level after trauma and proposed management may lead to unnecessary, insufficient, or even erroneous treatment planning. In particular, when injury to the TMJ is sustained during growth, the clinician must consider the presence of additional adaptive responses.

Interest has also been directed toward the response of the tissues in the TMJ. Forces that are required to irreparably damage the tissues vary, including the magnitude, direction, and duration of the force. The articular cartilage is distinctive in composition and biomechanical properties and has been reported as a viscoelastic tissue, which shows specific traits of gliding, hysteresis, and tensile stress. A combination of forces acting on the cartilage comprises shear and strain. Biomechanical properties of the articular cartilage derive from extracellular matrix configuration, which is heterogeneous throughout its lining. Normally, cartilage responds to anteroposterior shear forces, resulting in randomly arranged fiber bundles with higher tensile and shear stiffness of the cartilage in the anteroposterior direction.[23] Hence, condylar cartilage shows anisotropy, with the fibrous zone being comparable with the fibrocartilaginous temporomandibular disk. However, compression forces seem to be the primary mode of loading on the osseous portion of the condyle.[24] The temporomandibular disk, on the other hand, is more organized in terms of biochemical features than the mandibular condyle,

because it is under complex forces, including impact, excessive strain, and sustained loads. Because of obvious knowledge limitations of human temporomandibular disk, retrodiskal tissue, condyle, and cartilage, a consensus on their biomechanics is lacking.

ANATOMIC CONSIDERATIONS

Generally, in displaced condyle fracture, shortening of the ramus/condyle unit occurs as a result of traumatic impact, which also causes occlusal changes. The initial displaced location may further change as a result of pterygoid muscle resting tone, and the flexed position of the condyle after injury is most common in adult cases. This condition is shown by slight to severe inclination of the condylar fragment. In addition, mandibular movements under the influence of related musculature may further affect the position of the fractured condyle. In the event of even a slight override of the ipsilateral premature occlusal contact, a mandibular shift and anterior open bite take place. Resultant alterations may manifest in a spectrum of mild to severe clinical forms depending on the height loss of the ipsilateral ascending ramus. In bilateral fractures, mandibular posterior rotation, retrognathic appearance, and anterior open bite are common clinical findings.

Morphology of the condyle may also dictate the resultant injury.[25] In children, the thin cortical layer over the condylar head predisposes it to injuries at this level, whereas the slender neck in adulthood along with thickened cortex over the condylar head means that neck fractures are more likely (**Figs. 1** and **2**). In addition, the thin cortical layer is more likely to give rise to comminuted-type condylar head fractures. In adulthood, condylar head fractures are usually sagittal and more commonly involve the medial pole. Another anatomic variation that may affect the traumatic insult is the round versus elongated shapes of

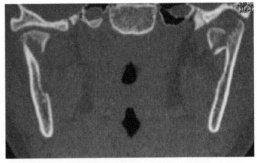

Fig. 1. Computed tomography (CT) of a patient aged 6 years with bilateral condylar head fracture.

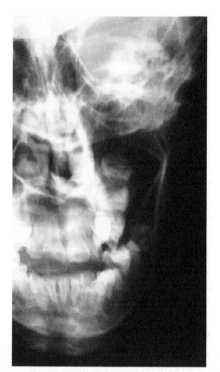

Fig. 2. Plane radiograph revealing a left-sided condylar neck fracture.

the condylar head. A small and diminished surface area with a rounded condylar head when subjected to a cranially directed force may penetrate through thin glenoid fossa then into the middle cranial fossa (**Fig. 3**). The likelihood of this occurrence may also be attributed to thin condylar neck, highly pneumatized bone, and mandibular open position at the time of inflicted force.[26] Even although such extreme dislocation, with the potential factors

described, is less likely to result in condylar neck fractures, fracture is more likely when the forces are exerted in more angled vectors. Reported cases of middle cranial fossa dislocations may require closed reduction or open reduction with or without craniotomy.

CAUSE AND EPIDEMIOLOGY

Indirect trauma is the predominant cause of condylar fractures, in which forces transfer from the more resistant facial skeleton, usually as a result of an impact or blow to the chin region anteriorly and the mandibular body region laterally (**Fig. 4**).[27] Fractures caused by indirect forces may occur if the mouth is open, following along the trajectories to its weakest and less supported part.[25,28] Some investigators have reported that excessive forces are more likely to be associated with bilateral condyle as well as intracapsular fractures.[29,30] On the other hand, when the mouth is closed, most of the impacted force is absorbed at the occlusal level by the teeth, which increases the likelihood of intracapsular injuries.[28]

In adults, the incidence is stated to be lower than that in children. In general, the incidence varies from 19% to as high as 67%.[29,31–36] Although both mandibular condyles can be fractured, most cases are unilateral, ranging in ratio from 1:5 to 1:3.[37] The left side is affected more than the right by a ratio of approximately 3:2. Males are reported to sustain these injuries more than females both in adult and pediatric populations, with the ratio being as high as 4.65:1.[37–39] In children, the boy/girl ratio is 1:0.7, with a mean distribution curve present at the mixed dentition period around 6 to 12 years. However, in

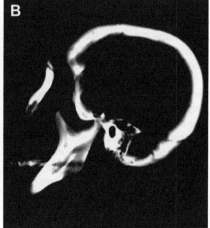
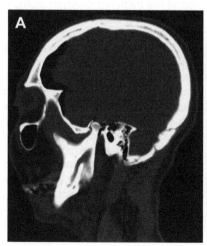

Fig. 3. CT of the left condyle penetrated to the middle cranial fossa (*A*) before treatment (*B*) 2 months after closed reduction.

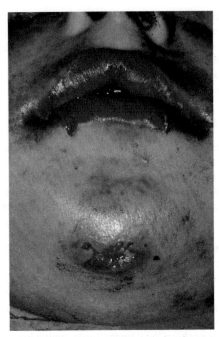

Fig. 4. Clinical view after a blow to the chin in a patient aged 6 years with bilateral condylar head fracture.

adulthood, the gender incidence difference ranges from between 2-fold and 3-fold in males over females.[30] Some studies showed that the male/female ratio nearly triples between the ages of 21 and 30 years when compared in patients aged from 11 to 20 years.[38]

Geography may play a role in the cause of condylar fractures when violence outweighs other factors in certain regions.[32,40] Road traffic accidents are reported to be a frequent cause, but this is independent of income per capita.[30,38,41] Physical falls, on the other hand, may be more related to cultural habits and population movements.[42,43]

Determinants of the resultant fracture include the direction of the force, the position of the mandible during impact (open or closed) and the status of the dental occlusion, all of which are crucial for determination of degree and direction of fracture displacement (**Box 2**). In younger ages, it is more likely for patients to sustain fractures above the condylar neck level, which present as high condylar or condylar head fractures, contrary to elderly patients, in whom condylar fractures are unlikely to be detected above the ascending ramus. Infrequently, traumatic insults induce condylar dislocations without occurrence of any fractures but dislodging the mandibular condyle into the infratemporal fossa, although lateral, posterior, and superior dislocations have

---

Box 2
Determinants of condylar fracture and injury pattern
Direction of the force
Magnitude of energy
Position of the mandible during impact (open or closed)
Muscle pull
Status of dentition and dental occlusion
Age
Extent of soft tissue involvement

also been reported. Anatomy of the condyle, direction and nature of the insult, and vector of muscle pull have all been defined as attributing factors.[44–46]

CLASSIFICATION

Several studies have been conducted regarding classification of condylar fractures, and the earliest reports used criteria such as anatomic site, degree of displacement, fracture level, relationship to capsule, and types of insult. These criteria were predicated on closed reduction treatment considerations, which almost always reflected the choice of management. Introduction of advanced imaging modalities incited clinically more relevant nomenclature systems to be used and the commonly used classification of Spiessl and Schroll proposed 6 classes of fractures at the condylar head and condylar neck with various types of displacements.[47] Lindhall[48] furthered a classification system addressing the level of fracture and position of the fractured condylar stump in relation to corresponding stump inferiorly and to the glenoid fossa superiorly. Low condylar neck fractures analogous to fracture of the ascending ramus were added by Krenkel.[49]

Most recently, a classification described by Loukota and colleagues[50] was adopted for the Strasbourg Osteosynthesis Research Group (SORG), based on 3 distinct anatomic levels, which involve the condylar head, condylar neck, and condylar base. SORG also addressed a common misnomer regarding intracapsular fractures, which are not always confined within the joint capsule itself but sometimes can occur such that they are popped out in a sagittal-inferior direction.[51] This situation can lead to an alteration, with a more clinically relevant definition of condylar head fractures with ramus shortening or condylar head fractures without ramus shortening.[52]

MANAGEMENT

Surgical treatments with open reduction techniques are almost always reported to produce unsightly scars.[3,53] Persistent facial nerve palsy, despite well-described techniques, continues to exist as a surgical consequence of open reduction.[8,54–58] Intraoral approaches to surmount some of these inconveniences were introduced, but with inevitable restrictions, including difficulty in visualization and fixation.[59] On the other hand, maxillomandibular fixation rarely achieves reduction of the fractured bones.[2] This technique causes vertical shortening of the ipsilateral ramus with or without noticeable facial midline shift. The maxillomandibular immobilization period is reported to be associated with subsequent impairment in bite force and reduction in vertical mouth opening.[60–62]

FUNCTIONAL AND CLOSED MANAGEMENT (NONSURGICAL)

Typically, the aim of closed treatment alternatives is to obtain favorable functional adaptation. This method is still a preferred treatment in certain cases, supported by patient survey reports that revealed statistically acceptable results in terms of pain as a typical outcome.[27] Some comparative studies have reported minimal or even unchanged occlusal disturbances when comparing closed and open methods.[39,63,64] Furthermore, functionally reasonable outcomes have been reported in which preinjury symmetry, occlusion, and painless mandibular range of movement were regained.[64] Some evidence exists that shows that the condylar position is not static but may tilt in certain cases and thus is compatible with the results of open methods.[64,65]

A wide range of closed treatment modalities have been reported for selected patients (**Box 3**).

Box 3
Supportive and closed treatment options for condylar fractures

Dietary restrictions (liquid, soft)

Medication (pain)

Partial immobilization (7–15 days)

Total immobilization (not exceeding 20 days)

Continuous passive motion

Functional appliances

Orthodontic therapy

Physical therapy

Data from Refs.[4,7,27,106,118–121]

Functional treatments, elastic guidance, vertical mandibular movement exercises to maintain midline, and soft diet regimes may be chosen either as a supportive therapy or as a primary choice of treatment. Physiotherapy is recommended when patient comfort permits, usually by straight mouth opening exercises but also by exerting tongue force on the palatal surface anteriorly, as well as manually, and assisted maneuvers for incremental increase for jaw opening. Functional therapy is a nonoperative modality to maintain dental occlusion, enabling early mobilization and recovery of intra-articular physiology, especially in children, in order to eliminate intracapsular sources, which might limit future mandibular mobility and normal facial growth. In children, remodeling is believed to result after functional or restorative adaptation with enhanced structural remodeling ability.[18,66]

Closed treatment with or without maxillomandibular fixation may still be selected in the presence of unilateral, isolated, and mild to moderately displaced condylar fractures, because it is considered to be safe, noninvasive and minimally complicated, outweighing the possible benefits of open operative methods. In cases with malocclusion, the main goal is to establish an acceptable bite and if semi-immobilization with allowance for limited function is chosen, then close monitoring is required. It is usually recommended to reduce the duration of maxillomandibular fixation as much as possible to minimize deleterious and sometimes irreversible effects on the TMJ.

OPERATIVE MANAGEMENT STRATEGIES

Controversies still exist around the operative management of condylar fractures for open reduction and internal fixation.[3,7,8,18,53,67–69] According to reports,[7] the choice of open operative treatment, irrespective of the method of internal fixation used, was found to be superior in terms of functional parameters. Anatomic reduction of the fracture to allow primary bony healing and accelerated functional recovery after trauma reconstruction are the desirable goals. In addition, operative complications, temporomandibular functional embarrassment, and facial deformity can be avoided.

Soft Tissue Injuries

In open treatment, if not already lacerated, it is preferred not to use the joint capsule for surgical access. Operative handling restores the displaced disk and ligamentous attachments per se, and hence, intra-articular surgical manipulations may not be needed.[70] Determination of disk position may be misleading, because preoperative assessment tools of clinical, functional, and magnetic resonance imaging results are found to be discordant with operative observations.[70] On the other hand, failure of early disk repositioning is likely to be linked with postoperative dysfunction caused by contracture healing of the injured capsule and retrodiskal tissue.[71] In the case of dislocated yet intact condyles out of the fossa, nonoperative and closed manipulations are suggested for repositioning the condyle into its anatomic location. Only on rare occasions is surgical reduction required.[72] Soft tissue injuries can be found in as many as 97.6% of cases; the most common injury is inferomedial displacement of the disk along with the condylar segment in dislocated condylar fractures.[73] Retrodiskal tear is another common finding, whereas capsular tear can be detected in around half of the cases.[74] In operative treatment of intracapsular fractures, soft tissue injuries are common, and a critical operative preference is given to the preservation of the lateral pterygoid muscle rather than stripping it off to facilitate reduction.[74] Furthermore, stripping off even more soft tissues around the condylar fracture site in order to ease visualization, reduction, and internal fixation can compromise vascular supply.[13,18]

Condyle Fractures in Children

The earlier the trauma to the condylar region, the greater the potential of disturbance to development of facial growth if an improper treatment is delivered or the injury goes unnoticed without any form of treatment (**Fig. 5**). In general, a soft diet or closed treatment modalities are advocated in children because of the local and functional remodeling capacity and regeneration potential of the mandibular condyle.[66,67,75–78] However, nonoperative treatments may result in various complications such as facial asymmetries in any case caused by distorted condylar growth

complicated by the degree of displacement of the condylar fracture.[79,80] Conservative treatments may also cause functional disturbances and incomplete remodeling, hence justifying operative treatments in dislocated condyle fractures for a favorable outcome.[15,81,82] Operative management is still not the first-line option unless in specific indications (**Box 4**).

Intracapsular Condylar Fractures

The outcome of intracapsular fractures is related to increased incidence of complications. A recent study[83] suggested that open reduction and internal fixation may cause aseptic necrosis, which may or may not be directly related to trauma. On the other hand, the use of closed modalities may not avoid complete remodeling, especially during and after puberty (**Fig. 6**).[84] A study[9] revealed that operative management improves Helkimo dysfunction index results, favoring open reduction and internal fixation. Many patients noted moderate and severe dysfunction when treated by closed approach, and occlusal disturbances were observed in many cases, whereas occlusal disturbances were not noted in open-operated patients.

Approaches

Mainly transoral or transcutaneous approaches have been proposed for operative management of condylar fractures (**Box 5**). Surgical options in either group pose several challenges related to access, exposure, and manipulation for anatomic reduction and internal fixation (**Box 6**).

In general, if transoral access with or without specialized instruments is deemed insufficient, then transcutaneous approaches should be used despite the possible increased operative risks involved. Preauricular or postauricular access may be selected if the fracture is located at a more cranial level (**Fig. 7**). Submandibular,

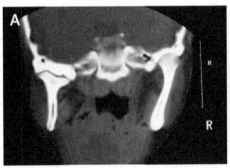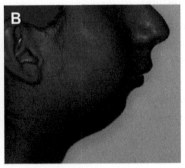

Fig. 5. Fifteen-year-old patient with a childhood history of trauma who developed a right-sided temporomandibular ankylosis. (A) Coronal CT of the patient at (B) clinical presentation with severe mandibular retrusion.

Box 4
Relative operative indications in children
Dislodgement of the condylar segment out of the fossa
Dislocation into:
Tympanic wall
Cranial fossa
External auditory meatus
Infratemporal fossa
Presence of foreign bodies
Bilateral fractures with unmanageable occlusion by closed therapies complicated by concomitant mandibular and maxillary fractures
Open wounds

Box 5
Operative approaches
Transcutaneous
Existing lacerations or scars
Transmasseteric
Anteroparotid
Transparotid
Retromandibular
Submandibular
Periangular
Extended temporal
Preauricular
Retroauricular
Hemicoronal/bicoronal
Endoscopic
Transoral
Posterior vestibular
Endoscopic
Data from Refs.[93,110,122–133]

periangular, or retromandibular approaches may be needed if the fracture site is at a more caudal location. Submandibular and periangular approaches are designed to follow the lower border in a straight line or the angle of the mandible in a more curved fashion (**Fig. 8**). A modification of submandibular access is an incision placed higher, aiming for more direct visualization of the ascending ramus and subcondylar region through the parotid and masseter muscle between the marginal mandibular and buccal branches, retracted caudally and cranially, respectively. The incision is made just below the perimandibular border at the angle region for about 5 cm in length.[85] Retromandibular access is essentially located at the posterior border of the mandible. Among some modifications, 1 of the 2 commonly used routes involves cutting through parotid capsule, which should be marked to ease the location and complete closure at the end of the surgery. Then blunt dissection is carried out through the parotid gland, taking into consideration the position of the facial nerve branches by transposing and appropriate retraction in order to reach the underlying masseter muscle. The muscle is then dissected along its fibers or transected down to the mandibular periosteum, which is incised and elevated to visualize the bony fracture site. Anther preferred route is by retracting the parotid gland anteriorly and superiorly after dissection of the fascia toward the sternocleidomastoid muscle and elevating the gland medially off the masseter muscle by keeping the facial nerve branches within. Then the periosteum underneath the muscle sling is incised and elevated off the bone (**Fig. 9**).

Transoral approaches, obviating facial scars, may be used in selected cases.[86–88] The approach has limited visualization but it can be reserved for those fractures in which reduction and internal fixation is achievable, especially with the introduction of newer technologies and instruments. Angled handpieces for drilling holes, special screwdrivers, and endoscopic assistance broaden the indications for transoral approaches.[89,90] Access is maintained through incised vestibular mucosa over the anterior ridge of the ascending ramus followed by dissection of the masseter muscle and

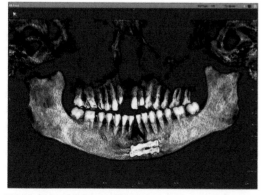

Fig. 6. Incomplete condylar remodeling at both sides of bilateral intracapsular fracture with symphyseal fracture.

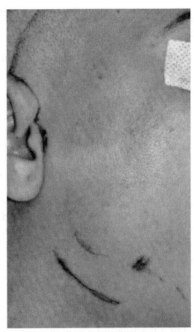

Fig. 8. Periangular incision around the angle and lower border of the mandible.

mandibular periosteum. Internal fixation may be carried out by transcutaneous trocar and angled screwdriver with or without the assistance of endoscopy (**Fig. 10**). Some of the possible advantages of using endoscopy involve minimized marginal mandibular branch injury and improved visualization of the anatomic reduction. However, endoscopy may not necessarily overcome the inherent shortcomings of the transoral approach.[88]

Alternative access may be planned away from the fracture location with the convenience of specially designed reduction techniques and instruments.[91] Lag screw techniques provide stable and rigid fixation with fewer surrounding soft tissues manipulations, which in turn reduces the likelihood of interference with blood supply.

Advances in Internal Fixation

Osteosynthesis materials and techniques have dramatically facilitated implementation of open reduction and internal fixation of condylar fractures. Titanium plates and screws are considered the most reliable materials if proper site selection, sufficient quantity or rigidity, and handling and placement techniques are used. One plate, 2 plates, specially designed condylar plates (eg, delta, trapezoidal), lag screws, and resorbable fixation systems might be selected as the materials to be used for internal fixation.[92] Some recent studies proposed that using 2 4-hole plates is a more biomechanically stable fixation than other methods.[53,93] Open reduction and internal fixation by dual plates might be executed at the condylar base or lower level condylar neck fractures to overcome tension and compression trajectories and if warranted, should be applied at the posterior and anterior borders of the condylar neck. On the other

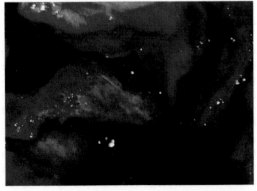

Fig. 7. Preauricular approach to the condylar head.

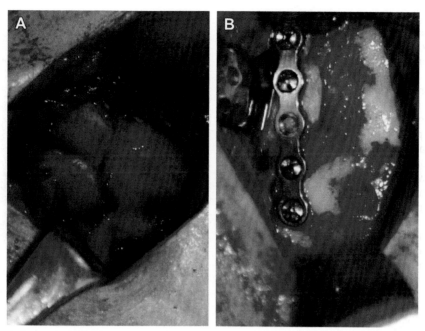

Fig. 9. Modified retromandibular route to a late comminuted fracture of the left condyle. (*A*) Intraoperative appearance; (*B*) internal fixation.

hand, condylar segment or fragmented segments, including the condylar head, sometimes barely allow placement of a single plate or screws, even when this is the sole option for internal fixation. If 1 plate is chosen, then at least 2 screws on each side of the fractures are needed.

Resorbable osteosynthesis materials have been introduced for internal fixation of condylar base and condylar head fractures.[94–97] Despite long-term reliability and biocompatibility, titanium hardware still poses shortcomings and may require removal, thus causing a re-entry operation, with its own added esthetic, functional, and financial risks. Recently, resorbable materials with fewer manipulation and handling requirements were introduced both to overcome the relative

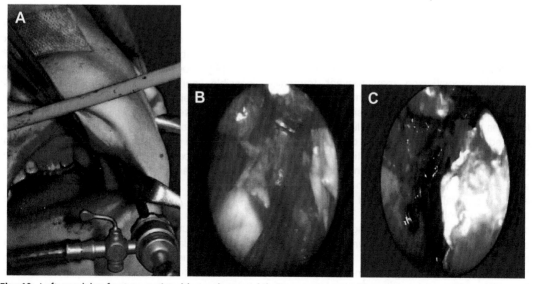

Fig. 10. Left condylar fracture assisted by endoscopy (*A*). Transoral access (*B*) snapshot image of condylar neck fracture reduction. (*C*) Snapshot image of internal fixation.

disadvantages of titanium hardware as well as those of resorbable materials that need tapping, particularly in a location in which the area may require management with strong retractions and difficult or restricted operative angulations.[98] A novel resorbable technology was recently developed and instead of screw insertion, ultrasonic welding and smelting of resorbable pins are used. The pin is inserted into the drilled hole and melts laterally with the cancellous bone, and therefore, anchorage is enhanced for improved fixation. Pins fuse with the plates together to form a solid unit, which improves stability.[99,100] Diacapitular fractures are considered challenging in terms not only of access and repositioning but also of stabilization. Such fractures are managed favorably, provided an exact repositioning can be achieved using only miniscrews. If adequate stabilization is achieved, these resorbable pins have fewer complications than metal screws and have shown promising results, both clinically and in experimental models.[101,102]

Complications

Complications can arise from any injury or associated treatment of condylar fractures. Persistent pain, hypomobility, malocclusion, osteonecrosis, and growth disturbances are some of the reported complications and the aim is to avoid functional, esthetic, and neurosensory deficits.[18,103–105] Clinical progression of condylar fractures may result in skeletal changes, including condylar remodeling, temporal bony region changes, or loss of vertical height of the ramus. Such fractures may fuse with the opposing bony segments, leading to cross-unions, which interfere with mandibular mobility (**Fig. 11**). Certain types of condylar fractures such as sagittal and comminuted types predispose the patient to TMJ ankylosis. An additional risk factor is the displacement of the articular disk, but early repositioning may prevent trauma-induced TMJ ankylosis.[106] Condylar fractures when treated by closed methods show several deformities and compensations, including ipsilateral reduced ramus height, occlusal cant, and tilted bigonial planes.[107] Reconstruction of certain condylar fractures using the condylar fractured segment as a free graft have been described, although generally it is preferred to use a technique that avoids endangering vascularity by means of such maneuvers during the reduction and internal fixation of the fracture.[58,108] The reported incidence of facial nerve injury after the transcutaneous route ranges from 3% to 43%. A search for modifications with an optimal exposure and precise anatomic reduction and internal

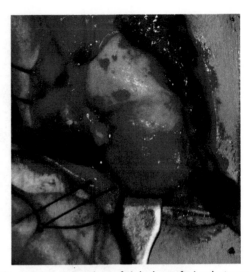

Fig. 11. Operative view of right bony fusion between condyle and temporal bone in a patient with trauma history.

fixation, yet minimizing facial nerve paralysis, is an ongoing effort for improved outcomes.[109] Most commonly, the marginal mandibular branch is injured as a result of extracranial branching patterns, so surgical modifications have been proposed to avoid its course and rather dissect the parotid gland anteriorly above or below the buccal branches (which have been shown to have numerous cross-unions) with less vulnerability for permanent injuries.[110] TMJ ramifications are noteworthy and internal derangements are not uncommon in nonsurgically treated patients over the long-term. Acute effects may include inflammation, disk perforation, capsular ruptures, retrodiskal tears, and diskal detachments.[70] Intra-articular bleeding and hematoma formation, if suspected, despite animal studies in prolonged maxillomandibular immobilization, interfere with TMJ physiology (**Fig. 12**).[74,111,112] Among other possible complications, arteriovenous fistula have been reported.[105] Although rare, infections can occur after trauma as a result of penetration of the neurocranium (auditory canal, petrous bone, middle cranial fossa), and with subsequent *Staphylococcus* infection, this circumstance can be life threatening (see **Fig. 3**).

FRACTURES OF THE CORONOID PROCESS

Coronoid fractures constitute an uncommon incidence of facial injuries, and among the reported studies, occurrence among mandibular fractures is also infrequent.[113,114] Coronoid process fractures can be isolated or they can occur in combination with other bones, especially with overlying

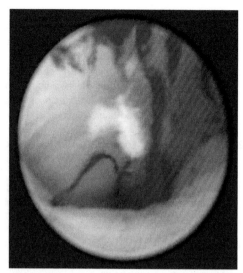

Fig. 12. Bleeding and hematoma in the right superior joint space of a patient with acute trauma history without any fracture.

zygomatic arch fractures. Physical falls, traffic accidents, violence, iatrogenic, or reflex-type fractures are accounted as the causes.[114–116] Bilateral involvement is extremely infrequent, and usually occurrence is unilateral (**Fig. 13**). Clinical findings may include swelling and tenderness over the cheek, preauricular, temporal, and intraoral buttress areas on the affected side. Earache, malocclusion, and submucosal bleeding around the zygomatic buttress or superiorly along the anterior ridge have also been reported. Limited mouth opening is an occasional finding, although asymptomatic cases are also reported without limitation of mouth opening.[113]

Management

Management is related to patient discomfort and severity of limitation of mouth opening. The principal goal is to avoid limitation of mouth opening

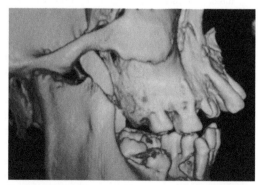

Fig. 13. Three-dimensional CT of right coronoid process fracture.

as early as possible, especially if open operative option is not considered. Otherwise, progression into adhesions can occur between the coronoid process and surrounding soft tissue, which become harder and more troublesome to manage in later stages.

Usually, conservative approaches adopted include short maxillomandibular immobilization, passive exercises, and soft diet followed by active exercises. Operative treatments may also be considered in cases with severe clinical symptoms, malocclusion, and severe displacements, which interfere with patient comfort and good function. One commonly applied surgical technique is the removal of the fractured segment and immediate postoperative exercises. However, reduction and internal fixation have also been described by intraoral and extraoral access.[115–117]

REFERENCES

1. Eckelt U. History of treatment concepts. In: Kleinheinz J, Meyer C, editors. Fractures of the mandibular condyle. Surrey (United Kingdom): Quintessence; 2009. p. 41–6.
2. Brandt MT, Haug RH. Open versus closed reduction of adult mandibular condyle fractures: a review of the literature regarding the evolution of current thoughts on management. J Oral Maxillofac Surg 2003;6:1324–32.
3. Ellis E III, Simon P, Throckmorton GS. Occlusal results after open or closed treatment of fractures of the mandibular condylar process. J Oral Maxillofac Surg 2000;58:260–8.
4. De Riu G, Gamba U, Anghinoni M, et al. A comparison of open and closed treatment of condylar fractures: a change in philosophy. Int J Oral Maxillofac Surg 2001;30:384–9.
5. Baker AW, McMahon J, Moos KF. Current consensus on the management of fractures of the mandibular condyle. A method by questionnaire. Int J Oral Maxillofac Surg 1998;27:258–66.
6. Vesnaver A. Open reduction and internal fixation of intra-articular fractures of the mandibular condyle: our first experiences. J Oral Maxillofac Surg 2008; 66:2123–9.
7. Eckelt U, Schneider M, Erasmus F, et al. Open versus closed treatment of fractures of the mandibular condylar process–a prospective randomized multi-center study. J Craniomaxillofac Surg 2006; 34:306–14.
8. Worsaae N, Thorn JJ. Surgical versus nonsurgical treatment of unilateral dislocated low subcondylar fractures: a clinical study of 52 cases. J Oral Maxillofac Surg 1994;52:353–61 [discussion: 360–1].
9. Hlawitschka M, Loukota R, Eckelt U. Functional and radiological results of open and closed treatment of

intracapsular (diacapitular) condylar fractures of the mandible. Int J Oral Maxillofac Surg 2005;34: 597–604.

10. Schneider M, Erasmus F, Gerlach KL, et al. Open reduction and internal fixation versus closed treatment and mandibulomaxillary fixation of fractures of the mandibular condylar process: a randomized, prospective, multicenter study with special evaluation of fracture level. J Oral Maxillofac Surg 2008; 66:2537–44.

11. Danda AK, Muthusekhar MR, Narayanan V, et al. Open versus closed treatment of unilateral subcondylar and condylar neck fractures: a prospective, randomized clinical study. J Oral Maxillofac Surg 2010;68:1238–41.

12. Singh V, Bhagol A, Goel M, et al. Outcomes of open versus closed treatment of mandibular subcondylar fractures: a prospective randomized study. J Oral Maxillofac Surg 2010;68:1304–9.

13. Landes CA, Lipphardt R. Prospective evaluation of a pragmatic treatment rationale: open reduction and internal fixation of displaced and dislocated condyle and condylar head fractures and closed reduction of non-displaced, non-dislocated fractures. Part I: condyle and subcondylar fractures. Int J Oral Maxillofac Surg 2005;34:859–70.

14. Vesnaver A, Ahčan U, Rozman J. Evaluation of surgical treatment in mandibular condyle fractures. J Craniomaxillofac Surg 2012;40:647–53.

15. Landes CA, Day K, Glasl B, et al. Prospective evaluation of closed treatment of nondisplaced and nondislocated mandibular condyle fractures versus open reposition and rigid fixation of displaced and dislocated fractures in children. J Oral Maxillofac Surg 2008;66:1184–93.

16. Kermer CH, Undt G, Rasse M. Surgical reduction and fixation of intracapsular condylar fractures–a follow up study. Int J Oral Maxillofac Surg 1998; 27:191–4.

17. Nusbaum ML, Laslin DM, Best AM. Closed versus open reduction of mandibular condylar fractures in adults: a meta-analysis. J Oral Maxillofac Surg 2008;66:1087–92.

18. Ellis E III, Throckmorton GS. Treatment of mandibular condylar process fractures: biological considerations. J Oral Maxillofac Surg 2005;63:115–34.

19. Throckmorton GS, Groshan GJ, Boyd SB. Muscle activity patterns and control of temporomandibular joint loads. J Prosthet Dent 1990;63:685–95.

20. Ellis E III, Throckmorton GS. Bite forces after open or closed treatment of mandibular condylar process fractures. J Oral Maxillofac Surg 2001;59: 389–95.

21. Takenoshita Y, Ishibashi H, Oka M. Comparison of functional recovery after nonsurgical and surgical treatment of condylar fractures. J Oral Maxillofac Surg 1990;48:1191–5.

22. Silvennoinen U, Iizuka T, Oikarinen K, et al. Analysis of possible factors leading to problems after nonsurgical treatment of condylar fractures. J Oral Maxillofac Surg 1994;52:793–9.

23. de Bont LG, Boering G, Havinga P, et al. Spatial arrangement of collagen fibrils in the articular cartilage of the mandibular condyle: a light microscopic and scanning electron microscopic study. J Oral Maxillofac Surg 1984;42:306–13.

24. Herring SW, Liu ZJ. Loading of the TMJ: anatomical and in vivo evidence from the bones. Cells Tissues Organs 2001;169:193–200.

25. da Fonseca GD. Experimental study on fractures of the mandibular condylar process (mandibular condylar process fractures). Int J Oral Surg 1974; 3:89–101.

26. Musgrove BT. Dislocation of the mandibular condyle into the middle cranial fossa. Br J Oral Maxillofac Surg 1986;24:22–7.

27. Dimitroulis G. Condylar injuries in growing patients. Aust Dent J 1997;42:367–71.

28. Gassner R, Tuli T, Hächl O, et al. Craniomaxillofacial trauma in children: a review of 3,385 cases with 6,060 injuries in 10 years. J Oral Maxillofac Surg 2003;62:399–407.

29. Ellis E III, Moos KF, el-Attar A. Ten years of mandibular fractures: an analysis of 2137 cases. Oral Surg Oral Med Oral Pathol 1985;59:120–9.

30. De Luca S. Mandibular fracture and dislocation in a case study from the Jewish cemetery of Lucena (Cordoba), in South Iberian Peninsula (8th-12th AD). Int J Osteoarcheol 2011;23(4):485–504.

31. Zachariades N, Mezitis M, Mourouzis C, et al. Fractures of the mandibular condyle: a review of 466 cases. Literature review, reflections on treatment and proposals. J Craniomaxillofac Surg 2006;34: 421–32.

32. Cascone P, Leonardi R, Marino S, et al. Intracapsular fracture of mandibular condyle: diagnosis, treatment, and anatomical and pathological evaluations. J Craniofac Surg 2003;14:184–91.

33. Erol B, Tanrıkulu R, Gorgun B. Maxillofacial fractures. Analysis of demographic distribution and treatment in 2901 patients (25-year experience). J Craniomaxillofac Surg 2004;32:308–12.

34. Oikarinen KK, Thalib LL, Sàndor KB, et al. Differences in the location and multiplicity of mandibular fractures in Kuwait, Canada and Finland during the 1990s. Med Princ Pract 2005;14:10–5.

35. Dijkstra PU, Stegenga B, de Bont LG, et al. Function impairment and pain after closed treatment of fractures of the mandibular condyle. J Trauma 2005;59:422–8.

36. Marker P, Nielsen A, Bastian HL. Fracture of the mandibular condyle. Part 1: patterns of distribution of types and causes of fractures in 348 patients. Br J Oral Maxillofac Surg 2000;38:417–21.

37. Sawazaki R, Júnior SM, Asprino L, et al. Incidence and patterns of mandibular condyle fractures. J Oral Maxillofac Surg 2010;68:1252–9.

38. Zhou HH, Liu Q, Cheng G, et al. Aetiology, pattern and treatment of mandibular condylar fractures in 549 patients: a 22-year retrospective study. J Craniomaxillofac Surg 2013;41:34–41.

39. Marker P, Nielsen A, Bastian HL. Fracture of the mandibular condyle. Part 2: results of treatment of 348 patients. Br J Oral Maxillofac Surg 2000;38: 422–6.

40. Silvennoinen U, Iizuka T, Lindqvist C, et al. Different patterns of condylar fractures: an analysis of 382 patients in a 3-year period. J Oral Maxillofac Surg 1992;50:1032–7.

41. Fridrich KL, Pena-Velasca G, Olson RA. Changing trends with mandibular fractures: a review of 1067 cases. J Oral Maxillofac Surg 1992;50:586–9.

42. Larsen OD, Nielsen A. Mandibular fractures. An analysis of their etiology and location in 286 patients. Scand J Plast Reconstr Surg 1976;10: 213–8.

43. Amaratunga NA. A study of condylar fractures in Sri Lankan patients with special reference to the recent views on treatment, healing and sequelae. Br J Oral Maxillofac Surg 1987;25:391–7.

44. Ferguson JW, Stewart IA, Whitley BD. Lateral displacement of the intact mandibular condyle. Review of literature and report of case with associated facial nerve palsy. J Craniomaxillofac Surg 1989; 17:125–7.

45. Ohura N, Ichioka S, Sudo T, et al. Dislocation of the bilateral mandibular condyle into the middle cranial fossa: review of the literature and clinical experience. J Oral Maxillofac Surg 2006;64: 1165–72.

46. Bu SS, Jin SL, Yin L. Superolateral dislocation of the intact mandibular condyle into the temporal fossa: review of the literature and report of a case. Oral Surg Oral Med Oral Pathol Oral Radiol Endod 2007;103:185–9.

47. Wermker K. Incidence, etiology and classification of condylar fractures. In: Kleinheinz J, Meyer C, editors. Fractures of the mandibular condyle. Basic considerations and treatment. Surrey (United Kingdom): Quintessence; 2009. p. 29–40.

48. Lindahl L. Condylar fractures of the mandible. I. Classification and relation to age, occlusion and concomitant injuries of teeth and teeth-supporting structures, and fractures of the mandibular body. Int J Oral Surg 1977;6:12–21.

49. Krenkel C. General principles of osteosynthesis. Chicago: Quintessence; 1994. p. 39–72.

50. Loukota RA, Eckelt U, De Bont L, et al. Subclassification of fractures of the condylar process of the mandible. Br J Oral Maxillofac Surg 2005;43: 72–3.

51. Bos RR, Ward-Booth RP, de Bont LG. Mandibular condyle fractures: a consensus. Br J Oral Maxillofac Surg 1999;37:87–9.

52. Loukota RA, Neff A, Rasse M. Nomenclature/classification of fractures of the mandibular condylar head. Br J Oral Maxillofac Surg 2010;48:477–8.

53. Haug RH, Assael LA. Outcomes of open versus closed treatment of mandibular subcondylar fractures. J Oral Maxillofac Surg 2001;59:370–5.

54. Konstantinovic VS, Dimitrijevic B. Surgical versus conservative treatment of unilateral condylar process fractures: clinical and radiographic evaluation of 80 patients. J Oral Maxillofac Surg 1992; 50:349–52.

55. Widmark G, Bagenholm T, Kahnberg KE, et al. Open reduction of subcondylar fractures. A study of functional rehabilitation. Int J Oral Maxillofac Surg 1996;25:107–11.

56. Chossegros C, Cheynet F, Blanc JL, et al. Short retromandibular approach of subcondylar fractures: clinical and radiologic long-term evaluation. Oral Surg Oral Med Oral Pathol Oral Radiol Endod 1996;82(3):248–52.

57. Eckelt U, Hlawitschka M. Clinical and radiological evaluation following surgical treatment of condylar neck fractures with lag screws. J Craniomaxillofac Surg 1999;27:235–42.

58. Raveh J, Vuillemin T, Ladrach K. Open reduction of the dislocated, fractured condylar process: indications and surgical procedures. J Oral Maxillofac Surg 1989;47:120–7.

59. Ellis E III, Dean J. Rigid fixation of mandibular condyle fractures. Oral Surg Oral Med Oral Pathol 1993;76:6–15.

60. Ellis E, Carlson DS. The effects of mandibular immobilization on the masticatory system. A review. Clin Plast Surg 1989;16:133–46.

61. Ellis ED, Dechow PC, Carlson DS. A comparison of stimulated bite force after mandibular advancement using rigid and nonrigid fixation. J Oral Maxillofac Surg 1988;46:26–32.

62. Palmieri C, Ellis E III, Throckmorton G. Mandibular motion after closed and open treatment of unilateral mandibular condylar process fractures. J Oral Maxillofac Surg 1999;57:764–75.

63. Santler G, Kärcher H, Ruda C, et al. Fractures of the condylar process: surgical versus nonsurgical treatment. J Oral Maxillofac Surg 1999;57:392–7.

64. Villarreal PM, Monje F, Junquera LM, et al. Mandibular condyle fractures: determinants of treatment and outcome. J Oral Maxillofac Surg 2004;62:155–63.

65. Cascone P, Sassano P, Spallacia F, et al. Condylar fractures during growth: follow-up of 16 patients. J Craniofac Surg 1999;10:87–92.

66. Defabianis P. TMJ fractures in children and adolescents: treatment guidelines. J Clin Pediatr Dent 2003;27:191–9.

67. Zhang Y, He DM. Clinical investigation of early post-traumatic temporomandibular joint ankylosis and the role of repositioning discs in treatment. Int J Oral Maxillofac Surg 2006;35:1096–101.

68. Türp JC, Stoll P, Schlotthauer U, et al. Computerized axiographic evaluation of condylar movements in cases with fractures of the condylar process: a follow up over 19 year. J Craniomaxillofac Surg 1996;24:46–52.

69. Umstadt HE, Ellers M, Muller HH, et al. Functional reconstruction of the TM joint in cases of severely displaced fractures and fracture dislocation. J Craniomaxillofac Surg 2000;28:97–105.

70. Lindahl L, Hollender L. Condylar fractures of the mandible. II. Radiographic study of remodeling processes in the temporomandibular joint. Int J Oral Surg 1977;6:153–65.

71. Ellis E III, Palmieri C, Throckmorton G. Further displacement of condylar process fractures after closed treatment. J Oral Maxillofac Surg 1999;57:1307–16.

72. Hoving J, Boering G, Stegenga B. Long-term results of nonsurgical management of condylar fractures in children. Int J Oral Maxillofac Surg 1999;28:429–40.

73. Andersson J, Hallme F, Eriksson L. Unilateral mandibular condylar fractures: a 31-year follow-up of non-surgical treatment. Int J Oral Maxillofac Surg 2007;36:310–4.

74. Schneider A, Zahnert D, Klengel S, et al. A comparison of MRI, radiographic and clinical findings of the position of the TMJ articular disc following open treatment of condylar neck fractures. Br J Oral Maxillofac Surg 2007;45:534–7.

75. Takaku S, Yoshida M, Sano T, et al. Magnetic resonance images in patients with acute traumatic injury of the temporomandibular joint: a preliminary report. J Craniomaxillofac Surg 1996;24:173–7.

76. Brusati R, Paini P. Facial nerve injury secondary to lateral displacement of the mandibular ramus. Plast Reconstr Surg 1978;62:728–33.

77. Wang P, Yang J, Yu Q. MR imaging assessment of temporomandibular joint soft tissue injuries in dislocated and nondislocated mandibular condylar fractures. AJNR Am J Neuroradiol 2009;30:59–63.

78. Chen M, Yang C, He D, et al. Soft tissue reduction during open treatment of intracapsular condylar fracture of the temporomandibular joint: our institution's experience. J Oral Maxillofac Surg 2010;68:2189–95.

79. Strobl H, Emshoff R, Rothler G. Conservative treatment of unilateral condylar fractures in children: a long-term clinical and radiological follow-up of 55 patients. Int J Oral Maxillofac Surg 1999;28:95–8.

80. Dahlström L, Kahnberg KE, Lindahl L. 15 years follow-up on condylar fractures. Int J Oral Maxillofac Surg 1989;18:18–23.

81. Norholt SE, Krishnan V, Sindet-Pedersen S, et al. Pediatric condylar fractures: a long-term follow-up study of 55 patients. J Oral Maxillofac Surg 1993;51:1302–10.

82. Kaban LB, Mulliken JB, Murray JE. Facial fractures in children: an analysis of 122 fractures in 109 patients. Plast Reconstr Surg 1977;59:15–20.

83. Myall RW. Condylar injuries in children: what is different about them?. In: Worthington P, Evans JR, editors. Controversies in oral and maxillofacial surgery, vol. 17 Philadelphia: WB Saunders; 1994. p. 191–200.

84. Lund K. Mandibular growth and remodeling processes after condylar fracture. A longitudinal roentgencephalometric study. Acta Odontol Scand 1974;32(Suppl):3–11.

85. Choi J, Oh N, Kim IK. A follow-up study of condyle fracture in children. Int J Oral Maxillofac Surg 2005;34:851–8.

86. Schoen R, Gellrich NC, Schmelzeisen R. Minimally invasive open reduction of a displaced condylar fracture in a child. Br J Oral Maxillofac Surg 2005;43:258–60.

87. Wysocki J, Reymond J, Krasucki K. Vascularization of the mandibular condylar head with respect to intracapsular fractures of mandible. J Craniomaxillofac Surg 2012;40:112–5.

88. Gundlach K, Lammers E, Schwipper E. Growth of the mandibular condyle: histological findings in rodents relevant to the treatment of fractures of the condyle. In: Hörting-Hansen E, editor. Oral and maxillofacial surgery. Chicago: Quintessence; 1985. p. 200.

89. Haug RH, Dodson TB, Morgan JP. Trauma surgery. In: Haug RH, editor. Parameters and pathways: clinical practice guidelines for oral and maxillofacial surgery. Philadelphia: WB Saunders; 2001. p. 1–58.

90. Wilk A. High perimandibular approach/modified Risdon-Strasbourg approach. In: Kleinheinz J, Meyer C, editors. Fractures of the mandibular condyle. Basic considerations and treatment. Surrey (United Kingdom): Quintessence; 2009. p. 143–53.

91. Hammer B, Schier P, Prein J. Osteosynthesis of condylar neck fractures: a review of 30 patients. Br J Oral Maxillofac Surg 1997;35:288–91.

92. Vesnaver A, Gorjanc M, Eberlinc A, et al. The preauricular transparotid approach for open reduction and internal fixation of condylar fractures. J Craniomaxillofac Surg 2005;33:169–79.

93. Devlin MF, Hislop WS, Carton AT. Open reduction and internal fixation of fractured mandibular condyles by a retro-mandibular approach: surgical morbidity and informed consent. Br J Oral Maxillofac Surg 2002;40:23–5.

94. Dunaway DJ, Trott JA. Open reduction and internal fixation of condylar fractures via an extended

bicoronal approach with a masseteric myotomy. Br J Plast Surg 1996;49:79–84.

95. Ellis E III, Reynolds ST, Park HS. A method to rigidly fix high condylar fractures. Oral Surg Oral Med Oral Pathol 1989;68:369–74.

96. Choung PH, Nam JW. An intraoral approach to treatment of condylar hyperplasia or high condylar process fractures using the intraoral vertico-sagittal ramus osteotomy. J Oral Maxillofac Surg 1998;56:563–70.

97. Anastassov GE, Rodriguez ED, Schwimmer AM, et al. Facial rhytidectomy approach for treatment of posterior mandibular fractures. J Craniomaxillofac Surg 1997;25:9–14.

98. Choi BH, Yoo JH. Open reduction of condylar neck fractures with exposure of the facial nerve. Oral Surg Oral Med Oral Pathol Oral Radiol Endod 1999;88:292–6.

99. Guerrissi JO. A transparotid transcutaneous approach for internal rigid fixation in condylar fractures. J Craniofac Surg 2002;13:568–71.

100. Wilson AW, Ethunandan M, Brennan PA. Transmasseteric antero-parotid approach for open reduction and internal fixation of condylar fractures. Br J Oral Maxillofac Surg 2005;43:57–60.

101. Miloro M. Endoscopic-assisted repair of subcondylar fractures. Oral Surg Oral Med Oral Pathol Oral Radiol Endod 2003;96:387–91.

102. Chen CT, Lai JP, Tung TC, et al. Endoscopically assisted mandibular subcondylar fracture repair. Plast Reconstr Surg 1999;103:60–5.

103. Schön R, Schramm A, Gellrich NC, et al. Follow-up of condylar fractures of the mandible in 8 patients at 18 months after transoral endoscopic-assisted open treatment. J Oral Maxillofac Surg 2003;61:49–54.

104. Undt G, Kermer C, Rasse M, et al. Transoral mini-plate osteosynthesis of condylar neck fractures. Oral Surg Oral Med Oral Pathol Oral Radiol Endod 1999;88:534–43.

105. Silverman SL. A new operation for displaced fractures at the neck of the mandibular condyle. Dental Cosmos 1925;67:876–7.

106. Lachner J, Clanton JT, Waite PD. Open reduction and internal rigid fixation of subcondylar fractures via an intraoral approach. Oral Surg Oral Med Oral Pathol 1991;71:257–61.

107. Schneider M, Lauer G, Eckelt U. Surgical treatment of fractures of the mandibular condyle: a comparison of long-term results following different approaches–functional, axiographical, and radiological findings. J Craniomaxillofac Surg 2007;35: 151–60.

108. Krenkel C. Axial 'anchor' screw (lag screw with biconcave washer) or 'slanted-screw' plate for osteosynthesis of fractures of the mandibular condylar process. J Craniomaxillofac Surg 1992; 20:348–53.

109. Schön R, Gutwald R, Schramm A, et al. Endoscopy assisted open treatment of condylar fractures of the mandible: extraoral vs intraoral approach. Int J Oral Maxillofac Surg 2002;31:237–43.

110. Lauer G, Schmelzeisen R. Endoscope-assisted fixation of mandibular condylar process fractures. J Oral Maxillofac Surg 1999;57:36–9.

111. Lauer G, Pradel W, Schneider M, et al. A new 3-dimensional plate for transoral endoscopic-assisted osteosynthesis of condylar neck fractures. J Oral Maxillofac Surg 2007;65:964–71.

112. Suzuki T, Kawamura H, Kasahara T, et al. Resorbable poly-l-lactide plates and screws for the treatment of mandibular condylar process fractures: a clinical and radiologic follow-up study. J Oral Maxillofac Surg 2004;62:919–24.

113. Lauer G, Pradel W, Leonhardt H, et al. Resorbable triangular plate for osteosynthesis of fractures of the condylar neck. Br J Oral Maxillofac Surg 2010; 48:532–5.

114. Bos RR, Boering G, Rozema FR, et al. Resorbable poly(l-lactide) plates and screws for the fixation of zygomatic fractures. J Oral Maxillofac Surg 1987; 45:751–3.

115. Eckelt U, Nitsche M, Müller A, et al. Ultrasound aided pin fixation of biodegradable osteosynthetic materials in cranioplasty for infants with craniosynostosis. J Craniomaxillofac Surg 2007;35:218–21.

116. Schneider M, Seinige C, Pilling E, et al. Ultrasound-aided resorbable osteosynthesis of fractures of the mandibular condylar base: an experimental study in sheep. Br J Oral Maxillofac Surg 2012;50:528–32.

117. Meissner H, Pilling E, Richter G, et al. Experimental investigations for mechanical joint strength following ultrasonically welded pin osteosynthesis. J Mater Sci Mater Med 2008;19:2255–9.

118. Buijs GJ, van der Houwen EB, Stegenga B, et al. Mechanical strength and stiffness of the biodegradable SonicWeld Rx osteofixation system. J Oral Maxillofac Surg 2009;67:782–7.

119. Schneider M, Eckelt U, Reitemeier B, et al. Stability of fixation of diacapitular fractures of the mandibular condylar process by ultrasound-aided resorbable pins (SonicWeld Rx System) in pigs. Br J Oral Maxillofac Surg 2011;49:297–301.

120. Abdel-Galil K, Loukota R. Fixation of comminuted diacapitular fractures of the mandibular condyle with ultrasound activated resorbable pins. Br J Oral Maxillofac Surg 2008;46:482–4.

121. Talwar RM, Ellis E III, Throckmorton GS. Adaptations of the masticatory system after bilateral fractures of the mandibular condylar process. J Oral Maxillofac Surg 1998;56:430–9.

122. Long X, Goss AN. A sheep model of intracapsular condylar fracture. J Oral Maxillofac Surg 2007;65: 1102–8.

123. Long X, Cheng Y, Li X, et al. Arteriovenous fistula after mandibular condylar fracture. J Oral Maxillofac Surg 2004;62:1557–8.

124. Ellis E III, Throckmorton GS. Facial symmetry after closed and open treatment of fractures of the mandibular condylar process. J Oral Maxillofac Surg 2000;58:719–28.

125. Zhang X, Obeid G. A comparative study of the treatment of unilateral fractured and dislocated mandibular condyles in the rabbit. J Oral Maxillofac Surg 1991;49:1181–90.

126. Tang W, Gao C, Long J, et al. Application of modified retromandibular approach indirectly from the anterior edge of the parotid gland in the surgical treatment of condylar fracture. J Oral Maxillofac Surg 2009;67:552–8.

127. Jones JK, Van Sickles JE. A preliminary report of arthroscopic findings following acute condylar trauma. J Oral Maxillofac Surg 1991;49: 55–60.

128. Goss AN, Bosanquet AG. The arthroscopic appearance of acute temporomandibular joint trauma. J Oral Maxillofac Surg 1990;48:780–3.

129. Delantoni A, Antoniades I. The iatrogenic fracture of the coronoid process of the mandible. A review of the literature and case presentation. Cranio 2010;28:200–4.

130. Philip M, Sivarajasingam V, Shepherd P. Bilateral reflex fracture of the coronoid process of the mandible. A case report. Int J Oral Maxillofac Surg 1999;28:195–6.

131. Rapidis AD, Papavassiliou D, Papadimitriou J. Fractures of the coronoid process of the mandible. An analysis of 52 cases. Int J Oral Surg 1985;14:126–30.

132. Shen L, Li J, Li P, et al. Mandibular coronoid fractures: treatment options. Int J Oral Maxillofac Surg 2013;42:721–6.

133. Yaremchuk MJ. Rigid internal fixation of a displaced mandibular coronoid fracture. J Craniofac Surg 1992;3:226–9.

Management of Mandibular Angle Fracture

Daniel Cameron Braasch, DMD,
A. Omar Abubaker, DMD, PhD*

KEYWORDS

- Angle fracture • Mandible • Biomechanics • Miniplate • Treatment

KEY POINTS

- The angle fracture is one of the most common fractures of the mandible and is associated with the highest complication rates.
- Treatment of angle fractures has incorporated better understanding of the biomechanics of the mandible, the evolution in the patterns, and types of fixation and advances in surgical techniques treating these fractures.
- Several techniques are acceptable to treat mandibular fractures, and the most common technique for isolated mandibular angle fracture is a single miniplate placed at the superior border.
- Routine use of postoperative antibiotics and removal of teeth in line of fracture is less advocated and best judged on a case-by-case basis.

INTRODUCTION

Fractures through the angle of the mandible are one of the most common facial fractures. The management of such fractures has been controversial, however. This controversy is related to the anatomic relations and complex biomechanical aspects of the mandibular angle. The debate has become even more heated since the evolution of rigid fixation and the ability to provide adequate stability of the fractured segments. This article provides an overview of the special anatomic and biomechanical features of the mandibular angle and their impact on the management of these fractures.

ETIOLOGY

Angle fractures are the most common mandibular fracture, accounting for 30% of all mandibular fractures.[1] The majority of such fractures occur as a result of interpersonal violence or motor vehicle accidents. Other potential causes of mandibular fractures include falls, sporting or work-related accidents, gunshot wounds, and pathology. Fractures occur more frequently in the male population and are often associated with alcohol consumption.[2] Although most fractures occur as a result of a traumatic event, some may occur due to preexisting pathology. Pathologic fractures result from such conditions as osteoradionecrosis, bisphosphonates-related osteonecrosis, and benign or malignant tumors or cysts that weaken the structure of the angle to the point where a fracture occurs from minimal or no trauma (**Fig. 1**).

CLASSIFICATION AND PATTERNS OF MANDIBULAR ANGLE FRACTURES

The mandibular angle is best described as an anatomic region rather than a precise anatomic location. This region is designated as a triangular area with the superior edge being the junction of

Dr Braasch is currently in private practice in 33 Trafalgar Square, Nashua, NH 03603.
Disclosures: The authors have nothing to disclose.
Department of Oral and Maxillofacial Surgery, School of Dentistry, VCU Medical Center, Virginia Commonwealth University, 521 North 11th Street, PO Box 980566, Richmond, VA 23298-0566, USA
* Corresponding author.
E-mail address: abubaker@vcu.edu

Oral Maxillofacial Surg Clin N Am 25 (2013) 591–600
http://dx.doi.org/10.1016/j.coms.2013.07.007
1042-3699/13/$ – see front matter © 2013 Elsevier Inc. All rights reserved.

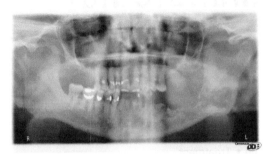

Fig. 1. Pathologic fracture through the left angle due to osteoradionecrosis.

the horizontal body and vertical ramus, usually where the third molar is or was located. The anterior border of the masseter muscle forms the anterior border and the posterior border of the triangle is formed by an oblique line extending from the third molar region to the posterior superior attachment of the masseter muscle (**Fig. 2**).[3]

Fractures through the mandibular angle can be classified in a variety of ways. First, they can be described as either closed or open fractures. A closed fracture does not communicate to the outside environment; whereas an open fracture is partially or completely exposed intraorally or extraorally through the overlying tissues. Extraoral open fractures rarely occur except in high-velocity or penetrating injuries. Intraoral open fractures are more common due to tearing of the gingiva overlying the angle at its superior border. Connection of the fracture to the mouth through the periodontal ligament also creates an open fracture.

Angle fractures can also be classified as simple or comminuted. Simple fractures involve only a single break through the bone whereas comminuted fractures display multiple breaks. The latter are more often caused by high impact trauma, such as gunshot wounds and high-speed motor vehicles accidents.

The degree of fracture separation is another basis for classification. Complete fractures occur when there is disruption of both the medial and lateral cortices (**Fig. 3**). Greenstick fractures, which are rare, occur when there is disturbance of only one cortex.

Mandibular angle fractures can also be described as favorable or unfavorable. A favorable fracture occurs when the masseter and medial pterygoid muscle action on the proximal and distal segments of the fracture help to reduce it. The more common unfavorable fracture involves separation of the proximal and distal segments due to muscle pull. An unfavorable fracture is further labeled as horizontally or vertically unfavorable. During a horizontally unfavorable fracture, the action of the masseter and medial pterygoid muscles distracts the proximal segment superiorly while the suprahyoid muscles act to distract the distal segment inferiorly (**Figs. 4** and **5**). A vertically unfavorable fracture occurs when the fracture pattern allows for the distal segment to be pulled medially by the medial pterygoid muscle (see **Fig. 3**; **Fig. 6**).

Mandibular angle fractures can occur in combination with many other facial or mandibular fractures. When angle fractures occur in combination with other mandibular fractures, the most common secondary fracture site is at the contralateral parasymphysis.[4] The presence of bilateral mandibular angle fractures is rare but, when present, requires special attention because the dentate segment can become displaced posteriorly, resulting in

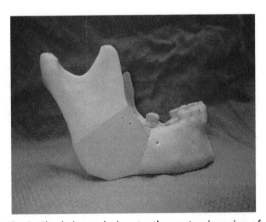

Fig. 2. Shaded area designates the anatomic region of the mandibular angle.

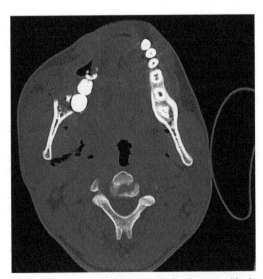

Fig. 3. Complete fracture through the mandibular angle.

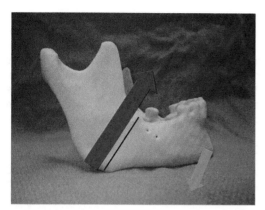

Fig. 4. Unfavorable fracture is created by the pull of the masseter (*lateral*) and medial pterygoid (*medial*) superiorly (*red arrow*) and suprahyoid muscles inferiorly (*blue arrow*).

airway compromise. Close observation of patients with these type of fractures is needed to prevent airway collapse.

BIOMECHANICAL CONSIDERATIONS

Understanding the biomechanics of mandibular angle fractures helps clinicians chose their proper management. Such biomechanics are based on the mandible acting as a class 3 lever. In this model, the muscles attached to the mandible create a tensile force at the superior border and a compressive force at the inferior border. A zone of no tension or compression is found between the superior and inferior borders. This zone is termed, *the neutral zone.* The anatomic location of the tensile zone corresponds to the mandibular alveolus and external oblique ridge. The compressive zone is located at the inferior border of the mandible.[5] The neutral zone is found at the level of the inferior alveolar nerve. **Figs. 7** and **8** demonstrate the superior tension zone and inferior compression zone, where separation at the superior border and reduction at the inferior border occur during a mandibular angle fracture under function.

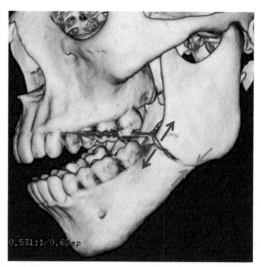

Fig. 6. Separation at the superior border demonstrated by the red arrows. Compression at the inferior border indicated by blue arrows.

Based on these considerations, Spiessel recommended the use of an arch bar when the fracture is within the dental arch.[6] The arch bar acts to prevent fracture displacement at the superior border. Along the alveolar ridge, when the fracture is beyond the dental arch, he recommended the use of a 2-hole tension band plate. Later, Schmoker and Spiessl[7] introduced another method of neutralizing the alveolar tensile forces by using an eccentric dynamic compression plate at the inferior border, where the design of the holes in the plate generated eccentric compression at the superior border similar to that of a tension band. This was expected to result in what was

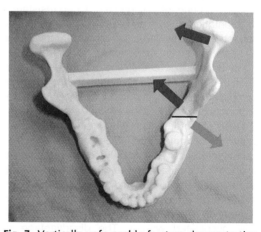

Fig. 7. Vertically unfavorable fracture demonstrating the potential medial displacement of the proximal segment due to the pull of the medial and lateral pterygoid muscles (*red arrows*) compared with the lesser lateral pull of the masseter (*blue arrow*).

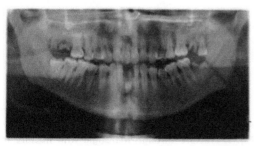

Fig. 5. Unfavorable left mandibular angle fracture.

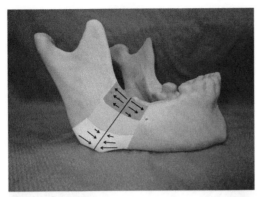

Fig. 8. Demonstration of the superior tension zone, middle neutral zone, and inferior compression zone. *Arrows* showing zone of tension superiorly and zone of compression inferiorly.

described as buttressing away from the plate. This technique, although initially accepted, never gained popular use, likely due to the technical difficulty. In the 1970s, however, Michelet and colleagues[8] and, later, Champy and colleagues[9] thoroughly studied the use of a minplate along the superior border of the mandible. The plate was placed transorally and secured with monocortical screws, thus minimizing possible risk to the teeth and inferior alveolar nerve. Subsequently, several additional biomechanical and clinical studies have shown the effectiveness of this technique.

TEETH IN THE LINE OF FRACTURE

The presence of impacted third molars has been shown to increase the risk of angle fractures.[10–12] This increased risk is related to the decreased amount of bone, resulting in a reduced resistance to traumatic forces. The depth and angulation of impaction is considered by most authors to not be associated with an increased risk of fracture.[11]

Management of teeth in line of fracture has also often been examined in relation to the incidence of complications with mandibular angle fracture. Although one study showed that there is an increased risk of infection when teeth are retained in the line of fracture, the difference was not statically significant.[13] Accordingly, the mere presence of a tooth in the fracture line does not necessitate its removal. The tooth should be removed, however, if it prevents reduction of the fracture, there is infection related to the tooth, or there is pathology associated with it. The disadvantage of routine removal of impacted or even erupted third molars in a mandibular angle fracture is related to the possibility of creating a soft tissue deficit at the extraction site. Furthermore, there is a risk of

converting a closed fracture to an open fracture, especially when a transoral approach is not used. Another disadvantage to removing an impacted tooth in the fracture site is the potential need to remove bone to facilitate its extraction. This may compromise the buttressing of bone and result in inadequate bone to place the tension band plate at the superior border (**Figs. 9 and 10**).

DIAGNOSIS
Physical Examination

With the routine use of CT scans in emergency departments, the importance of the physical examination is often overlooked. Extraoral examination should begin with a visual inspection. Swelling, ecchymosis, and step deformity and tenderness to palpation at the inferior border may be a sign of an angle fracture.[1] A thorough cranial nerve examination should be routine practice in any physical examination, with special attention to potential changes in the third division of the fifth cranial nerve. Fractures through the mandibular angle, especially when there is some degree of displacement, are likely to cause hypoesthesia, anesthesia, or dysesthesia of inferior alveolar nerve. Rarely is the facial nerve (cranial nerve VII) injured with angle fractures, but this can occur with penetrating trauma. It is imperative to document these findings in the preoperative evaluation as a baseline for postoperative monitoring.

Intraoral examination can reveal ecchymosis, gingival lacerations, and bleeding in the posterior buccal and lingual vestibules. Evaluation of the occlusion may show a malocclusion, with premature tooth contact on the fractured side and an open bite on the contralateral side. In cases of bilateral mandibular angle fractures, an anterior open bite and posterior displacement of the tooth-bearing segment can occur.

Radiographic Examination

When using plain films, at least 2 views of the mandible should be obtained. The radiographs

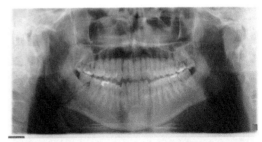

Fig. 9. Fracture through the angle with fracture of tooth #32.

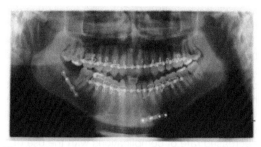

Fig. 10. Postoperative panoramic radiograph showing extraction of tooth #32 and placement of a superior border plate at the right mandibular angle.

should be 90° from each other to ensure proper evaluation. The use of plain films has fallen out of favor due to the accessibility of CT scans in most hospital emergency departments. Axial CT scans with sagittal and coronal reconstructions provide excellent visualization of all dimensions of the fracture and are becoming the gold standard. In the office setting and as an initial screening tool, a panoramic radiograph is still a valuable tool, especially when considering the ease of obtaining it, the low cost, and minimal radiation exposure to patients.

PRINCIPLES OF TREATMENT OF MANDIBULAR ANGLE FRACTURES

Although there has been considerable evolution in the treatment of mandibular angle fractures over the past 3 decades, there is still wide acceptance of the both closed and open treatment of these fractures. These alternatives are dictated by the nature of the fracture, patient age and medical and psychological status, cost, and occasionally surgeon preference and training. Thus, the initial discussion is focused on these 2 types of treatment, followed by a more detailed discussion of the open treatment.

Closed Treatment with Maxillomandibular Fixation

Closed reduction for mandibular angle fractures can only be used with favorable fracture patterns. In favorable fractures, the elevator muscles at the angle of the mandible are less likely to cause the proximal segment to rotate superiorly and anteriorly when the segment is not securely fixed to the dentate part of the mandible. In such cases, closed reduction is generally achieved with fixation screws. The use of arch bars provides no added stability of the proximal segment because, unlike in dentate portions of the mandible, an arch bar is unable to provide a superior tension

band at the angle. After use of closed reduction, an immediate postoperative panoramic radiograph should always be obtained to confirm the proper reduction of the segments.

Maxillomandibular fixation can also be used alone or in combination with external pin fixation when there is a comminuted fracture with several small bony segments that cannot be stabilized using standard plate and screw fixation.

Open Reduction and Internal Fixation

With the exception of these situations (discussed previously), open reduction and internal fixation are used to treat the majority of mandibular angle fractures. The variations in open reduction and internal fixation of the mandibular angle fracture stem from the surgical approach to the fractures and the method of rigid fixation. It is easy to understand these variations in treatment when viewed based on an understanding of fracture biomechanics and rigid fixation.

Approaches

Generally speaking, either a transoral or transfacial (extraoral) approach is used to access the fractured site. The recent increase in the popularity, however, of using a superior border plate technique has resulted in the use of a transoral approach becoming common. The transoral approach uses an incision over the external oblique ridge that is carried superiorly along the ascending ramus and anteriorly to the first molar. A 3-mm to 5-mm cuff of unattached tissue is left below the mucogingival junction to facilitate closure. This design allows complete access to the lateral and superior aspect of the mandible at the angle. If the Champy technique is planned, the incision is modified and carried slightly medial to the external oblique ridge, which allows better access to the retromolar area. Care must be taken to maintain a subperiosteal dissection to ensure protection of the lingual nerve.

When access to the inferior border is needed, a submandibular approach is required. This approach provides excellent access to the inferior border but it carries the risk of damage to the facial nerve and scarring. Posterior to the facial artery and vein, the course of the marginal mandibular branch of the facial nerve is found below the inferior border of the mandible in 19% to 53% of the time. The nerve can run as far as 1.2 cm below the inferior border of the mandible so the planned incision should be at least 2 cm below the inferior border of the mandible to prevent it being injured.[14,15]

Internal Fixation

Historically, a variety of techniques have been used for internal fixation of mandibular angle fractures. These techniques include wire osteosynthesis, a single superior border plate, a single inferior border plate (2.3 or 2.7 mm), 2 plates (1 at the superior border and 1 at the inferior border), or a lag screw. Since introduction of the technique for fixation of mandibular angle fractures described by Michelet and colleagues,[8] however, there has been a great deal of controversy regarding the most appropriate method.

The treatment of mandibular angle fractures is based on the theory of providing a superior tension band and an inferior compression band. **Fig. 7** demonstrates the displacement at the superior border that occurs in an angle fracture. At the angle, displacing forces are present at the superior border, which is perpendicular to the line of fracture. Placement of a superior border plate can provide resistance to such displacing forces.

The method of fixation must provide adequate stability at the fracture site to allow for proper healing and a low complication rate. The different methods and techniques of fixation for isolated mandibular angle fractures are discussed. When there are additional associated fractures in the mandible, in addition to angle fractures, the treatment may best be adjusted to minimize possible complications. Recently, Ellis[16] showed that when there is a fracture of the angle and an associated body or symphysis fractures, at least one of these fractures must be rigidity fixed to minimize complications of these fractures. Such rigid fixation may include locking/nonlocking reconstruction bone plates, multiple bone plates at the fracture site, single strong nonreconstruction bone plates, or multiple lag screws.

Single Plate: Superior Border

The position and number of plates to fix a mandibular angle fracture have been extensively researched and reported in the literature. Most investigators agree on the use of a single noncompression miniplate at the superior border for treatment of noncomminuted mandibular angle fractures. Gear and colleagues[17] looked at the current practice of North American and European AO/ISF (Arbeitsgemeinschaft für Osteosynthesefragen/Association for the Study of Internal Fixation) faculty and showed that the most common practice (51% of surveyed faculty) was the placement of a single superior border plate. Although many surgeons have accepted the superior border plate as the method of treatment of angle fractures,

there are several other treatments options that can be used.

A single plate can be placed at the superior border along the lateral aspect of the mandible to act as a tension band.[8,9] This has a low complication rate of 12% to 16%.[18,19] Several studies have shown no increased risk of complications when comparing the use of 1 plate with 2 plates whereas other studies have actually shown a decreased rate of complications with the use of 1 superiorly placed noncompression plate.[20–23]

The superior border and Champy techniques traditionally use a 2.0-mm plate to provide fixation. The use of a more malleable plate would allow for easier plate adaptation, potentially lower rates of dehiscence, and result in shorter operating times. Potter and Ellis[24] showed a complication rate of only 15% when a 1.3-mm miniplate was used, but the incidence of plate fracture was high. Microplates were shown to successfully treat angle fractures, but this required maxillomandibular fixation for 6 weeks after open reduction.[4,25] As a result, a 2.0 miniplate is recommended by most investigators. This plate still allows for easy adaptation but provides an adequate amount of stability to allow for proper healing (**Figs. 11** and **12**).

Two-Plate Technique

The 2-plate technique involves placement of 1 plate at the superior border to act as a tension band and 1 plate at the inferior border to act as a compression band. In vitro studies have demonstrated that 2-plate fixation is a more stable method, with lower stress at the fracture site compared with a single superior border plate placed in the Champy style.[26] Choi showed a low complication rate with the 2 noncompression miniplate technique, reporting only 4 complications (2 postoperative infections and 2 occlusal disturbances) in 40 patients.[26,27] Conversely, in

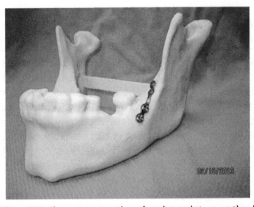

Fig. 11. Champy superior border plate method fixation.

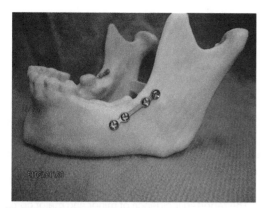

Fig. 12. Superior border plate.

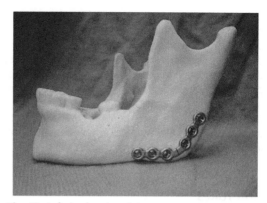

Fig. 13. Inferior border plate.

1994, Ellis and Walker[28] showed the use of two 2.0-mm noncompression miniplates had an unacceptable complication rate of 28%. A prospective randomized study by Danda and coworkers[29] indicated no difference in the rate of malocclusion, infection, and wound dehiscence between a single plate placed with the Champy technique versus 2 plates. This suggests that the use of a second plate at the inferior border is not necessary for proper fixation and healing. Furthermore, the placement of the inferior plate increases operating time and often requires an extraoral approach, which introduces the risk of facial nerve damage and scarring.

Single Plate: Inferior Border

The use of a single plate at the inferior border often requires an extraoral approach to allow for proper placement. A larger, 2.3-mm plate or a reconstruction plate is used to provide more rigid fixation in the compression zone. With the success and ease of access using a superior border plate, the use of inferior border plates has declined. An inferior border plate is still indicated, however, when there is a lack of adequate bone at the superior border, which may occur with comminuted fractures, previously failed hardware, or pathologic fractures (**Fig. 13**).

Lag Screw Fixation

The major advantages of lag screws are the high degree of compression at the fracture site, superior stability, decreased equipment cost, and reduced operating time.[30,31] Due to the technical difficulty of lag screw fixation at the angle, this method has not gained popular use.

3-D/Matrix Plate

Recently, a new plate configuration has been introduced for the treatment of mandibular angle fractures. The 3-D or matrix plate is a straight or curved ladder plate that uses monocortical screws to provide stabilization along the lateral aspect of the mandible. This plate configuration has been shown to have similar stability compared with the 2.0 miniplate but superior resistance to out-of-plane movements.[32] Several in vivo studies have shown the success of the 3-D plate for treatment of angle fractures.[32–34] In these studies, there have been low complication rates, with no reports of malunion or nonunion. When complications occurred, they included wound dehiscence and surgical site infection, which did not have a significant impact on healing at the fracture site.[33,34]

Bioresorbable Plates

There are few studies involving the use of bioresorbable plates in the treatment of mandibular angle fractures. In vitro studies have shown no statistically significant difference in breaking and displacement forces when comparing 2.0-mm titanium plates and resorbable plates.[35,36] Limited studies with small sample sizes have shown that bioresorbable plates can be used to successfully treat angle fractures, with no reports of malunion or nonunion. These studies also demonstrated a low complication rate with bioresorbable plates.[37–39] Although these studies have shown the efficacy of bioresorbable plates, more studies are required before routine use is recommended.

ANTIBIOTICS FOR TREATMENT OF MANDIBULAR FRACTURES

The use of preoperative antibiotics in the treatment of mandibular angle fractures is an accepted practice by a majority of surgeons. The use of postoperative antibiotics, however, continues to be debated. There have been several studies evaluating the incidence of infection in mandibular fractures treated with postoperative antibiotics compared with those treated without the use of postoperative antibiotics. Prospective, randomized studies have shown no difference in the incidence of infection in mandibular fracture patients treated with postoperative penicillin versus no postoperative antibiotics.[40,41] Other studies have shown similar results with different classes of antibiotics.[42,43] To date, there continues to be no good evidence in the literature to support the use of long-term postoperative antibiotics.

COMPLICATIONS OF MANDIBULAR ANGLE FRACTURES

Postoperative complications associated with mandible fractures are most common in the angle region. The variety of reported complications is most likely due to variations in the method of fixation, patient-related factors, and how these 2 variables interact with the complex biomechanics of the mandibular angle.

Although prospective randomized studies on complications of mandibular angle fractures are scarce, there is an emerging consensus from the retrospective studies, clinical review articles, and the meta-analyses on this topic.[3,18,19,23,44–52] This consensus involves lower complications rates with the use of noncompression, moncortical, single-plate fixation placed at the superior border of the mandible. Although the use of 3-D grid plates and the locking miniplates have also shown good clinical results with low complication rates, there are too few clinical studies evaluating the use of these plates.[34] The use of biodegradable plates for fixation of mandibular angle fractures has been shown to be a stable method of fixation but may require the use of additional means of fixation to provide adequate stability of the fractured segments.[53] Finally, the use of a reconstruction plate for fixation of comminuted angle fractures still represents the optimal choice for such fractures.

Postoperative complications of mandibular angle fractures are often divided into minor and major complications. Minor complications can be managed in the office, without the need for hospitalization or operating room procedures. Minor complications include localized wound infections, wound dehiscence, loosening of the fixation screws or plate, and fracture of the plate. Major complications after angle fractures are less common but often result in hospitalization and additional procedures. These complications include severe infections requiring incision and drainage, malocclusion, nonunion, malunion, nerve injury, and extensive wound débridement with or without bone grafting.

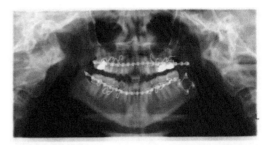

Fig. 14. Hardware failure and malunion of the left angle.

The reported incidence of minor and major complications in the literature varies widely, but minor complications constitute the majority.[20] Minor complication, such as localized infections, wound dehiscence, hardware exposure, and plate loosening, are frequently related to each other. These complications are generally managed by removal of the loose screws and plate. When they occur in the early postoperative period, however, they can often be managed by placing the patient on oral antibiotics and chlorhexidine rinses. In addition, maxillomandibular fixation can be used to further stabilize the fracture until healing occurs. If swelling or drainage continues after the healing period is complete, the screws and plate then can be removed under local anesthesia in the office.

Major complications are uncommon after treatment of mandibular angle fractures, especially with the use of single miniplate fixation. These complications are more common with the use of 2 miniplates, extraoral placement, and use of an inferior border plate and bicortical screws. The rate of major complications in one study constituted 28% of all complications of mandibular angle fractures.[19] Treatment of major complications varies depending on the nature of the complication. Potential treatment options include simple removal of the existing hardware and débridement of the necrotic and infected bone. More extensive treatment may be required, however, including

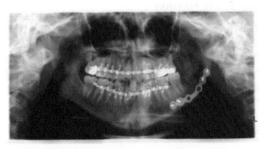

Fig. 15. Removal of the failed hardware and placement of new hardware at the inferior border.

resetting the fracture and applying new internal fixation. If a large defect remains after débridement, bone grafting is required (**Figs. 14** and **15**).

SUMMARY

The angle fracture is still one of the most common fractures of the mandible and continues to be associated with the highest complication rates. Treatment of these fractures has witnessed a significant change over the past 3 decades. This change has incorporated better understanding of the biomechanics of the mandible, the evolution in the patterns and types of fixation, and advances in surgical techniques treating these fractures. Currently, several techniques are considered acceptable to treat mandibular fractures; the most commonly accepted technique for isolated mandibular angle fracture is a single miniplate placed at the superior border. When angle fractures are associated with another mandibular fracture, the same technique can be used for the angle but preferably with rigid fixation of the other fracture or fractures. Routine use of postoperative antibiotics and removal of teeth in line of fracture is less advocated and best judged on a case-by-case basis.

REFERENCES

1. Aleysson PO, Abuabara A, Passeri LA. Analysis of 115 mandibular angle Fractures. J Oral Maxillofac Surg 2008;66:73–6.
2. Fonseca RJ, Barber HD, Powers MP, et al, editors. Oral and maxillofacial trauma. 3rd edition. 2012.
3. Ellis E. Management of fractures through the mandibular angle. Oral Maxillofac Surg Clin North Am 2009;21:163–74.
4. Levy FE, Smith RW, Odland RM, et al. Monocortical miniplate fixation of mandibular angle fractures. Arch Otolaryngol Head Neck Surg 1991;117:149–54.
5. Rudderman RH, Mullen RL, Phillips JH. The biophysics of mandibular fractures: an evolution toward understanding. Plast Reconstr Surg 2008;121(2):596–607.
6. Spiessl B. Trauma. In: Kruger E, Schilli W, editors. Textbook of oral and maxillofacial traumatology, vol. I. Berlin: Quintessence Publishing; 1982.
7. Schmoker R, Spiessl B. Excentric-dynamic compression plate. Experimental study as contribution to a functionally stable osteosynthesis in mandibular fractures. SSO Schweiz Monatsschr Zahnheilkd 1973;83(12):1496–509 [in German].
8. Michelet FX, Deymes J, Dessus B. Osteosynthesis with miniaturized screwed plates in maxillofacial surgery. J Maxillofac Surg 1973;1:79.
9. Champy M, Lodd JP, Schmitt R, et al. Mandibular osteosynthesis by miniature screwed plates via a buccal approach. J Maxillofac Surg 1978;6:14.
10. Duan DH, Zhang Y. Does the presence of mandibular third molars increase the risk of angle fracture and simultaneously decrease the risk of condylar fracture. Int J Oral Maxillofac Surg 2008;37:25–8.
11. Meisami T, Sojat A, Sàndor GK, et al. Impacted third molars and risk of angle fracture. Int J Oral Maxillofac Surg 2002;31:140–4.
12. Máaita J, Alwrikat A. Is the mandibular third molar a risk factor for mandibular angle fracture? Oral Surg Oral Med Oral Pathol 2000;89:143–6.
13. Ellis E. Outcomes of patients with teeth in the line of mandibular angle fractures treated with stable internal fixation. J Oral Maxillofac Surg 2002;60:863–5.
14. Dingman RO, Grabb WC. Surgical anatomy of the mandibular ramus of the facial nerve based on the dissection of 100 facial halves. Plast Reconstr Surg Transplant Bull 1962;29:266–72.
15. Ziarah HA, Atkinson ME. The surgical anatomy of the mandibular distribution of the facial nerve. Br J Oral Surg 1981;19(3):159–70.
16. Ellis E. Open reduction and internal fixation of combined angle and body/symphysis fractures of the mandible: how much fixation is enough? J Oral Maxillofac Surg 2013;71:726–33.
17. Gear AJ, Apasova E, Schmitz JP, et al. Treatment modalities for mandibular angle fractures. J Oral Maxillofac Surg 2005;63:655–63.
18. Barry CP, Kearns GJ. Superior border plating technique in the management of isolated mandibular angle fractures: a retrospective study of 50 consecutive patients. J Oral Maxillofac Surg 2007;65:1544–9.
19. Ellis E, Walker L. Treatment of mandibular angle fractures using one noncompression miniplate. J Oral Maxillofac Surg 1996;54:864–71.
20. Danda AK. Comparison of a single noncompression miniplate versus two noncompression miniplates in the treatment of mandibular angle fractures: a prospective, randomized clinical trial. J Oral Maxillofac Surg 2010;68:1565–7.
21. Seemann R, Schicho K, Wutzl A, et al. Complication rates in the operative treatment of mandibular angle fractures: a 10-year retrospective. J Oral Maxillofac Surg 2010;68:647–50.
22. Siddiqui A, Markose G, Moosc KF, et al. One miniplate versus two in the management of mandibular angle fractures: a Prospective Randomized Study. Br J Oral Maxillofac Surg 2007;45:223–5.
23. Regev E, Shiff JS, Kiss A, et al. Internal fixation of mandibular angle fractures: a meta-analysis. Plast Reconstr Surg 2010;125(6):1753–60.

24. Potter J, Ellis E. Treatment of mandibular angle fractures with a malleable noncompression miniplate. J Oral Maxillofac Surg 1999;57:288–92.

25. Haug R, Morgan JP III. Microplate and screw technique for intraoral open reduction of mandibular angle fractures. J Oral Maxillofac Surg 1995;23:218–9.

26. Choi BH, Kim KN, Kang HS. Clinical and in vitro evaluation of mandibular angle fracture fixation with the two miniplate system. Oral Surg Oral Med Oral Pathol Oral Radiol 1995;79:692–5.

27. Choi BH, Yoo JH, Kim NK, et al. Stability testing of a two miniplate fixation technique for mandibular angle fractures. An in vitro Study. J Craniomaxillofac Surg 1995;23(2):123–5.

28. Ellis E, Walker L. Treatment of mandibular angle fractures using two noncompression miniplates. J Oral Maxillofac Surg 1994;52:1032–6.

29. Danda AK, Muthusekhar MR, Narayanan V, et al. Open versus closed treatment of unilateral subcondylar and condylar neck fractures: a Prospective, Randomized Clinical Study. J Oral Maxillofac Surg 2010;68(6):1238–41.

30. Ellis E, Ghali GE. Lagscrew fixation of mandibular-angle fractures. J Oral Maxillofac Surg 1991;49(3): 234–43.

31. Farris PE, Dierks EJ. Single oblique lagscrew fixation of mandibular angle fractures. Laryngoscope 1992;102(9):1070–2.

32. Feledy J, Caterson EJ, Steger S, et al. Treatment of mandibular angle fractures with a matrix miniplate: a preliminary report. Plast Reconstr Surg 2004; 114(7):1711–6.

33. Zix J, Lieger O, Iizuka T. Use of straight and curved 3-dimensional titanium miniplates for fracture fixation at the mandibular angle. J Oral Maxillofac Surg 2007;65:1758–63.

34. Guimond C, Johnson JV, Marchena JM. Fixation of mandibular angle fractures with a 2.0-mm 3-dimensional curved angle strut plate. J Oral Maxillofac Surg 2005;63:209–14.

35. Bregagnolo LA, Bertelli PF, Ribeiro MC, et al. Evaluation of in vitro resistance of titanium and resorbable (poly-L-DL-lactic acid) fixation systems on the mandibular angle fracture. Int J Oral Maxillofac Surg 2011;40(3):316–21.

36. Bayram B, Araz K, Uckan S, et al. Comparison of fixation stability of resorbable versus titanium plate and screws in mandibular angle fractures. J Oral Maxillofac Surg 2009;67(8):1644–8.

37. Bayat M, Garajei A, Ghorbani K, et al. Treatment of mandibular angle fractures using a single bioresorbable miniplate. J Oral Maxillofac Surg 2010; 68(7):1573–7.

38. Laughlin RM, Block MS, Wilk R, et al. Resorbable plates for the fixation of mandibular fractures: a Prospective Study. J Oral Maxillofac Surg 2007; 65(1):89–96.

39. Vazquez-Morales DE, Dyalram-Silverberg D, Lazow SK, et al. Treatment of mandible fractures using resorbable plates with a mean of 3 weeks maxillomandibular fixation: a Prospective Study. Oral Surg Oral Med Oral Pathol Oral Radiol 2013; 115(1):25–8.

40. Abubaker AO, Rollert MK. Postoperative antibiotic prophylaxis in mandibular fractures: a preliminary randomized, double-blind, and placebo-controlled Clinical Study. J Oral Maxillofac Surg 2001;59(12):1415–9.

41. Miles BA, Potter JK, Ellis E III. The efficacy of postoperative antibiotic regimens in the open treatment of mandibular fractures: a prospective randomized trial. J Oral Maxillofac Surg 2006;64:576–82.

42. Lovato C, Wagner JD. Infection rates following perioperative prophylactic antibiotics versus postoperative extended regimen prophylactic antibiotics in surgical management of mandibular fractures. J Oral Maxillofac Surg 2009;67:827–32.

43. Hindawi YH, Oakley GM, Kinsella CR Jr, et al. Antibiotic duration and postoperative infection rates in mandibular fractures. J Craniofac Surg 2011;22: 1375–7.

44. Ellis E. A prospective Study of 3 Treatment Methods for Isolated Fractures Mandibular Angle. J Oral Maxillofac Surg 2010;68(11):2743–54.

45. Wald RM Jr, Abemayor E, Zemplenyi J, et al. The transoral treatment of mandibular fractures using noncompression miniplates: a Prospective Study. Ann Plast Surg 1988;20(5):409–13.

46. Ellis E. Treatment methods for fractures of the mandibular angle. J Craniomaxillofac Trauma 1996;2(1):28–36.

47. Ellis E, Karas N. Treatment of mandibular angle fractures using two mini dynamic compression plates. J Oral Maxillofac Surg 1992;50:958–63.

48. James RB, Fredrickson C, Kent JN, et al. Prospective Study of Mandibular Fractures. J Oral Surg 1982;39:275–8.

49. Iizuka T, Lindqvist C, Hallikainen D, et al. Infection after rigid internal fixation of mandibular fractures. A Clinical and Radiological Study. J Oral Maxillofac Surg 1991;49:585–93.

50. Gabrielli MA, Gabrielli MF, Marcantonio E, et al. Fixation of mandibular fractures with 2.0-mm miniplates: review of 191 cases. J Oral Maxillofac Surg 2003;61:430–6.

51. Lamphier J, Ziccardi V, Ruvo A, et al. Complications of Mandibular Fractures in an Urban Teaching Center. J Oral Maxillofac Surg 2003;61:745–9.

52. Chrcanovic BR. Fixation of mandibular angle fractures: clinical studies. Oral Maxillofac Surg 2012. [Epub ahead of print].

53. Dorri M, Nasser M, Oliver R. Resorbable versus titanium plates for facial fractures. Cochrane Database Syst Rev 2009;(1):CD007158.

Management of Fractures of the Mandibular Body and Symphysis

Reginald H.B. Goodday, DDS, MSc, FRCD(C), FICD

KEYWORDS

- Mandible • Body • Symphysis • Fracture • Trauma • Fixation • Complications

KEY POINTS

- Mandibular fracture, specifically in the symphysis and body region, is very common and often multiple.
- The benefit of open reduction with internal fixation to eliminate interfragment mobility is considered greater than the cost of interrupting periosteal blood supply.
- The introduction of locking plates decreases the probability of bone resorption, screw loosening, hardware failure, and fracture displacement.
- Open reduction of fractures of the atrophic edentulous mandible achieves the best outcome.
- When body and/or symphysis fractures exist, the best surgical outcome will be achieved by the combination of a correct diagnosis, proper treatment plan, and the appropriate operation.

INTRODUCTION

Mandibular fracture is among the most common injury seen in the emergency room. In a 2008 review of all hospitalizations in the United States, Nalliah[1] found that 21,244 patients underwent facial fracture reduction as a primary procedure. The most frequently performed operation was open reduction in mandibular fractures (52.2%). Oral and maxillofacial surgeons have extensive knowledge of mandibular anatomy, function, and occlusion, which is essential when treating any injury that disrupts the bone and tooth or denture-bearing region of the mandible. The application of this knowledge will result in the correct diagnosis, appropriate treatment plan, and desired surgical outcome.

INCIDENCE OF SYMPHYSIS AND BODY FRACTURE

One classification of mandibular fracture is by the anatomic area of involvement. Using the classification by Dingman and Natvig,[2] the region of the symphysis is bound by vertical lines just distal to the lower canine teeth. Fractures in this location are also commonly referred to as parasymphyseal. The region of the body comprises the mandible from the canine line to a line coinciding to the anterior border of the masseter muscle (**Fig. 1**).

Incidence and etiology of mandibular fractures vary from one country to another because of social, cultural, and environmental factors. Therefore, international comparisons are difficult. In North America, assault is the most common cause of mandibular trauma, followed by motor vehicle accidents.[1,3,4] The use of drugs and alcohol abuse along with economic disparity seems to have a direct influence on interpersonal violence. Changes in seat-belt legislation and incorporation of air bags and other safety features have resulted in motor vehicle accidents playing a decreasing role in facial trauma.

Ogundare and colleagues[3] reviewed the pattern of mandibular fractures in an urban major trauma

The author has nothing to disclose.
Department of Oral and Maxillofacial Sciences, Faculty of Dentistry, Dalhousie University, 5981 University Avenue, Halifax, Nova Scotia B3H 4R2, Canada
E-mail address: Reginald.Goodday@dal.ca

Oral Maxillofacial Surg Clin N Am 25 (2013) 601–616
http://dx.doi.org/10.1016/j.coms.2013.07.002

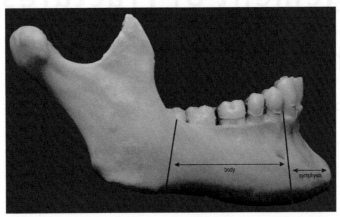

Fig. 1. The body comprises the mandible from the canine line to a line coinciding to the anterior border of the masseter muscle. The symphysis is bound by vertical lines just distal to the lower canine teeth.

center in the United States. The most common location of mandibular fracture in 1267 patients was the angle region (36%), followed by the body (21%) and symphysis (17%). Fifty-two percent of patients presented with more than 1 fracture site. Lamphier and colleagues[5] analyzed 594 mandibular fractures in an American urban teaching center, and found the incidence of fractures in the symphysis and body region to be 25% and 24%, respectively. A review of 134 patients in a United States suburban trauma center found symphysis fractures to be the most frequent (35%); body fractures were the second most common at 21%, and 68% of patients sustained fractures in multiple sites.[4] These studies confirm the common occurrence of symphysis and body fractures and that all patients should be suspected of having a second fracture site. The clinician needs to assess the patient to both determine the presence of a fracture and confirm the absence of others.

DIAGNOSIS

The diagnosis of symphysis and/or body fractures is based on the patient's history followed by a clinical and appropriate radiographic evaluation.

Patient History

When taking the history, it is important to ask the patient to describe the traumatic event, as the magnitude and direction of the force will influence the number and location of fractures. Any change in occlusion is highly suggestive of either a mandibular fracture or hemarthrosis of the temporomandibular joint. Conscious patients should be asked "how does your bite feel"? If "fine" or "normal," it is highly unlikely that a displaced fracture is present. Patients should be asked if they

have paresthesia or anesthesia of the lip and chin. Numbness in the distribution of the inferior alveolar nerve after trauma is suggestive of a displaced fracture distal to the mandibular foramen in the mandibular body. The finding of normal sensation, however, does not eliminate the presence of a fracture. Presence and severity of pain increases the suspicion of a possible fracture.

Clinical Examination

Extraoral

The surgeon should examine the patient for skin abrasion and lacerations to help determine the direction and force of the trauma (**Fig. 2**A). A body fracture could result in a flattened appearance of the lateral aspect of the face. A loss of anteroposterior projection of the chin can be caused by a bilateral parasymphyseal fracture. A facial asymmetry may be the result of an underlying displaced mandibular fracture or associated edema. The mandible should be palpated along the inferior border of the mandible to detect any step defects.

Intraoral

Common signs of a symphysis or body fracture include:

- Gingival laceration (**Fig. 2**B)
- Step defect in the occlusion (**Fig. 3**A)
- Ecchymosis in the floor of the mouth (**Fig. 4**)

The mandible should be manipulated using both hands, with the thumb on the teeth and fingers on the inferior border of the mandible. By slowly and carefully placing pressure between the two hands, mobility can be noted in a fracture.

Radiographic examination

Radiographic imaging is an essential component of the management of mandibular trauma. From

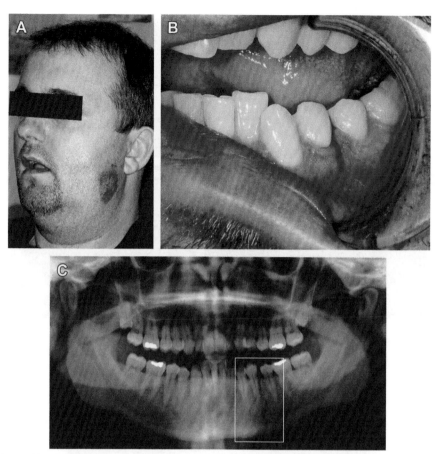

Fig. 2. Patient with a left body fracture of the mandible. (*A*) Skin abrasion secondary to blunt trauma fracturing mandible. (*B*) Gingival laceration overlying fracture. (*C*) Pretreatment panoramic radiograph highlighting oblique body fracture.

the point of view of diagnosis it should confirm the presence and magnitude of fracture displacement. The radiograph is reviewed when considering treatment options and assessing outcomes (**Fig. 5**A, B).

Single or combinations of plain films are considered as a good screening tool for the initial assessment of traumatic events involving the maxillofacial complex.[6]

Information gained from conventional plain radiographs is limited by the 3-dimensional anatomy of the imaged area being compressed into a 2-dimensional image. This limitation is overcome by using a combination of different conventional plain films being taken on different planes. Advanced imaging modalities such as medical computed tomography (CT) and cone-beam CT (CBCT) are able to generate images easily on the sagittal, coronal, and axial planes, eliminating superimposition of anatomic structures. Using volumetric data, 3-dimensional reconstruction allows the virtual visualization of the area of trauma (**Fig. 6**).

The most informative radiograph used in diagnosing mandibular fractures is the panoramic radiograph showing the entire mandible (**Fig. 2**C).

Advantages:
- Simplicity of technique
- Availability
- Cost effective
- Lower radiation exposure compared with CT or CBCT
- Ability to visualize the entire mandible in one radiograph
- Provides generally good detail

Disadvantages:
- Technique usually requires the patient to be upright, which may make it impractical in the severely traumatized patient
- It is a 2-dimensional image, making it difficult to appreciate buccal lingual bone displacement
- Fine details may be lacking in the symphysis region, owing the thickness of bone

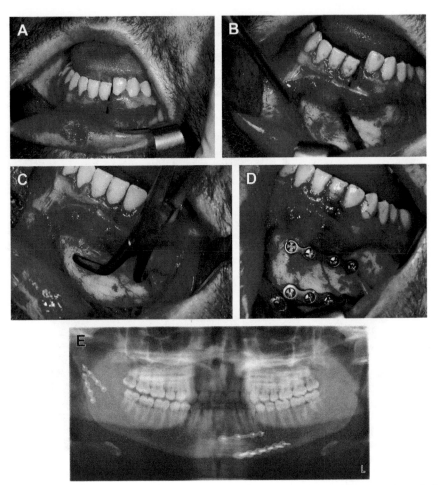

Fig. 3. Patient with symphysis fracture of the mandible. (*A*) Occlusal step defect. (*B*) Intraoral surgical exposure. (*C*) Use of bone-reducing forceps to achieve bony reduction. (*D*) Use of 2 miniplates to stabilize bone segments. (*E*) Postsurgery radiograph.

The occlusal topographic radiograph can be used as a supplement to the panoramic film to identify buccal lingual displacement of fractures in the body or symphysis region. This radiograph

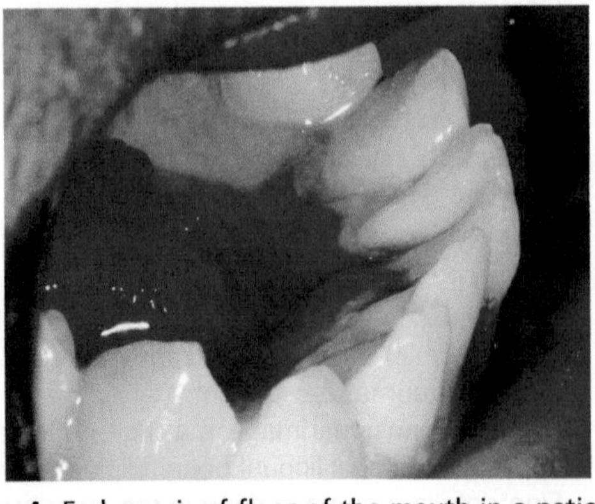

Fig. 4. Ecchymosis of floor of the mouth in a patient with symphysis fracture.

can confirm proper reduction of the fracture after surgery (**Fig. 7**).

Patients with signs and symptoms of a mandibular fracture that are not visible on conventional 2-dimensional radiographs may benefit from CBCT or medical CT scans, which have the following advantages[7]:

- Image-enhancing tools
- Better imaging quality
- Higher sensitivity in identification of fractures
- Decreased interpretation error
- Greater interphysician agreement in the identification of mandibular fractures
- Possible in the nonambulatory patient
- Three-dimensional appreciation of fracture

In CBCT the complete 3-dimensional volume of data is acquired in a single rotation of the scanner around the patient, which allows images acquired with lower acquisition time and radiation exposure

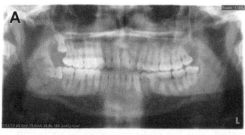 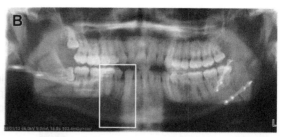

Fig. 5. (A) Pretreatment radiograph of patient with angle fracture. (B) Postsurgery radiograph highlighting undiagnosed body fracture.

compared with medical CT.[8] If further information is required, CBCT should be considered instead of medical CT because of its lesser costs and radiation dosage. If better soft-tissue detail is desired, a medical CT is preferable.

Deciding on the use of conventional and/or advanced imaging modalities to diagnose mandibular fractures should be decided after considering:

- Severity of the injury
- Structural superimposition
- Patient's functional restrictions
- Cost
- Availability
- Soft-tissue imaging requirements
- Need for 3-dimensional views

TREATMENT PLANNING
Sequence of Fracture Repair

In more than 50% of patients who have suffered mandibular trauma, examination will confirm the presence of more than 1 mandibular fracture.

The sequence of fracture repair can enhance the accuracy of reduction, decrease the length of surgery, facilitate restoration of the preinjury occlusion, and result in fewer complications. The most predictable result occurs when the least displaced mandibular fracture is treated first. The reduction of a tooth-bearing fragment should be performed before that of a tooth-free fragment.[9]

Tooth in the Line of Fracture

In the dentate patient, a fracture of the symphysis or body will most likely involve a tooth in the line of fracture. The management of this clinical scenario has been controversial. Historically the accepted treatment was to remove the tooth so as to eliminate a potential source of infection. This recommendation, however, was made by clinicians who typically performed closed reduction and used intermaxillary mandibular fixation (IMF) to stabilize the fracture. It is most likely that infections attributed to the presence of teeth in the line of fracture were actually caused by interbony fragment mobility. The use of rigid fixation for fracture

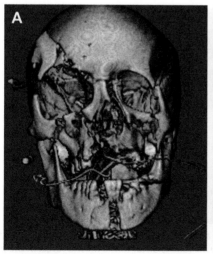 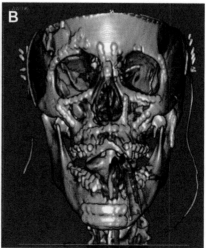

Fig. 6. (A) Preoperative medical computed tomography demonstrating multiple fractures. (B) Postoperative medical computed tomography demonstrating 3-dimensional fracture repairs.

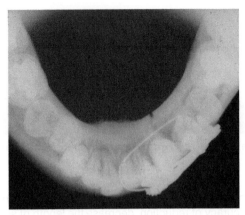

Fig. 7. Postsurgery occlusal radiograph confirming reduction of fracture.

- Has a compromised periodontium (mobile tooth)
- Has an extensive periapical lesion (infection)

Before extraction, the tooth may be used to aid in the reduction of the fracture. After applying the plate across the fracture, the reduction is confirmed and the occlusion checked. The plates and screws can then be removed, the tooth extracted, and the plate reapplied by replacing the screws in the initial holes.

Biomechanics

From a biomechanical aspect, the mandible represents 2 Class III levers joined in the midline with the fulcrum at the summit of each condyle, muscle force applied distal to the fulcrum, and occlusal force applied distal to the muscle force (**Fig. 8**). Understanding of the muscle attachments and forces imposed on the mandible are useful in assisting the surgeon when planning treatment.

Champy and colleagues[12] used this biomechanical approach when describing the ideal lines of osteosynthesis (**Fig. 9**). In the body of the mandible, the masticatory forces create strains of tension along the alveolar bone superior to the mandibular canal, and compression strains along the inferior border of the mandible. With a fracture in the mandibular body, the zone of compression is favorable in maintaining bony contact; however, the zone of tension strives to pull the bone apart (see **Fig. 8**). This force must be neutralized when applying fixation. In the anterior mandible there are moments of torsion that are highest in the mandibular symphysis.

According to Champy and colleagues,[12] one miniplate proximal to the first premolar below the

stabilization has greatly reduced the incidence of infection.

Gerbino and colleagues[10] have demonstrated that when using miniplates for fixation, incidence of complications increases when the tooth in the line of fracture is extracted rather than left in place. The presence of a tooth can constitute an occlusal reference and provide a posterior stop. Freitag and Landau[11] have shown that the presence of teeth at the fracture site does not impede bone healing and has a stabilizing effect on the fracture. Conserving the tooth facilitates fracture reduction in many cases, making it more accurate, quicker, and easier.

Extracting a tooth in the line of fracture is indicated when the tooth:

- Makes the reduction of the fracture difficult or impossible
- Has fractured roots

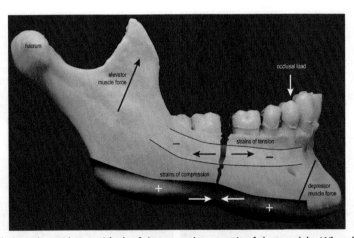

Fig. 8. The mandible is a Class III lever with the fulcrum at the summit of the condyle. When biting, the elevator muscle force is applied distal to the fulcrum and the occlusal load is distal to the muscle force. In the presence of a body fracture, masticatory forces create strains of tension above the mandibular canal pulling the bone apart and strains of compression along the inferior border of the mandible promoting bony contact.

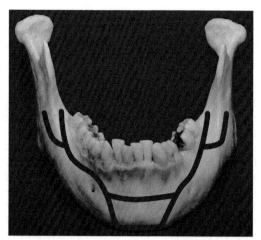

Fig. 9. Champy's ideal lines of osteosynthesis.

apices of the teeth and above the inferior alveolar nerve is sufficient to treat a body fracture. In symphysis the placement of 2 miniplates separated by 4 to 5 mm is necessary to neutralize the moments of torsion (**Fig. 3**D).

TREATMENT OPTIONS

The primary treatment objective is to restore form and function by achieving anatomic reduction and fixation that eliminates mobility of the bone fragments. Failure to achieve these objectives may result in a malocclusion that will predispose the patient to chronic pain, significant problems with mastication, and poor facial esthetics.

Closed Reduction

Intermaxillary mandibular fixation
IMF reestablishes the patient's presurgery occlusion, and in certain cases can sufficiently stabilize the bone to allow healing to take place.

Indications
- When the fracture line and vector of the muscle pull is favorable and keeps the fracture appropriately reduced
- Patient has a healthy dentition with sufficient teeth to obtain a stable occlusion
- Comminuted fractures with multiple small bone fragments that could become displaced with periodontal stripping
- Patient is compliant and is amenable to immobilization of the jaw for 2 to 6 weeks

IMF can be accomplished by attaching Erich arch bars to the remaining dentition using circumdental wires. The patient is then placed in preinjury occlusion, and interarch wires or elastics are placed to stabilize the occlusion (**Fig. 10**).

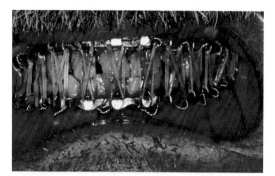

Fig. 10. Erich arch bars with elastic fixation.

Advantages of Erich Arch Bars:
- Ease of application
- Low cost
- Minimize the distraction of bone at the healing site
- Maintain intact periosteum over bone
- Restore normal occlusion

Disadvantages:
- Increase surgical time
- Require a second procedure to remove the arch bars
- Only semirigid fixation
- Risk to surgeon from penetration injuries caused by circumdental and IMF wires[13]
- Promote poor oral hygiene
- Pain from loose circumdental wires
- Delayed healing due to loose IMF wires

IMF Self-tapping screws
These screws are placed in sound bone in the anterior and posterior vestibular regions, and provide a bone anchor for elastics or wires for IMF when establishing and/or maintaining the patient's occlusion (**Fig. 11**).

Advantages Over Arch Bars:
- Ease of application
- Decrease in surgical time

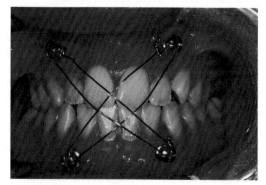

Fig. 11. Intermaxillary mandibular fixation screws.

- Low risk of inadvertent skin puncture
- Stable anchorage promoting realignment of the occlusion
- Do not loosen with time
- Promote better oral hygiene
- Suitable when dentition has been heavily restored with crown and bridge restorations
- Easy to remove

Disadvantages:
- Risk of tooth-root damage
- Cannot be used to splint dental alveolar fractures or stabilize loose teeth
- Maxilla needs to be intact
- Soft-tissue burying of screw heads in the anterior vestibule
- Require sound bone stock clear of tooth roots
- Interarch wiring may cause orthodontic movement of teeth or cracking of enamel where it crosses the incisal tip

In pediatric patients with developing tooth buds and lack of dental anchorage, IMF skeletal suspension wires can be placed within sound bone in the zygomatic buttress or piriform aperture region. Circummandibular wires can be placed proximal and distal to the fracture and on the contralateral side, and then secured to the maxillary skeletal fixation with connector wires.

Most adult mandibular fractures require 4 to 6 weeks of stabilization. For those patients with minimally displaced mandibular fractures in the tooth-bearing area, 2 weeks may be sufficient.[14]

Contraindications to IMF include:

- Noncompliant patient
- Alcoholic patient
- Seizure disorders
- Severe pulmonary dysfunction
- Intellectual disability
- Psychosis
- Poor nutrition
- Pregnancy
- Patient with multiple system injuries

External fixation
This treatment modality is seldom used but may be considered for a patient who has a nonhealing infected body fracture that requires stabilization. Once the infection is eliminated and soft tissues are healthy, definitive treatment can take place and fixation removed.

Open Reduction

Open reduction allows the surgeon to visualize the fracture and control the reduction so that the anatomy is restored to its presurgery form, and is followed by the application of rigid fixation. This procedure eliminates the need for prolonged or, in many cases, any maxillomandibular fixation, and allows return to early function.

Surgical approach
The intraoral approach to the symphysis and body region of the mandible provides excellent access to the fracture and the ability to observe the occlusion during the reduction and application of rigid fixation. Of importance is that the risks associated with extraoral incision, including nerve damage and cosmesis, can be avoided. Typically the incision is made in the vestibule and placed approximately 5 to 7 mm inferior to the mucogingival junction to facilitate ease of closure and prevent wound dehiscence (**Fig. 3**B). Care should be taken to avoid close proximity of the mental nerve with the incision. This nerve is identified when dissecting in the premolar region, and the nerve sheath is carefully skeletonized to allow mobility, to prevent possible avulsion by the surgical retractors. After exposure of all fractures, they are mobilized and any trapped soft tissue is removed. The patient's occlusion can be stabilized with IMF using either arch bars or IMF screws, or the surgical assistant can hand-hold the occlusion, with predictable results.[15] Bone-reducing forceps can be used in the transoral approach to assist bony reduction (**Fig. 3**C). The fixation of choice is applied, the occlusion verified, and the incision closed with mentalis muscle reconstruction as required.

Internal fixation
A fracture is a result of a mechanical overload that is greater than the stiffness of bone and causes an interruption in the structural integrity. There is associated soft-tissue damage, specifically the interruption of intracortical blood vessels. For successful healing, minimal requirements of both a mechanical and biological nature must be met. The objective of internal fixation is to limit interfragmentary motion to achieve these requirements.[16] Healing time is directly related to the size of the gap between bone and interfragment motion. Two goals of rigid internal fixation are to stabilize bone fragments to minimize movement, in conjunction with having the smallest gap possible between the fracture margins (see **Fig. 3**D). There is common agreement that fixation which is truly rigid results in a low incidence of infection.[17–20]

Many choices for internal fixation of body and symphysis fractures are available, including lag screws, miniplates, trauma plates, and reconstruction plates. The application of any of these can be considered "rigid" fixation, indicating stability sufficient to prevent interfragment motion under function.

Champy suggests that the use of plates to initiate compression of the bone fragments is no longer advisable because:

- There is a natural strain of compression along the inferior border
- Compression may be excessive and can cause bone lysis
- It makes the reestablishment of normal occlusion more difficult
- It may require access through an extraoral approach

Since the 1978 publication by Champy and colleagues[12] of 103 cases of mandibular osteosynthesis, the use of miniplates placed along the lines of osteosynthesis have been indicated as an effective treatment modality.

When treating a body fracture, Champy's technique in its purest form places a single plate in the zone of tension while taking advantage of the compressive strains along the inferior border of the mandible. In the symphysis 2 plates are used, separated by 4 to 5 mm, to neutralize the moments of torsion (**Fig. 3**E).

To guarantee restoration of the preinjury occlusion it is necessary to bend these plates so that they lie passively on bone before monocortical screws are placed. When there is lack of bony contact following fracture reduction because of bone loss or there is significant comminution, rigid plates may be placed along the inferior border of the mandible using bicortical screws. The thicker the plate, the more difficult it is to bend, so that it will lie flush with the bone on either side of the fracture. If the plate is not passively adapted to the underlying bone, the engaging of the screw will create pressure that displaces the fracture, resulting in a poor reduction and malocclusion. Moreover, the bone underlying the plate can resorb and the fixation become loose before adequate

fracture healing, resulting in possible mobility around the fracture site and delayed healing.

The introduction of locking plates and screws overcomes the need for passive adaptation. The screw locks into the plate, creating a rigid functional unit, and removes unfavorable pressure from the bone. This procedure decreases the probability of bone resorption, screw loosening, hardware failure, and fracture displacement.

In a retrospective study of 682 patients, Ellis[17] compared the outcomes of treating mandibular symphysis/body fractures using 2 miniplates or 1 stronger plate. Each technique showed no statistically significant difference in occlusal or osseous healing outcomes. Of note, however, is his finding that although infrequent, there was more wound dehiscence, plate exposure, tooth-root damage, and need for plate removal with the 2-plate system.[17]

Lag screws

Using lag screws to provide rigid fixation in oblique fractures of the mandibular body and parasymphysis has been well documented.[20–27] If a fracture occurs in the body region in a sagittal plane with splitting of the buccal and lingual cortices, the fracture is amenable to treatment with 2 or 3 lag screws. Ellis[28] reviewed 31 patients and demonstrated that lag-screw fixation of mandibular body fractures is extremely simple and rigidly secures bone fragments, permitting continuous function during healing with essentially no complications.

Lag screws can also be used to counteract moments of torsion in the symphysis (**Fig. 12**). The anterior mandible is especially suited to this technique because:

- The curvature of the anterior mandible allows placement of screws across the symphysis
- The bony cortices are very thick
- Vital structures are absent below the apices of the anterior teeth

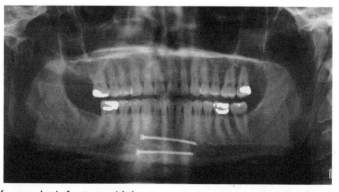

Fig. 12. Treatment of a symphysis fracture with lag screws to counteract moments of torsion.

A retrospective study by Ellis[21] analyzed 196 patients with fractures of the anterior mandible who were treated using bone screws, and demonstrated good stability in all fractures except 6. Lag-screw fixation is his first choice for providing rigid internal fixation of mandibular fractures unless there is significant comminution, or compression that would cause displacement of bone fragments, overriding of the segments, and/or shortening of the fracture gap, all of which can alter the occlusion. Ellis' preference is based on the following advantages:

- Rapid application
- Eliminates need to adapt a bone plate
- Minimal displacement of bone segments
- May enhance the fracture reduction
- Is truly rigid

Transosseous wiring

Transosseous wiring can be used to reduce mandibular fractures; however, it commits such patients to several weeks of postoperative intermaxillary fixation and a higher incidence of post-treatment infection.

MANAGEMENT OF FRACTURES OF THE EDENTULOUS MANDIBLE

Fractures of the severely resorbed edentulous mandible are not common, with an incidence of less than 1% to 5% of all mandibular fractures.[29–33] The region of greatest alveolar bone resorption in the mandible following the extraction of teeth is the body. The most common site of fracture in the edentulous mandible is this region.

A recent Cochrane review looking at all available data confirms there is inadequate evidence to support the effectiveness of any single approach, either open or closed, in the management of fractured atrophic edentulous mandibles and that, until high-level evidence is available, treatment decisions should continue to be based on the clinician's prior experience.[34]

Basic principles of fracture management (anatomic reduction and rigid immobilization) to restore form and function may be difficult in the edentulous mandible for several reasons.

Patient Factors
- Medically compromised
- Effects of general anesthetic of greater concern
- Decreased osteogenesis
- Lifestyle not conducive to good healing (alcohol abuse, poor oral hygiene)
- Present and future nutritional status
- Difficulty tolerating IMF
- Noncompliant with postoperative instructions

Anatomic Factors
- Decreased bone stock on either side of the fracture
- Lack of bone to apply rigid fixation
- Decreased quality of bone: osteoporosis
- Unfavorable position of the inferior alveolar nerve
- Requirement to place rigid fixation away from the denture-bearing area

Significant complications (such as nonunion, chronic infection, or fracture of hardware) have been widely reported in the management of atrophic mandible fractures, with an incidence from 4% to 20%.[30,35–40]

Closed Reduction Options

- Isolated mandibular fixation using the patient's complete lower denture with circummandibular wires to stabilize the fracture
- Using upper and lower dentures to secure maxillomandibular fixation
- Customized gunning splints (**Fig. 13**)
- External pin fixation (**Fig. 14**)

The use of various closed techniques using splints does not allow the clinician to confirm adequate reduction of the fracture nor does it provide adequate resistance to the distraction forces of the muscles of mastication, giving rise to nonunion or malunion. External pin fixation is difficult if there is insufficient bone available to achieve approximation of the margins of the fractures. Patients may be unwilling to accept the appearance of an extraoral external fixator.[41]

Open Reduction Options

Clayman and Rossi[42] reviewed the results of placing miniplates at the inferior border of the

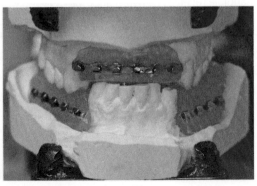

Fig. 13. Custom gunning splints.

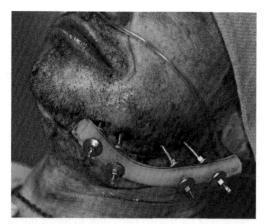

Fig. 14. External pin fixation to stabilize a nonhealing body fracture.

edentulous mandible to treat 23 body fractures. All patients achieved clinical union of their fractures. Other surgeons support the use of miniplates in achieving good results for the treatment of fractures of the atrophic mandible.[30,43–45]

The application of load-bearing fixation, using reconstruction bone plate spanning the area of fracture and secured in the areas of the mandible where the bone is stable and healthy, can succeed (**Fig. 15**A, B).[39,46–48] Ellis and Price[49] showed good outcomes after treating body fractures of the edentulous mandible by open reduction, with plating systems of different size, and immediate bone grafting when required. This review of 32 patients, 26 of whom had bilateral fractures, revealed 23 who received immediate bone grafts, and all patients healed uneventfully.

Many surgeons promote closed reduction of edentulous fractures because of concern that raising periosteum will decrease the healing potential at the fracture site. Luhr and colleagues[50] recommend application of plates over periosteum to avoid disturbing the periosteal blood supply to the area around the fracture. Ellis and Price[49] disagree, and state that the atrophic mandible receives its blood supply by the vessels perforating the periosteum; it is the soft tissues overlying the periosteum that provide the blood supply. Performing a supraperiosteal dissection to apply a plate will, therefore, disrupt the vascular supply to the periosteum overlying the bone.[49]

Much of the blood supply to the bone can be sacrificed for the advantage of providing stable internal fixation. Elimination of interfragment mobility is of the highest priority, and the periosteal blood supply issue is minor compared with the importance of achieving rigid internal fixation.[36,38,40,46,47,49]

MANAGEMENT OF MANDIBULAR FRACTURES IN CHILDREN

As mandibular fractures in children are less frequent, there is a lack of prospective studies identifying the effectiveness of any single approach to injury. The consensus in the literature is that children have a significant capacity for healing in a short time with minimal complications.

Facial fractures in the pediatric group account for about 5% of all facial fractures.[51] The most common requiring hospitalization involves the mandible with the condyle and angle more than the mandibular body.[52]

Management of pediatric mandibular fractures differs from that in adults, because of the need to consider growth and the developing dentition. In children, growth can work in favor of the objective of restoring form and function. Treatment should be designed to support, and not interfere with, this biological process.

A panoramic radiograph is usually sufficient to diagnose a body or symphysis fracture in the pediatric patient. If the patient is very young and cannot tolerate a panoramic radiograph, a CT scan is an option. When the clinician suspects a fracture in the symphysis region that is not obvious on a panoramic radiograph, an occlusal and/or periapical radiograph may help in confirming the diagnosis.

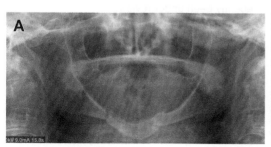
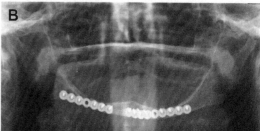

Fig. 15. (*A*) Bilateral body fractures of an atrophic edentulous mandible. (*B*) Use of 2 reconstruction plates spanning the areas of fracture and secured to stable bone.

In adolescent patients the treatment objective is to establish the best alignment of bony fragments with the least invasive technique. As growth will assist the restoration of form and function, it is important to minimize interference with the natural biology associated with bone growth and development of the permanent dentition.

Closed Reduction

Because of the high elasticity of the pediatric mandible, there typically is minimal displacement of the fracture fragments, and the injury is amenable to a closed reduction. Types of fixation would include:

- Circumdental wires applied to teeth across the line of fracture
- Application of a mandibular arch bar across the fracture
- Lingual splints
- IMF (IMF screws or arch bars)

In the very young patient 2 weeks of immobilization is sufficient, and up to puberty 3 or 4 weeks will suffice in most circumstances.[53]

Open Reduction

The benefit of open reduction with internal fixation in adult patients is well known, but this treatment modality for displaced fractures of the symphysis/body region of the adolescent is controversial. There are no prospective, randomized controlled trials assessing the effect of bone plates and screws on mandibular growth in children. Yaremchuk and colleagues[54] suggest that rigid fixation affects the craniofacial growth of rhesus monkeys, although the application of fixation was across cranial sutures. Schilli, writing on mandibular fractures in children, states that research shows that "titanium implants most probably do not interfere with the growth of the membranous skeletal bones."[55]

Although the greatest numbers of fractures are minimal to nondisplaced, it is considered that displaced fractures are better served with open reduction and internal rigid fixation. There is debate about whether resorbable plates have an advantage over titanium. Bos[56] supports the use of titanium because there is insufficient clinical scientific evidence regarding the short-term (mechanical properties) and long-term (bioresorbability) characteristics of the various resorbable osteosynthesis systems. Bos chooses small titanium plates and screws for fixation of pediatric fractures because they have superior mechanical properties, smaller dimensions, and can be removed if necessary after many years.[56]

Eppley[57] promotes of the use of resorbable plates and screws in pediatric facial fractures. His study of 29 displaced fractures of the symphysis, body, and ramus in patients younger than 10 years concluded that resorbable plates and screws can be an effective fixation method for facial fractures in children in the primary and secondary dentition periods.

Turvey and colleagues[58] recently reviewed their 10-year experience using biodegradable fixation for 761 craniomaxillofacial operations in all age groups. Successful outcomes were found in a variety of surgical applications, and the investigators acknowledged that there is a learning curve and a requirement for trained personnel to assist during the operation because of the complexity of the polylactate systems. Moreover, the cost of the material is not yet competitive with alternative means of rigid fixation.[58]

Laughlin and colleagues[59] published a prospective study looking at the use of resorbable plates for the fixation of mandibular fractures in adults. Clinical and radiographic evaluation of 50 consecutive mandibular fractures, of which more than 50% were in either the body or symphysis, demonstrated union in all fractures. Their surgical technique included the placement of all patients in maximum intercuspation and IMF using elastics for a 2-week period. The need for IMF may limit the use of this technique in children.

COMPLICATIONS
Infection

Mandibular fractures of the body and symphysis that involve the tooth-bearing segments are considered to be contaminated at the time of fracture. The use of preoperative and perioperative antibiotics is the standard of care supported by the literature.[60–67] Incidence of infection in patients with compound fractures of the mandible in whom no antibiotics were used has been reported to be as high as 50%. Use of prophylactic antibiotics has reduced this incidence to as low as 6%.[68] Duration of antibiotic prophylaxis has recently been under review.

Abubaker and Rollert[69] conducted a prospective, randomized, double-blind clinical study using a placebo control in 30 patients with uncomplicated fractures of the mandible. Their results demonstrated no benefit of a postoperative course of oral antibiotics. Miles and colleagues[70] conducted a much larger prospective study that looked at the effectiveness of postoperative antibiotics in 181 patients treated by open reduction with internal fixation of their mandibular fractures involving the tooth-bearing segment. Their results were similar to those of Abubaker and Rollert in finding no statistically significant difference in the rate of infection in groups that did or did not receive antibiotics after surgery. This study showed an increase in the risk of infection postoperatively in those patients who abused tobacco and alcohol concomitantly. As alcohol abuse alone approached statistical significance, a larger sample would reveal this as an individual risk for postoperative infections. Of importance was the statistically significant increase in time between fracture repair and the diagnosis of postoperative infection in patients who received postoperative antibiotics compared with those who did not.

Nonunion of the Mandible

A review of the literature reveals considerable variability in the rate of nonunion (2%–32%) depending on the surgical technique and patient population studied.[71,72] Overall this complication has been rare. Mathog and colleagues[73] published a retrospective review of 1432 mandibular fractures, and found 25 nonunion complications for an incidence of 2.8%. This rate is similar to that of studies by Bochlogyros[74] and Haug and Schwimmer[75] (3.2%).

There seems to be agreement that the site of most nonunions is in the mandibular body. Predisposing factors that contribute to this condition include:

- Multiple fracture sites
- Delayed treatment
- Inadequate reduction
- Inadequate fixation
- Noncompliance of the patient (premature release of IMF, poor oral hygiene)
- Alcohol or drug abuse (poor nutrition)
- Systemic disease (diabetes)
- Misdiagnosis

When nonunion has occurred, a successful outcome is typically achieved with stabilization of the mandible with either internal or external rigid fixation, with a bone graft if a bony defect has developed.

Neurosensory Changes

The literature indicates that the prevalence of postinjury/pretreatment inferior alveolar nerve (IAN) injury ranges from 5.7% to 58.5%.[76] The prevalence of IAN neurosensory deficit after fracture treatment ranges from 0.4% to 91.3%.[76–78]

In a prospective study, Halpern and colleagues[79] documented perioperative neurosensory changes in the IAN in 97 fractures located between the lingula and symphysis of the

mandible. There was an abnormal neurosensory examination of the IAN in 81% of the cases before treatment. In 85% of these patients, the degree of neurosensory deficit was either unchanged or improved immediately after treatment. In 15% of the cases the IAN neurosensory score was worse after treatment than before treatment. A fracture displaced 5 mm or greater, a normal preoperative neurosensory score, and open reduction/internal fixation were associated with a 6-, 25-, and 40-fold increase, respectively, in risk for worsening of the IAN neurosensory score after treatment of mandibular fracture. In this study, a surprising finding was how frequently patients with fractures distal to the mental foramen had abnormal postinjury/pretreatment IAN neurosensory examinations (76%). As the postoperative evaluation was performed within 7 days following surgery, the neurosensory changes noted in this study could certainly be temporary, because the long-term outcome was not studied and is unknown. Another clinically relative observation in this study is the finding that patients with a normal postinjury neurosensory score had an increased risk for worsening of their IAN neurosensory score after treatment, regardless of the treatment choice or degree of fracture displacement. Fortunately, however, the results of this study suggest that for most patients the neurosensory status is unchanged or improved after treatment of mandibular fracture.[79]

SUMMARY

Mandibular fracture, specifically in the symphysis and body region, is very common and frequently multiple. Patients with signs and symptoms of mandibular fracture that are not visible on 2-dimensional radiographs will benefit from CBCT or medical CT scans.

When treating multiple fractures, the most predictable outcome occurs when the least displaced fracture is treated first and the tooth-bearing fragment is reduced before the tooth-free fragment. A tooth in the line of fracture should be retained whenever possible. Biomechanical principles need to be considered when deciding on treatment options.

The benefit of open reduction with internal fixation to eliminate interfragment mobility is considered greater than the cost of interrupting periosteal blood supply. Fixation that is truly rigid results in a low incidence of infection. The introduction of locking plates decreases the probability of bone resorption, screw loosening, hardware failure, and fracture displacement. Lag screws provide rigid fixation in oblique fractures of the mandibular body, are useful in counteracting moments of torsion in the symphysis, and have a very low complication rate.

Open reduction of fractures of the atrophic edentulous mandible achieves the best outcome. Management of pediatric mandibular fractures differs from that in adults because of the need to consider mandibular growth and the developing dentition. The treatment objective is to establish the best alignment of bony fragments with the least invasive techniques. The use of resorbable plates and screws continues to be controversial.

The protocol of prescribing a postoperative course of oral antibiotics in patients with uncomplicated fractures of the mandible is not supported in the literature. The site of most nonunions is in the mandibular body, although the incidence is rare. When this complication occurs, successful treatment is achieved with stabilization of the mandible by internal or external rigid fixation, with a bone graft if a bony defect has developed.

In conclusion, when body and/or symphysis fractures exist, the best surgical outcome will be achieved by the combination of a correct diagnosis, proper treatment plan, and the appropriate operation.

REFERENCES

1. Nalliah R. Economics of facial fracture reductions in the United States over 12 months. Dent Traumatol 2012. http://dx.doi.org/10.1111/j.1600-9657.2012.01137.x.
2. Dingman RO, Natvig P. Occlusion and intermaxillary fixation. In: Dingman RO, Natvig P, editors. Surgery of facial fractures. Philadelphia: WB Saunders; 1964. p. 143.
3. Ogundare B, Bonnick A, Bayley N. Pattern of mandible fractures in an urban major trauma center. J Oral Maxillofac Surg 2003;61:713–8.
4. King R, Scianna J, Petruzzelli G. Mandibular fracture patterns: a suburban trauma center experience. Am J Otolaryngol 2004;25:301–7.
5. Lamphier J, Ziccardi V, Ruvo A, et al. Complications of mandibular fractures in an urban teaching center. J Oral Maxillofac Surg 2003;61:745–9.
6. Scarfe WC, Farman AG, Sukovic P. Clinical applications of cone-beam computed tomography in dental practice. J Can Dent Assoc 2006;72:75–80.
7. Roth FS, Kokoska MS, Awward EE, et al. The identification of mandible fractures by helical computed tomography and panorex tomography. J Craniofac Surg 2005;16:394–9.
8. Werner S, Venturin J, Azevedo B, et al. Applications of cone-beam computed tomography in fractures of the maxillofacial complex. Dent Traumatol 2009;25:358–66.
9. Dell G, Orabona A, Iaconetta G, et al. Bifocal mandibular fractures: which should be treated first? J Craniofac Surg 2012;23:1723–7.
10. Gerbino F, Tarello M, Fasolis M, et al. Rigid fixation with teeth in the line of mandibular fractures. Int J Oral Maxillofac Surg 1997;26:182–6.
11. Freitag V, Landau H. Healing of dentate or edentulous mandibular fractures treated with rigid or semirigid fixation plate fixation—an experimental study in dogs. J Craniomaxillofac Surg 1996;24:83–7.
12. Champy M, Lodde J, Schmitt J, et al. Mandibular osteosynthesis by miniature screwed plates via a buccal approach. J Maxillofac Surg 1978;6:14–21.
13. Avery CM, Johnson PA. Surgical glove perforation and maxillofacial trauma: to plate or wire? Br J Oral Maxillofac Surg 1992;30(1):31–5.
14. Adeyemi M, Adeyemo W, Mobolanle O, et al. Is healing outcome of 2 weeks intermaxillary fixation different from that of 4 to 6 weeks intermaxillary fixation in the treatment of mandibular fractures? J Oral Maxillofac Surg 2012;70(8):1896–902.
15. Bell RB, Wilson DM. Is the use of arch bars or interdental wire fixation necessary for successful outcomes in the open reduction and internal fixation of mandibular angle fractures? J Oral Maxillofac Surg 2008;66(10):2116–22.
16. Assael LA, Klotch DW, Manson PN, et al. Scientific and technical background. In: Prein J, editor. Manual of internal fixation in the craniofacial skeleton. Berlin: Springer-Verlag; 1998. p. 7–9.
17. Ellis E. A study of 2 bone plating methods for fractures of the mandibular symphysis/body. J Oral Maxillofac Surg 2011;69:1978–87.
18. Cawood JI. Small plate osteosynthesis of mandibular fractures. Br J Oral Maxillofac Surg 1985;23:77–91.
19. Nakamura S, Takenoshita Y, Oka M. Complications of miniplate osteosynthesis for mandibular fractures. J Oral Maxillofac Surg 1994;52:233–8.
20. Scolozzi P, Richter M. Treatment of severe mandibular fractures using AO reconstruction plates. J Oral Maxillofac Surg 2003;61:458–61.
21. Ellis E. Lag screw fixation of mandibular fractures. J Craniomaxillofac Trauma 1997;3(1):16–26.
22. Kallela I, Tateyuki I, Laine P, et al. Lag-screw fixation of mandibular parasymphyseal and angle fractures. Oral Surg Oral Med Oral Pathol Oral Radiol Endod 1996;81:510–6.
23. Brons R, Boering G. Fractures of the mandibular body treated by stable internal fixation: a preliminary report. J Oral Surg 1970;28:407.
24. Niederdellmann H, Schilli W, Duker J, et al. Osteosynthesis of mandibular fractures using lag screws. Int J Oral Surg 1976;5:117–21.
25. Niederdellmann H, Akuamoa-Boateng E, Uhlig G. Lag-screw osteosynthesis: a new procedure for

treating fractures of the mandibular angle. J Oral Surg 1981;39:938–40.

26. Leonard MS. The use of lag screws in mandibular fractures. Otolaryngol Clin North Am 1987;20: 479–93.

27. Ellis E, Ghali GE. Lag screw fixation of anterior mandibular fractures. J Oral Maxillofac Surg 1991;49:13–21.

28. Ellis E. Use of lag screws for fractures of the mandibular body. J Oral Maxillofac Surg 1996;54: 1314–6.

29. Ellis E, Moos KF, El-Attar A. Ten years of mandibular fractures. An analysis of 2137 cases. J Oral Surg 1985;59:120–9.

30. Iatrou I, Samaras C, Theologre-Lygidakis N. Miniplate osteosynthesis for fractures of the edentulous mandible: a clinical study. J Craniomaxillofac Surg 1998;26:400–4.

31. Newman I. The role of autogenous primary rib grafts in treating fractures of the atrophic edentulous mandible. Br J Oral Maxillofac Surg 1995;33: 381–7.

32. Zacchariades N, Papavassilou D, Triantafyllou D, et al. Fractures of the facial skeleton in the edentulous patient. J Maxillofac Surg 1984;12:262–6.

33. Marciani Rd, Hill OJ. Treatment of the fractured edentulous mandible. J Oral Surg 1979;37:569–77.

34. Nasser M, Fedorowicz Z, Ebadifar A. Management of the fractured edentulous atrophic mandible. Cochrane Database Syst Rev 2007;1:CD006087.

35. Bruce RA, Strachan DS. Fractures of the edentulous mandible: the Chalmers J. Lyons Academy study. J Oral Surg 1976;34:973–9.

36. Bruce RA, Ellis E. The second Chalmers J. Lyons Academy study of fractures of the edentulous mandible. J Oral Maxillofac Surg 1993;51:904–11.

37. Buchbinder D. Treatment of fractures of the edentulous mandible, 1943 to 1993: a review of the literature. J Oral Maxillofac Surg 1993;51:1174–80.

38. Luhr HG, Reidick T, Merten HA. Results of treatment of fractures of the atrophic edentulous mandible by compression plating. J Oral Maxillofac Surg 1996;54:250–4.

39. Eyrich GK, Gratz KW, Sailer HF. Surgical treatment of fractures of the edentulous mandible. J Oral Maxillofac Surg 1997;55:1081–7.

40. Kunz C, Hammer B, Prein J. Fractures of the edentulous atrophic mandible: management and complications. Mund Kiefer Gesichtschir 2001;5: 227–32 [in German].

41. Madsen M, Haug R, Christensen B, et al. Management of atrophic mandible fractures. Oral Maxillofac Surg Clin North Am 2009;21:175–83.

42. Clayman L, Rossi E. Fixation of atrophic edentulous mandible fractures by bone plating at the inferior border. J Oral Maxillofac Surg 2012;70: 883–9.

43. Mugino H, Takagi S, Oya R, et al. Miniplate osteosynthesis of fractures of the edentulous mandible. Clin Oral Investig 2005;9:266–70.

44. Frost D, Tucker M, White R. Small plate fixation for fixation of mandibular fractures. In: Tucker MR, Terry BC, White RP, et al, editors. Rigid fixation in maxillofacial surgery. Philadelphia: Lippincott; 1991. p. 104.

45. Thaller SR. Fractures of the edentulous mandible: a retrospective review. J Craniofac Surg 1993;4: 91–4.

46. Spiessl B. Internal fixation of the mandible. New York: Springer-Verlag; 1989. p. 223.

47. Schilli W, Stoll P, Bähr W, et al. Mandibular fractures. In: Prein J, editor. Manual of internal fixation in the cranio-facial skeleton: techniques recommended by the AO/ASIF Maxillofacial Group. New York: Springer; 1998. p. 87.

48. Alpert B. Discussion of Eyrich GK, Gratz KW, Sailer HF: surgical treatment of fractures of the edentulous mandible. J Oral Maxillofac Surg 1997;55: 1087–8.

49. Ellis E, Price C. Treatment protocol for fractures of the atrophic mandible. J Oral Maxillofac Surg 2008;66:421–35.

50. Luhr HG, Reidick T, Merten HD. Results of treatment of fractures of the atrophic edentulous mandible by compression plating. A retrospective evaluation of 84 consecutive cases. J Oral Maxillofac Surg 1996;59:250–4.

51. John B, John R, Stalin A, et al. Management of mandibular body fractures in pediatric patients: a case report with review of literature. Contemp Clin Dent 2010;1(4):291–6.

52. Aizenbud D, Hazan-Molina H, Emodi O, et al. The management of mandibular body fractures in young children. Dent Traumatol 2009;25:565–70.

53. Amaratunga N. The relation of age to the immobilization period required for healing of mandibular fractures. J Oral Maxillofac Surg 1987;45: 111–3.

54. Yaremchuk MJ, Fiala TG, Barker F, et al. The effects of rigid fixation on craniofacial growth of rhesus monkeys. Plast Reconstr Surg 1994;93:1–11.

55. Schilli W. Mandibular fractures. In: Prein J, editor. Manual of internal fixation in the cranio-facial skeleton. Berlin: Sringer-Verlag; 1998. p. 92.

56. Bos R. Treatment of pediatric facial fractures: the case for metallic fixation. J Oral Maxillofac Surg 2005;63:382–4.

57. Eppley B. Use of resorbable plates and screws in pediatric facial fractures. J Oral Maxillofac Surg 2005;63:385–91.

58. Turvey T, Proffit W, Phillips C. Biodegradable fixation for craniomaxillofacial surgery: a 10-year experience involving 761 operations and 745 patients. Int J Oral Maxillofac Surg 2011;40:244–9.

59. Laughlin R, Block M, Wilk R, et al. Resorbable plates for the fixation of mandibular fractures: a prospective study. J Oral Maxillofac Surg 2007; 65:89–96.

60. Burke JF. The effective period of preventive antibiotic action in experimental incisions and dermal lesions. Surgery 1961;50:161–8.

61. Mile AA, Miles EM, Burke J. The value and duration of defence reaction of the skin to the primary lodgment of bacteria. Br J Exp Pathol 1957;38:79–96.

62. Uluap K, Condon RE. Antibiotic prophylaxis for scheduled operative procedures. Infect Dis Clin North Am 1992;6:613–25.

63. Condon RE, Wittmann DH. The use of antibiotics in general surgery. Curr Probl Surg 1991;28:801–949.

64. Burdon DW. Principles of antibiotic prophylaxis. World J Surg 1982;6:262–7.

65. Zallen RD, Curry JT. A study of antibiotic usage in compound mandibular fractures. J Oral Surg 1975;33:431–4.

66. Greenberg RN, James RB, Marier RI, et al. Microbiologic and antibiotic aspects of infections in the oral and maxillofacial region. J Oral Surg 1979; 37:873–84.

67. James RB, Fredrickson C, Kent J. Prospective study of mandibular fractures. J Oral Surg 1981; 39:275–81.

68. Chole RA, Yee J. Antibiotic prophylaxis for facial fractures. Arch Otolaryngol Head Neck Surg 1987;113:1055–7.

69. Abubaker A, Rollert M. Postoperative antibiotic prophylaxis in mandibular fractures: a preliminary randomized, double-blind, and placebo-controlled clinical study. J Oral Maxillofac Surg 2001;59:1415–9.

70. Miles B, Potter J, Ellis E. The efficacy of postoperative antibiotic regimens in the open treatment of mandibular fractures: a prospective randomized trial. J Oral Maxillofac Surg 2006;64:576–82.

71. Ellis E, Walker LR. Treatment of mandibular angle fractures using one noncompression miniplate. J Oral Maxillofac Surg 1996;54:864–71.

72. Kellman RM. Repair of mandibular fractures via compression plating and more traditional techniques: a comparison of results. Laryngoscope 1984;94:1560–7.

73. Mathog RH, Toma V, Clayman L, et al. Nonunion of the mandible: an analysis of contributing factors. J Oral Maxillofac Surg 2000;58:746–52.

74. Bochlogyros PN. Non union of fractures of the mandible. J Maxillofac Surg 1985;13:189–93.

75. Haug RH, Schwimmer A. Fibrous union of the mandible: a review of 27 patients. J Oral Maxillofac Surg 1994;52:832–9.

76. Thurmuller P, Dodson TB, Kaban LB. Nerve injuries associated with facial trauma: natural history, management and outcomes of repair. Oral Maxillofac Surg Clin North Am 2001;13:283–94.

77. Itzuka T, Lindquist C. Rigid internal fixation of mandible fractures: an analysis of 270 fractures using the AO/ASIF method. Int J Oral Maxillofac Surg 1992;21:65–9.

78. Itzuka T, Lindquist C. Rigid internal fixation of fractures in the angular region of the mandible: an analysis of fractures contributing to different complications. Plast Reconstr Surg 1993;91:265–71.

79. Halpern L, Kaban L, Dodson T. Perioperative neurosensory changes associated with treatment of mandibular fractures. J Oral Maxillofac Surg 2004;62:576–81.

Management of Fractures of the Zygomaticomaxillary Complex

Rodrigo Otávio Moreira Marinho, DDS, MSc, FDSRCS[a,b,]*,
Belini Freire-Maia, DDS, MSc[c,d,e]

KEYWORDS

- Zygomatic fractures • Zygomaticomaxillary fractures • Orbital fractures • Orbital floor fractures
- Surgery • Fixation • Reduction • Complications

KEY POINTS

- A thorough eye assessment is an imperative part of the examination for all fractures of the zygomaticomaxillary complex (ZMC).
- Computed tomography is the gold-standard imaging modality to aid in the diagnosis of ZMC fracture.
- Accurate 3-dimensional fracture reduction is the most important component of the surgical treatment of ZMC fractures.
- The zygomaticosphenoid suture at the lateral orbital wall seems to be the most reliable site for assessment of adequate reduction in complex fractures.
- Surgical exploration of a fractured orbital floor should only be performed in the presence of a clear clinical and/or radiologic indication.
- Well-designed clinical studies that will ultimately produce evidence-based guidelines for the management of ZMC fractures are needed.

INTRODUCTION

The zygomaticomaxillary complex (ZMC) functions as a major buttress for the face and, because of its prominent convex shape, is frequently involved in facial trauma.[1–8] The most common etiologic factors involved in these injuries are interpersonal violence, road traffic accidents, falls, and sports injuries.[1,4,6,8–10]

The ZMC occupies a key position in the anterolateral aspect of the face, contributing to set the midface width, and to define the shape and contour of the inferior and lateral orbital borders as well as the cheek prominence. It is a tetrapod structure relating to (**Fig. 1**):

- Maxilla at the zygomaticomaxillary buttress (ZMB) and at the inferior orbital rim (IOR)

The authors have no financial associations that might create a conflict of interest with information presented in this article.

a Oral and Maxillofacial Surgery, Hospital Lifecenter, Avenida Contorno, 4747, sala 1311, Funcionários, Belo Horizonte, Minas Gerais 30110-921, Brazil; b Oral and Maxillofacial Surgery, Hospital HGIP/IPSEMG, Belo Horizonte, Minas Gerais, Brazil; c Oral Surgery, School of Dentistry, Pontifícia Universidade Católica de Minas Gerais, Belo Horizonte, Minas Gerais, Brazil; d Oral and Maxillofacial Surgery, Hospital da Baleia, Belo Horizonte, Minas Gerais, Brazil; e Oral and Maxillofacial Surgery, Hospital Lifecenter, Avenida Contorno, 4747, sala 1011, Funcionários, Belo Horizonte, Minas Gerais 30110-921, Brazil
* Corresponding author. Oral and Maxillofacial Surgery, Hospital Lifecenter, Avenida Contorno, 4747, sala 1311, Funcionários, Belo Horizonte, Minas Gerais, Brazil.
E-mail address: rodmarinho@yahoo.com

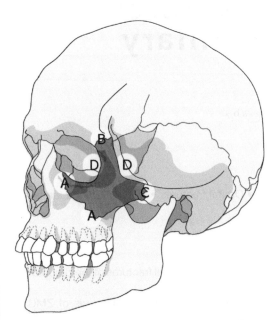

Fig. 1. Zygomatic bone articulations: A, maxilla; B, frontal bone; C, temporal bone; D, sphenoid bone.

- Frontal bone at the frontozygomatic suture (FZS)
- Temporal bone forming the zygomatic arch (ZA)
- Sphenoid bone at the zygomaticosphenoid suture (ZSS)

This tetrapod configuration lends itself to complex injuries, as fractures here rarely occur in isolation.[11] Fractures often, but not always, occur across the buttress-related sutures where the zygomatic bone meets the maxilla, frontal, temporal, and sphenoid bones. Failure of recognition and treatment of these injuries may result in significant cosmetic and functional morbidity.

CLASSIFICATION

Several anatomic, clinical, and radiologic classification systems for ZMC fractures have been proposed.[3,12–14] The classification presented by Zingg and colleagues[3] is used here, mainly because of its simplicity of description and its suitability for the planning of treatment of these injuries (**Fig. 2**):

Type A: Incomplete zygomatic fracture. Isolated fractures involving only one zygomatic pillar:
Type A1: Isolated ZA fracture (see **Fig. 2**A)
Type A2: Lateral orbital wall fracture (see **Fig. 2**B)
Type A3: Infraorbital rim fracture (see **Fig. 2**C)

Type B: Complete monofragment zygomatic fracture (tetrapod fracture). All 4 pillars of the zygomatic bone are fractured (see **Fig. 2**D).
Type C: Multifragment zygomatic fracture. Same as type B, but with fragmentation, including the body of the zygoma (see **Fig. 2**E).

GENERAL MANAGEMENT

There is an enormous amount of published material involving all aspects of the management of ZMC fractures, but very few systematic reviews compiling the research evidence on the subject have been produced to date.[15–18] These reviews looked at specific aspects of the management of facial fractures, including the use of prophylactic antibiotics,[15] the use of resorbable in comparison with titanium plates,[16] the diagnostic role of ultrasonography,[17] and ocular injury, visual impairment, and blindness associated with facial fractures.[18] With the exception of the review on the diagnostic role of ultrasonography,[17] a general conclusion of these publications is that there was very limited high-quality data addressing the studied issues.

There is a clear need for better designed prospective clinical studies for the production of evidence-based guidelines for the management of ZMC fractures, and in the meantime the decisions on the management of these injuries have to be made cautiously.[8]

DIAGNOSIS

The appropriate diagnosis of ZMC fractures should be based on a careful history of the trauma and medical condition of the patient, methodical and thorough physical examination, and the use of suitable special investigations, especially imaging of the fracture and associated structures.

History

An accurate history of the injury itself is extremely important when dealing with trauma cases. In cases of loss of consciousness, confusion, or whenever the patient is unable to narrate the accident, information regarding the injury mechanism and the subsequent management of the patient must be obtained from third parties such as a rescue team, eye-witnesses, or medical personnel that may have been involved in the early care of the victim. The past and present medical history must also be obtained, as it may interfere in the immediate and future management of the patient.

Physical Examination

A thorough examination of any trauma patient must be carried out by the consulting surgeon,

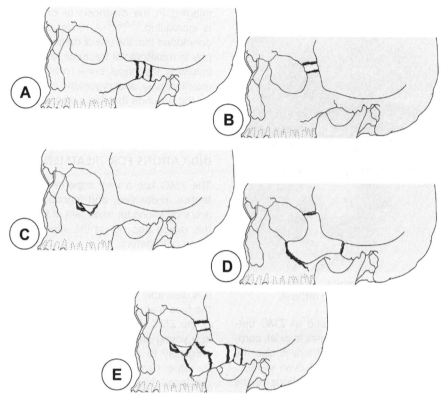

Fig. 2. Classification of ZMC fractures. (*A*) Type A1: isolated zygomatic arch fracture. (*B*) Type A2: lateral orbital wall fracture. (*C*) Type A3: infraorbital rim fracture. (*D*) Type B: complete monofragment zygomatic fracture. (*E*) Type C: multifragment zygomatic fracture. (*Modified from* Zingg M, Laedrach K, Chen J, et al. Classification and treatment of zygomatic fractures: a review of 1025 cases. J Oral Maxillofac Surg 1992;50(8):779; with permission.)

including a general physical examination to rule out the presence of any important associated injury that may need more urgent attention. The presence of pain, in addition to gross facial swelling and hematoma associated with ZMC fractures, makes the initial examination of the patient difficult and uncomfortable, and may also obscure important signs of the injury (**Fig. 3**).

Nevertheless, this initial examination is essential for the detection of early signs of important neurologic and ophthalmologic complications that require immediate treatment to avert serious consequences. The ZMC forms the lateral wall, inferior rim, and the floor of the orbit, and, consequently, most fractures involving this complex can be considered true orbital fractures. Therefore, a careful ocular examination including visual-acuity assessment and pupillary response carried out by the examining surgeon and/or a formal consultation with an ophthalmologist is a prudent routine when dealing with these injuries.[2,3,7,9,11,18–21] In fact, a systematic review of the literature on ocular injury, visual impairment, and blindness associated with facial fractures

identified several studies illustrating that ocular injuries can complicate midface fractures.[18]

The presenting signs and symptoms of a ZMC injury will vary according to the pattern and the severity of the fracture. The most common and most important signs and symptoms associated with ZMC fractures are listed in **Box 1**.

A reexamination of the facial injury must be carried out after the initial swelling, hematoma and other acute signs and symptoms of the trauma have subsided, so that the true severity of the fracture can be best evaluated, allowing a more accurate and definitive diagnosis of the injury (**Figs. 4** and **5**).

Imaging

Although plain radiographs, particularly the occipitomental (Water) view, may confirm the presence of a ZMC fracture, they are usually insufficient for appropriate diagnosis of the full extent of the injury.[20] Computed tomography (CT) is considered the gold-standard radiologic investigation for accurate diagnosis and treatment planning of ZMC fractures.[4,11,13,19–28] CT scans allow detailed

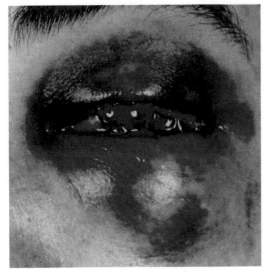

Fig. 3. Immediate circumorbital ecchymosis and edema, making initial examination difficult.

examination of the orbit walls and all ZMC buttresses and buttress-related sutures in axial, coronal, and sagittal views (**Fig. 6**). There is also the possibility of producing digital and even stereolithographic 3-dimensional reconstructions of the scan for easier spatial visualization of the sustained injury (**Fig. 7**). The use of ultrasonographic

Box 1
Signs and symptoms of ZMC fractures
Swelling or flattening of the cheek
Circumorbital ecchymosis
Subconjunctival hemorrhage and edema
Nose bleeding
Ecchymosis over zygomatic buttress intra-orally
Subcutaneous emphysema within the orbit or overlying soft tissues of the cheek
Step deformities and tenderness in the upper lateral orbital rim, IOR, and upper buccal sulcus
Restricted eye movements
Altered globe level
Lowering of the pupil level
Diplopia
Reduced visual acuity
Enophthalmos
Trismus or interference with normal range of mandibular movements
Pain
Altered sensation in distribution of infraorbital nerve

imaging in the diagnosis of craniofacial trauma is increasing.[17,26,29] A recent systematic review concluded that the use of diagnostic ultrasonography in maxillofacial fractures, especially fractures involving the nasal bone, orbital walls, anterior maxillary wall, and zygomatic complex, is justified on the grounds that the sensitivity and specificity of ultrasonography were considered generally comparable with those of CT.[17]

INDICATIONS FOR TREATMENT

The ZMC has a very important role in the aesthetics, protection, and function of the midface, and indications for treatment of fractures involving this region depend on the effect of the injury on these parameters.

Aesthetics

It is desirable to reestablish the typical contour of the face that may have been altered by a fracture of the ZMC. Even a minimally displaced fracture in a young and healthy patient should be treated surgically to restore perfect facial contours. On the other hand, sometimes even a more severely displaced fracture of the ZMC may be treated more conservatively in an elderly or medically compromised patient, as in these cases the effects of the actual treatment may cause more harm than good.

Protection

Because of its key anatomic location in the face, the ZMC has a vital absorbent function in the safeguard of more important structures such as the brain and the contents of the orbits. Surgical treatment is indicated in cases where this protective role is compromised by a fracture of the ZMC.

Functional Impairment

ZMC fractures may interfere with important ocular function and infraorbital nerve function as well as with normal mouth opening.

Normal ocular function
Normal ocular function may be interfered with by the presence of enophthalmos, diplopia, displacement of orbital contents and direct injury, entrapment or scarring of the extrinsic ocular musculature. Persistent diplopia and enophthalmos are clear indications for treatment. Rarely, blindness may occur in a dramatic case of retrobulbar hemorrhage and damage to the optical nerve. If retrobulbar hemorrhage is suspected, urgent medical (high-dose steroids, diuretics) and/or surgical (decompression)

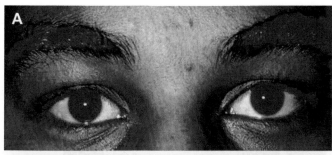

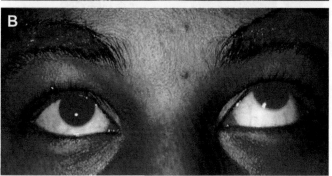

Fig. 4. Persistent restricted upward gaze of the right eye and diplopia after resolution of acute symptoms. (A) Normal gaze. (B) Upward gaze.

treatment is vital for the prevention of permanent visual impairment.

Infraorbital nerve

Most fractures of the ZMC will cause some damage to the infraorbital nerve, which may lead to temporary or permanent altered sensation on the distribution of this nerve. As far as nerve function is concerned, injuries caused by direct blunt trauma in an undisplaced fracture have a better prognosis and should be treated conservatively. Injuries caused by sharp trauma or entrapment by bony fragments have a more reserved prognosis and should be treated surgically, especially in the presence of a displaced fracture (**Fig. 8**). However, the surgical treatment itself carries the risk of causing further injury to the nerve.[8,30]

Restriction of the mandibular movements

Surgery is indicated when there is restricted mouth opening caused by the inward displacement of a fractured ZA and prevention of free movement of the coronoid process of the mandible (see **Fig. 6**C).

INITIAL TREATMENT

As part of the initial general management of patients sustaining ZMC fractures, the following aspects should be considered:

- Primary survey. The definitive treatment of a facial fracture is hardly ever an urgent procedure. As in any other traumatic injury, initial management of a patient with a midfacial injury includes establishment of airway patency with control of the cervical spine, appropriate ventilation, adequate circulation, and control of bleeding, including management of soft-tissue lacerations.
- Pain control. Although facial swelling and bruising can be dramatic, there is surprisingly little pain associated with ZMC fractures. Nonsteroidal anti-inflammatory drugs are the first choice for pain control. More powerful analgesic drugs that depress the level of consciousness should be avoided, as they may increase the risks of more severe complications.

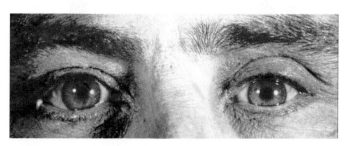

Fig. 5. Persistent enophthalmos of the left orbit after resolution of acute symptoms.

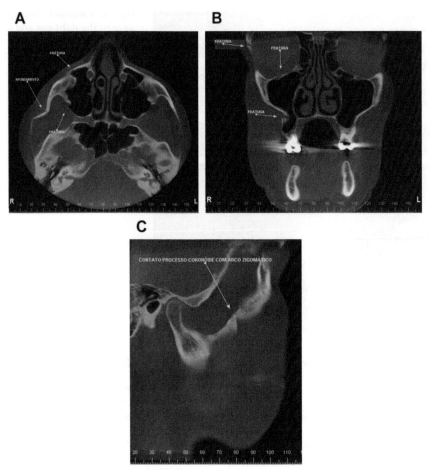

Fig. 6. CT scans of ZMC fractures. (*A*) Axial view of a type C fracture (*arrows*). (*B*) Coronal view of a type C fracture (*arrows*). (*C*) Sagittal view of a type A1 fracture with contact between the zygomatic arch and the coronoid process of the mandible (*arrow*).

- Infection control. Fractures of the ZMC usually involve the maxillary sinus, but the use of prophylactic antibiotics in these injuries is still controversial and unresolved.[31,32] In a systematic review published in 2006,[15] including 4 studies on prophylactic antibiotics in the surgical treatment of maxillofacial fractures, there was only 1 randomized study that incorporated ZMC fractures, which reported no infections in the treatment of 18 ZMC fractures irrespective of the use of antibiotics.[33]

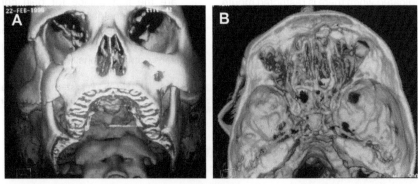

Fig. 7. 3-Dimensional reconstruction ZMC fractures. (*A*) Comminuted ZMC fracture in a type C fracture. (*B*) Isolated arch fracture in a type A1 fracture.

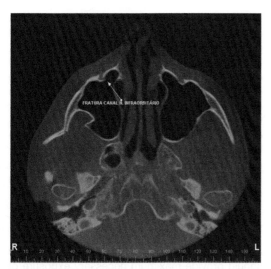

Fig. 8. Axial CT scan showing fracture through the infraorbital canal (*arrow*).

PRINCIPLES OF TREATMENT OF ZMC FRACTURES

A variety of methods, ranging from conservative treatment to surgical treatment by closed reduction of the fracture or open reduction with fixation, can be successfully used to treat ZMC fractures.[2–7,10,11,21,23–27,34–50]

Conservative Treatment

Conservative treatment is indicated if there is minimal or no displacement of the fractured bones, or in those cases involving more elderly or medically compromised patients for whom invasive surgical procedures and a general anesthetic may be contraindicated. Also, some patients may prefer to bear some permanent minor facial asymmetry rather than having to undergo surgery.[21]

Surgical Treatment

Surgical treatment is warranted in the presence of displacement, instability, or comminution of the bony fragments. The main objectives of the treatment are accurate anatomic reduction of the displaced bones and, where indicated, stable fixation of the reduced fractures to prevent postoperative aesthetic, sensory, or ocular complications.[3,11,20,26] Therefore, surgical treatment of ZMC fractures is either by fracture reduction without fixation or by open reduction and internal fixation (ORIF).

Fracture reduction without fixation
A precise reduction of the fractured ZMC is the first and most crucial step in the surgical treatment of these injuries. Some fractures may prove very stable after simple open or even closed reduction, and may not require any form of fixation. These injuries should be treated within the first 2 weeks of the trauma to allow better interdigitation of the fracture ends, thus improving stability. Often a type A1 fracture and, occasionally, a mildly displaced type B fracture can be treated by reduction only. The main advantage of this type of treatment is its simplicity: only a minimal surgical access is needed; general anesthesia may not be required; most patients can be treated in an outpatient setting; and fewer surgical complications are expected.

Open reduction and internal fixation
ORIF of a fractured ZMC is indicated when there is comminution or fracture instability. The main goal is to establish adequate 3-dimensional reduction and stable fixation.

Proper and accurate reduction of the fractured ZMC is of paramount importance for successful treatment, and as many sutures as necessary should be visualized to ensure anatomic reduction. A greater amount of fixation will not improve the final result in a fracture that has been poorly reduced in the first place. Ellis and Kittidumkerng[4] reported no perceptible change in ZMC position following adequate fixation with plates and screws in a series of ZMC fractures, and suggested that previous cases of reported asymmetry attributed to postoperative instability may have been primarily caused by unsatisfactory reduction.

In more challenging and displaced injuries, the application of fixation at several locations necessitates adequate exposure of the areas, which in turn allows direct visual assessment of the ZMC fracture at several points, thus improving accuracy of reduction.[4,51] In this respect, direct inspection of fracture reduction of the ZSS at the lateral orbital wall seems to be the most reliable assessment for adequate reduction.[3,11,20,23,50] Undetected axial rotation of the zygoma at the greater wing of the sphenoid during treatment of ZMC fractures has been associated with unsatisfactory outcomes.[3] Other important sites for checking adequacy of reduction include the ZMB and the IOR, whereas the FZS is considered as an unreliable site for visual judgment of reduction of the fracture.[3,6,11,23] Surgical reduction of a fractured ZA is usually achieved remotely without exposure of the fracture, and the arch is only directly surgically accessed if there is an indication for internal fixation of the fractured area.

Several reports in the literature have described the outcomes of ZMC fractures treated by ORIF with plates and screws.[2–7,10,26,27,34–42,44,46,48–50] Although these studies are not readily comparable, as they used different methodological designs, diverse locations and number of points of ORIF, and different methods for assessment of the outcome of their fixation models, the general conclusion is that regardless of the model of fixation used in the individual studies, the overall results were clinically satisfactory. Therefore, when fixation of the reduced ZMC fracture is indicated, the type, number, and location of the fixation will be determined by the fracture pattern and degree of displacement as well as by the surgeon's preference, as many combinations of fixation methods can provide enough resistance to displacement.[4,26,52] These techniques may range from 1-point to 3- or 4-point fixation using bone plates, but clearly not every articulation and/or buttress needs to be used.

As far as location is concerned, the FZS and ZMB are the first choices for fixation of ZMC fractures because they represent the main points of stability in reconstructing the vertical and horizontal buttresses of the midface. The IOR and/or the ZA are only used as fixation points in more unstable cases where additional fixation is needed. However, in a recently published randomized, prospective clinical trial comparing surgical treatment of zygomatic bone fractures using 2-point fixation versus 3-point fixation, the latter showed better inherent stability over the former for unstable and laterally displaced ZMC fractures.[50]

In cases of fracture comminution or where there is more marked displacement of the ZMC, one may decide preoperatively the location and amount of fixation required to stabilize the fracture. In this respect, a preoperative CT scan can help tremendously in the planning of the operative intervention (see **Figs. 6–8**). However, in many instances this decision has to be made intraoperatively by checking the stability of the fracture and adding further points of fixation if necessary. Several methods of testing intraoperative stability of reduction and consequent need for fracture fixation have been advocated, including digital pressure,[2,3] direct inspection and indirect palpation of keys areas,[7] and the use of special devices such as the Carroll-Girard screw.[4,11,20,21] More recently, intraoperative CT monitoring,[53–56] intraoperative ultrasonography,[26] and even navigation-guided reduction[57] have been used to assess and improve surgical reduction of facial fractures.

Metal miniplates and screws are the gold standard for fixation of facial fractures, as they provide more stable fixation of the reduced fractures with low complication rates.[2–7,11,20,21,23,35,37,38,40–43,47,50] Plates of different shapes, lengths, and thickness can be used depending on the location of the fixation, the pattern of the fracture, and the preference of the surgeon. The use of bioresorbable plates and screws alone[26,45,58] or in combination with metal plates[59] to treat ZMC fractures has been suggested. However, a systematic review conducted in 2009 concluded that there is insufficient evidence for the effectiveness of resorbable fixation systems in comparison with conventional titanium systems for facial fractures.[16] In addition, the results of a randomized trial published recently indicated that the benefits of using biodegradable systems (fewer plate-removal operations) should be confirmed during a follow-up of minimally 5 years, as part of a longer-running ongoing follow-up study.[58]

SURGICAL ACCESS

An ideal surgical access to treat ZMC fractures should provide maximum necessary exposure of the fracture segments, minimize potential for injury to facial structures, and enable good cosmetic results.[47] Some surgical accesses only permit closed reduction of the fractures, whereas other approaches allow ORIF of the fractures using the same surgical entry.

Accesses for Closed Reduction

For those cases whereby reduction without any form of internal fixation is anticipated as the sole treatment of a ZMC fracture, surgical approaches that are simple and/or allow good "closed" reduction of the fracture without direct exposure of the bony fragments can be used effectively. Good examples are the Gillies temporal and the percutaneous cheek approaches.

Gillies temporal access
With this surgical approach the body and arch of the zygomatic bone can be elevated and reduced via a temporal incision (**Fig. 9**). A 2.0-cm incision is made in the skin of the temporal region, followed by exposure and incision of the temporalis fascia. An instrument such as the Rowe or Bristow zygomatic elevator can then be inserted under the incised temporalis fascia and passed down on to the temporalis muscle beneath the zygomatic bone, allowing reduction of the fractured bone.[60] This approach is suitable for reduction of type A1 and type B fractures.

Percutaneous cheek access
This speedy surgical approach may be indicated as the sole method of treatment in cases of mildly displaced type A1 and type B fractures. After a minimal stab incision in the cheek skin, a bone hook is inserted percutaneously just below the zygomatic bone prominence or the ZA, to elevate and reduce the fracture (**Fig. 10**).[2,3,7,43]

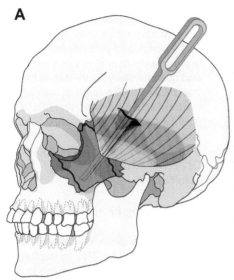

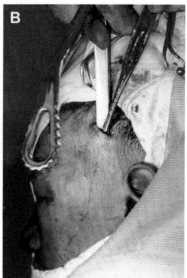

Fig. 9. Gillies access. (*A*) Schematic. (*B*) Intraoperative view.

Alternatively, a Carroll-Girard screw can be inserted percutaneously directly into the bone, and used for traction and reduction of the fracture (**Fig. 11**).[4,20] Care must be taken to avoid damaging the facial nerve when using this technique.

Accesses for Open Reduction and Internal Fixation

In those injuries where fixation of the fractured bone is necessary, a more direct, open surgical access to the fractured site, which allows the installation of the fixation hardware, is indicated. The ZMB, FZS, IOR, and ZA are the surgical sites used for ORIF of the ZMC fractures. Several surgical approaches have been described for accessing these sites (**Box 2**).

Zygomaticomaxillary buttress

The ZMB is the first choice for many authors as a surgical access for treating a fractured ZMC.[4,6,11,20,26,38,41,45] Placement of fixation devices at the ZMB buttress has increased with the advent of bone-plate fixation, even in the presence of comminution in this area.[4] In isolated ZMC fractures, stabilization at the ZMB effectively prevents medial rotation of the ZMC into the maxillary sinus, provided the maxilla itself is stable.[4,59] A large, strong, L-shaped plate secured with 2.0-mm diameter screws is ideal for this location,

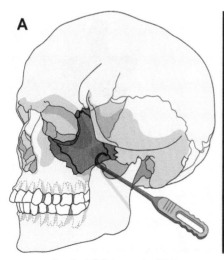

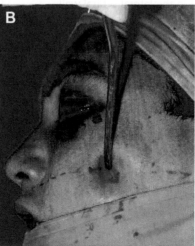

Fig. 10. Percutaneous hook. (*A*) Schematic. (*B*) Intraoperative view.

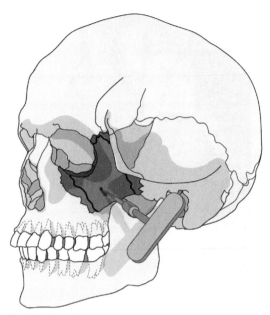

Fig. 11. Percutaneous screw.

as the tougher plate directly antagonizes the force of the masseter muscle.[23]

The area is readily accessible intraorally, where manipulation of the fracture is possible without the production of a visible scar.

Intraoral access This very simple and rapid approach exposes the maxilla, the ZMB, and the infraorbital rim. An intraoral buccal incision is placed just above the mucogingival junction in the maxillary molar area and carried through the oral mucosa and periosteum, allowing subperiosteal dissection and exposure of the zygomatic and nasomaxillary buttresses to the level of the infraorbital rim. One must be careful to protect the infraorbital nerve when using this approach. An instrument such as a large blunt elevator can be inserted upward under the zygomatic bone and arch, allowing its reduction, and a bone plate can be applied to the ZMB if the fracture requires fixation (**Fig. 12**).

Frontozygomatic and zygomaticosphenoid sutures

The FZS has been traditionally used as a main point of fixation for ZMC in fractures of types A2, B, and C.[2,3,5,7,23,37,38,60] Access to this area allows manipulation and reposition of the fractured ZMC by inserting an elevator in the infratemporal fossa, and permits a direct inspection to the very important ZSS area in the medial aspect of the lateral orbital wall, where accuracy of ZMC reduction can be best assessed.

The FZS is a suitable place for a strong and reliable fixation, as it is seldom comminuted in a fracture of the ZMC. The FZS is subject to a high degree of stress and stretch,[59] and fixation using one 2.0-mm miniplate with four 2.0-mm diameter

---

Box 2
Summary of surgical accesses for open reduction and fixation of ZMC fractures

ZMB

  Intraoral

FZS and ZSS in the lateral orbital wall

  Lateral eyebrow

  Lateral upper eyelid

  Extended transconjunctival with lateral canthotomy

  Coronal

IOR and orbital floor

  Subciliary (lower blepharoplasty)

  Subtarsal (mid-lid)

  Infraorbital

  Transconjunctival

  Coronal

ZA

  Coronal

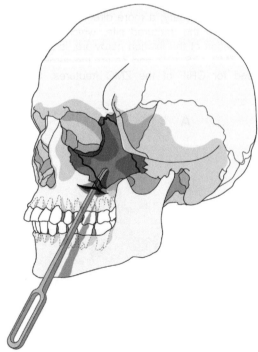

Fig. 12. Intraoral access.

screws have been advocated.[7] However, plates of lower profile that minimize the inconveniency of plate palpability have also been used successfully in this area.[4,14,20,21,23]

The FZS, ZSS, and lateral orbital wall can be accessed by eyebrow or upper-eyelid skin incisions (A, B in **Fig. 13**).

Lateral eyebrow access The so-called eyebrow incision is a relatively simple and quick operation that allows direct access to FZS and lateral orbital wall. The incision may be placed just above, just below, or through the eyebrow (A in **Fig. 13**). Incising through the eyebrow avoids the risk of a skin scar, but may lead to conspicuous hair loss in the brow.[20] The skin can be incised separately, with further dissection of the subcutaneous tissues, and a new periosteal incision performed to reach the bone. Alternatively the skin incision can be made directly to the depth of the periosteum in a full-thickness cut.

Upper eyelid access This approach, also called lateral upper-lid blepharoplasty, is the best choice to access the FZS because it provides good exposure to the whole lateral aspect of the orbit area and only leaves an inconspicuous scar.[20,61,62] A small incision is performed using a natural skin crease in the outer third of the upper eyelid well above the lid margin and the lateral canthus (B in **Fig. 13**). The incision is carried out through skin and orbicularis oculi muscle, followed by dissection deep to the muscle toward the periosteum, which is then incised just above the lateral aspect of the upper orbital rim with good exposure of the lateral orbital wall.

Inferior orbital rim

Although exposure of the IOR may be important to directly assess the accuracy of fracture reduction, the rim itself is not a reliable point for fixation of an unstable ZMC fracture.[4,23] The main indications for fixation of a fractured IOR are the maintenance of the reduced small fragments and restoration of the anatomy and contour of the IOR, as opposed to stabilization of the fractured ZMC. Because of the problem of hardware palpability and the reduced need for strong fixation at the IOR, low-profile plates and screws,[4,14,20,21,23] ligature wires,[3,23] and even absorbable sutures[3] may be used to stabilize a fractured IOR.

Access to the IOR and to the orbital floor can be gained transcutaneously via an infraorbital or a lower-eyelid incision, or transmucosally via a transconjunctival approach.

Infraorbital access Although very simple, rapid, and popular in the past, the approach using a skin incision placed below the IOR has been largely abandoned owing to the cosmetically objectionable scar and persistent lower-eyelid edema it may produce (E in **Fig. 13**). A commonly existing laceration located in this area can also be used as surgical access to the IOR and orbital floor (**Fig. 14**).

Lower eyelid skin access Lower-lid incisions include the subciliary (lower blepharoplasty), and the subtarsal (mid-lid) incisions.[61,63,64] The subciliary incision is placed 2 mm below the lower eyelash line (C in **Fig. 13**). The subtarsal incision is placed in a natural skin crease in the mid-lid region, below the tarsal plate (D in **Fig. 13**). The initial incision in both approaches is made through skin only, keeping the orbicularis oculi muscle intact. There is then the choice to either incise the muscle at the same level as the skin incision, or to carry out further subcutaneous dissection and divide the muscle 3 to 5 mm below the skin in a step incision. The former preserves a better blood supply to the thin skin flap, and the latter facilitates wound closure. This action

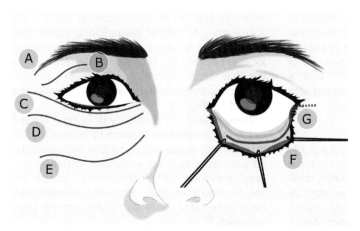

Fig. 13. Periorbital incisions. A, eyebrow; B, upper lateral eyelid; C, subciliary; D, subtarsal; E, infraorbital; F, transconjunctival; G, lateral canthotomy extension.

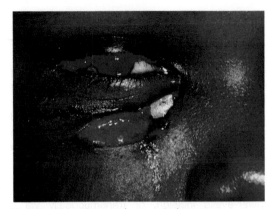

Fig. 14. Laceration used as surgical access.

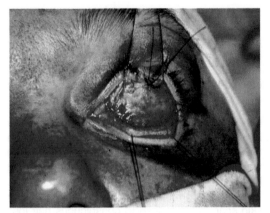

Fig. 15. Transconjunctival approach, intraoperative view.

is followed by dissection between the muscle and the orbital septum and incision of the periosteum to expose the IOR and orbital floor. Disadvantages of lid-skin incisions include an increased risk of postoperative lower-eyelid ectropion and scleral show,[2–4,6,20,64–67] and hypertrophic scarring.[64]

Transconjunctival access This access is a popular choice for the exposure of the IOR and orbital floor (F in **Fig. 13**).[2–4,11,61,62,66,68] It is a simple and rapid approach with the added advantage of producing a minimal scar that is hidden in the conjunctiva. The choice of a retroseptal[61,65] or preseptal[66,68,69] dissection exists. The former is a more direct approach but the latter avoids exposure of orbital fat. A lateral canthotomy (G in **Fig. 13**) may be added to enhance exposure of the IOR and orbital floor,[61,62,65,66] and even to gain access to the FZS.[20,21,68] When using the transconjunctival approach it is advisable to place a corneal shield for globe protection. The lower eyelid is then everted by traction sutures and a small incision is placed directly in the palpebral conjunctiva, 2 to 3 mm below the tarsal plate in the middle part of the lower eyelid.[61,69] The dissection continues inferiorly, toward the infraorbital rim, either in front of or behind the orbital septum (**Fig. 15**). Finally the infraorbital rim is palpated, and, with protection to the globe in place, the periosteum is incised and the subperiosteal dissection carried out to expose the rim and the orbital floor. A diminished risk of causing lower-lid ectropion[2,3,62,64–66,68] and a higher rate of entropion[64] has been reported with transconjunctival access.

Zygomatic arch
Occasionally the ZA needs to be directly surgically exposed for reduction and fixation of an unstable fracture located in the arch. Strong 2.0-mm mini-plates and screws can be used in the arch, as they are easily concealed in the region and provide further stability to this structure.[23] Alternatively, smaller plates and screws may also be used for fixation of ZA fractures, with good results.[4,14] Direct transcutaneous access to the arch is best avoided because of the risk of injury to the facial nerve, and those injuries that require fixation of the arch fragments are best approached via a coronal incision.

Coronal access This more extensive surgical approach exposes the upper and middle third of the face. The coronal approach allows excellent access to the lateral part of the ZMC, the ZA, and even the IOR and orbital floor when preauricular extensions and intraorbital dissections are also used.[61] Using this approach the long skin incision is hidden in the hairline and the facial nerve is protected. The initial incision is made through skin and subcutaneous tissue, down to the loose layer of areolar tissue from one temporal line to the other with preauricular extensions, to expose the ZA.[61] The dissection is continued in this plane until 3 cm above the superior orbital rims, where the periosteum is incised and the bone exposed. In the preauricular and temporal region the dissection is continued down to the temporalis fascia, where its superior layer is incised at about 1 cm above the ZA. Further dissection is carried out inferiorly in the lateral aspect of the fat tissue located between the two layers of the fascia, until the ZA is reached, where its periosteum is incised. The arch is then fully exposed via a subperiosteal dissection (**Fig. 16**).

There is also the possibility of using a smaller unilateral hemicoronal incision to access the ZA in unilateral fractures. A clinical trial involving 20 patients comparing a modified lateral orbitotomy approach with hemicoronal access for the treatment of ZMC fractures demonstrated more acceptable aesthetic results with the latter approach.[47]

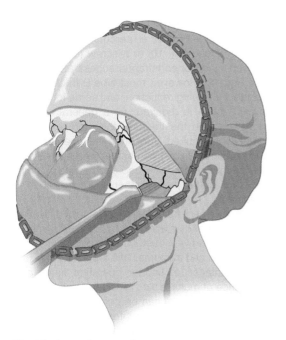

Fig. 16. Coronal approach.

TREATMENT OPTIONS FOR DIFFERENT TYPES OF ZMC FRACTURES

Undisplaced or even minimally displaced ZMC fractures may be treated conservatively without any surgical input. Fractures that are displaced, unstable, or comminuted will require some form of surgical treatment. The rationale for the surgical treatment of individual types of ZMC fractures not involving an orbital floor component is presented here.

Type A1 Fracture

The ZA arch may be fractured in isolation in a type A1 fracture (see **Figs. 2**A and **7**B; **Fig. 17**). Most of these injuries are fairly stable after closed reduction, as the V-shaped fracture tends to snap into place when mobilized, and is then stabilized by the interdigitation of the bone ends and by the natural splintage provided by adjacent muscles and fasciae.[3] Effective ways of reducing these types of injury include a closed reduction using a transcutaneous towel clip[3,14] or bone hook (see **Fig. 10**); or a more "surgical" approach that permits better control of the fracture, such as the Gillies temporal (see **Fig. 9**) or intraoral maxillary vestibular accesses (see **Fig. 12**).

In cases of instability, the reduced fracture can be immobilized with the aid of a splint secured with percutaneous sutures that embrace the arch (**Fig. 18**).[36]

Rarely a more complex and unstable type A1 fracture will require direct fixation of the arch fragments, and are best approached via a coronal

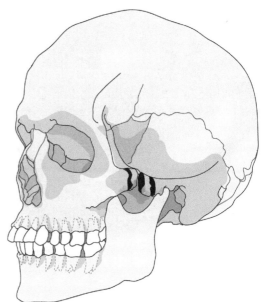

Fig. 17. Isolated arch fracture.

incision to avoid damage to branches of the facial nerve. Endoscopic techniques have been used in the surgical management of ZA fractures,[24] minimizing the dissection of the overlying soft tissues.

Type A2 Fracture

These fractures are of uncommon occurrence and are best treated by direct access to the fractured FZS for accurate reduction and internal fixation. The area may be surgically exposed via a lateral brow access or, ideally, by lateral upper-lid blepharoplasty incision, to minimize cosmetic inconvenience. Type A2 fractures can be safely fixed with plates of lower profile, as these isolated injuries are fairly stable following fixation.

Type A3 Fracture

Displaced type A3 fractures are mostly associated with orbital floor fractures,[3] and are best treated by open reduction and direct stabilization of the

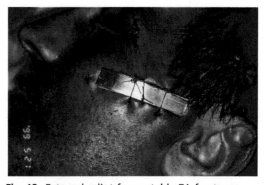

Fig. 18. External splint for unstable ZA fracture.

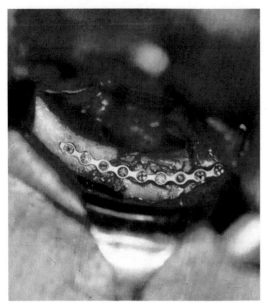

Fig. 19. Low-profile plate for alignment of IOR fracture.

reduced bony fragments to restore the contour of the IOR, and, if indicated, exploration of the orbital floor. Surgical access can be gained via a lower-lid incision, or preferably via a transconjunctival incision, to minimize the risk of ectropion. As there is diminished tendency for instability in these injuries, low-profile plates and screws can be used to stabilize the fractured IOR (**Fig. 19**).

Type B Fracture

Some of the mildly displaced type B fractures can be successfully treated by fracture reduction only, especially in the absence of extensive disruption of the IOR and orbital floor.[2,3] The reduction can be achieved by "closed" methods using the Gillies approach (see **Fig. 9**), or percutaneous insertion of a hook (see **Fig. 10**) or a screw (see **Fig. 11**), or even by an open intraoral access at the ZMB (see **Fig. 12**). However, most type B fractures are unstable following reduction, and some form of internal fixation is required. As a general rule the more unstable the fracture, the more extensive the fixation required. Very often the type, location, and amount of fixation is decided intraoperatively, and a sequential surgical approach based on post-reduction stability and further need of fixation is indicated.

In many type B fractures, a single point of fixation using plates and screws may be enough to ensure stability and prevent postoperative displacement in noncomminuted fractures. This 1-point fixation has the advantages of shorter operating times and avoidance of multiple skin incisions.

One-point fixation can be done by ORIF at the ZMB (**Fig. 20**A); using an intraoral access, or by ORIF at the FZS (see **Fig. 20**B) using brow or lateral upper-eyelid incisions. Alternatively, fracture reduction can be achieved remotely with a percutaneous hook or a Gillies temporal approach, and the fixation placed at the FZS via a separate incision.

In some more unstable type B fractures, fixation at both sites (FZS and ZMB) is necessary to ensure sufficient stability and to warrant accurate vertical positioning and anterior-posterior projection of the ZMC (**Fig. 21**). The IOR can be used as a second point of fixation in selected cases,[5,11,20] but fixation here is not as reliable as in the FZS or ZMB.

If the fracture still proves unstable following fixation at the ZMB and FZS, a greater degree of stabilization is indicated, and a third point of fixation can be placed at the IOR (**Fig. 22**) using a lower-lid skin incision or transconjunctival incision.

A

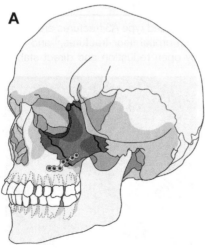

B

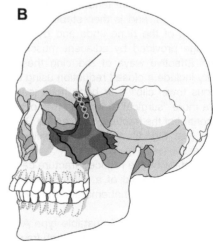

Fig. 20. One-point fixation. (*A*) ZMB. (*B*) FZS.

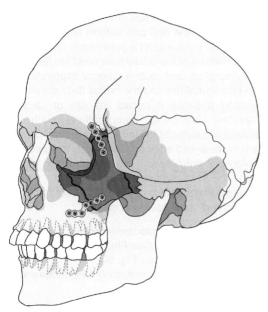

Fig. 21. Two-point fixation with ZMB and FZS.

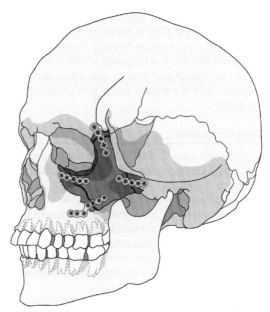

Fig. 23. Four-point fixation.

In some even more complex injuries where additional reduction and fixation of the fracture is required, the ZA can be approached via a coronal incision, with a fourth point of fixation created to ensure adequate stability of the reduced fracture **(Fig. 23)**.[4,5,14,23]

However, when the use of a coronal flap is anticipated for exposure of the ZA, the same approach can be used to approach the FZS and ZSS at the lateral wall of the orbit and even to access the IOR,[61] eliminating unnecessary skin incisions **(Fig. 24)**.

The order of placement of the different points of fixation used for these complex type B fractures is significant, as it may affect the final alignment of the fractured ZMC.[2,3,11,20] A suggested guideline for this order is as follows. After fracture mobilization and reduction, a small plate or a temporary wire ligature is placed at the FZS to set the vertical position of the fracture fragment while still allowing some rotational movement and further reduction if necessary.[20] The IOR is next approached, where, after appropriate reduction of the bony fragments, ligature wire or a low-profile plate is used for fixation while still checking for accurate reduction at all exposed sites, including the ZSS. Finally, a stronger plate is applied to the ZMB while constantly verifying fracture reduction at all exposed

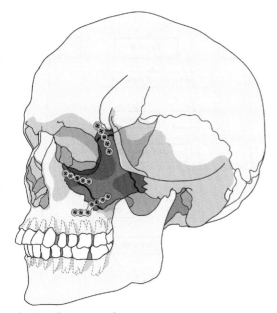

Fig. 22. Three-point fixation.

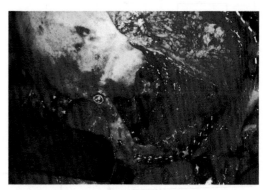

Fig. 24. Open reduction and internal fixation of ZA (*arrows*) using a coronal flap.

sites. At this time, any ligature wire that may have been used in the FZS is replaced by plates and screws for a more stable fixation. In cases where fixation of the ZA is anticipated, ORIF of the arch should be completed first to guarantee accurate definition of the midface width and projection of the ZMC.[20]

Type C Fracture

A displaced type C ZMC fracture represents an absolute indication for ORIF.[3] Liberal surgical exposure involving at least the ZMB, FZS, and IOR, and sometimes even the ZA, is indicated from the outset, as the enhanced exposure of 3 or 4 sites also helps tremendously in more accurate 3-dimensional reduction of these most challenging injuries. The same order of fixation described for the more complex type B fracture can be used for type C fractures.

The rationale for the treatment of ZMC fractures without an orbital-floor component is summarized in **Fig. 25**.

FRACTURES OF THE ORBITAL FLOOR

The ZMC forms most of the orbital floor, and fractures of this part of the orbit may occur in isolation or as part of a ZMC fracture. The treatment of these fractures is controversial, and is mainly decided according to the size and pattern of the fracture as well as the surgeon's preference. Clearly not every fracture of the orbital floor needs to be surgically repaired, and routine surgical exploration of the infraorbital rim and the orbital floor should be avoided because it carries the risk of causing important iatrogenic complications such as additional trauma to the infraorbital nerve,[7] persistent lower-eyelid edema,[2,3] epiphora,[19] worsening diplopia,[19] entropion,[2,3] scleral show and ectropion,[2–4,6,28,65,66] and even blindness.[19]

Surgical exploration of the orbital-floor fractures is indicated in the following cases:

- Nonresolving oculocardiac reflex[19]
- Primary diplopia (see **Fig. 4**)
- Enophthalmos (see **Fig. 5**)
- Mechanical entrapment of the extraocular muscles (**Fig. 26A**)
- Large defects (see **Fig. 26B**)
- CT evidence of a need to reconstruct the orbital floor or walls (see **Fig. 26C**)

When indicated, surgical repair of orbital-floor fractures should be done in the first 2 weeks of injury, as the immediate posttraumatic wound healing can make surgical repair more difficult.[19] Access to the orbital floor may be gained

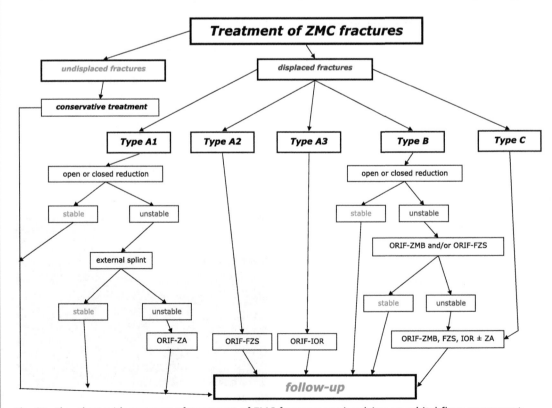

Fig. 25. Flowchart with summary of treatment of ZMC fractures not involving an orbital-floor component.

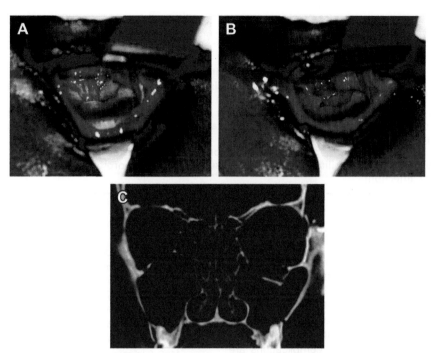

Fig. 26. Orbital-floor fractures. (*A*) Tissue entrapment. (*B*) Large defect. (*C*) CT image of large orbital-floor fracture.

transcutaneously via an infraorbital or a lower-eyelid incision or transmucosally via a transconjunctival approach. Alternatively, the orbital floor can be explored and repaired endoscopically, with less tissue disruption.[70,71]

A multitude of surgical techniques and materials have been used for the reconstruction of orbital-floor defects, depending on the size and type of the defect and on the surgeon's preference. Lyophilized dura,[2,3,10] cartilage,[2,3,72] temporal fascia,[71] bone grafts,[2,4,6,10,23] and different alloplastic implants[2,3,6,11,21,23,25,73] have all been used with variable degrees of success (**Fig. 27**).

SOFT-TISSUE SUSPENSION

Carefully placed skin and mucosal incisions, meticulous dissection, accurate wound closure,

and gentle handling of the soft tissues are vital when treating ZMC fractures surgically. Moreover, resuspension of incised, detached, or dissected tissues is critical in preventing postoperative cosmetic and functional defects such as ectropion and asymmetries. Soft-tissue suspension can be achieved by using suture ligation around the periosteum, drill holes in the surrounding bony structures, or attachment to the plates and screws used for fixation.[11,20,21]

FOLLOW-UP

Patients who have sustained ZMC fractures must be followed up closely for prevention and management of complications as well as to check on the appropriateness of treatment.

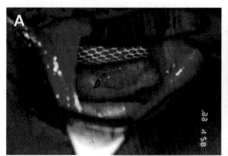
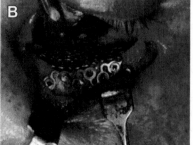

Fig. 27. Repair of orbital-floor fracture. (*A*) Reinforced silastic. (*B*) Titanium mesh.

Box 3		
Complications of ZMC fractures		
Persistent swelling	Persistent pain	Bleeding
Infection	Maxillary sinusitis	Oroantral fistula
Trismus	Facial nerve palsy	Altered sensation of infraorbital nerve
Diplopia	Gaze reduction	Decreased visual acuity
Blindness	Visible scarring	Bone malunion or nonunion
Facial asymmetry	Orbital dystopia	Enophthalmos/hypophthalmos
Ectropion	Entropion	Sclera show
Epiphora	Corneal abrasion	Persistent lid edema
Hardware problems (palpability, exposure, infection)	Thermal hypersensitivity	Meteorosensitivity

COMPLICATIONS

There are several possible complications associated with ZMC fractures that may be related to the trauma itself and/or its treatment. These complications may occur immediately after the injury or its treatment, or at a much later time. The most common and most important complications are summarized in **Box 3**.

As with most facial fractures, the best method of managing complications related to ZMC fractures remains the prevention of the complication itself, as some are extremely difficult to correct.[11] Prevention can take place preoperatively, with accurate assessment of the injury and formulation of a sound treatment plan; intraoperatively, with appropriate knowledge of the surgical anatomy and techniques in addition to correct understanding of the needs of adequate reduction and fixation; and postoperatively, with good wound care, rehabilitation, physiotherapy, and careful follow-up.

ACKNOWLEDGMENTS

The authors would like to thank Mr Rubens Fulgêncio Lima for his invaluable help with the production of the illustrations presented in this article.

REFERENCES

1. Ellis E 3rd, el-Attar A, Moos KF. An analysis of 2,067 cases of zygomatico-orbital fracture. J Oral Maxillofac Surg 1985;43:417–28.
2. Zingg M, Chowdhury K, Lädrach K, et al. Treatment of 813 zygoma-lateral orbital complex fractures. New aspects. Arch Otolaryngol Head Neck Surg 1991;117:611–20.
3. Zingg M, Laedrach K, Chen J, et al. Classification and treatment of zygomatic fractures: a review of 1,025 cases. J Oral Maxillofac Surg 1992;50:778–90.
4. Ellis E 3rd, Kittidumkerng W. Analysis of treatment for isolated zygomaticomaxillary complex fractures. J Oral Maxillofac Surg 1996;54:386–400.
5. Zachariades N, Mezitis M, Anagnostopoulos D. Changing trends in the treatment of zygomaticomaxillary complex fractures: a 12-year evaluation of methods used. J Oral Maxillofac Surg 1998;56: 1152–6 [discussion: 1156–7].
6. Olate S, Lima SM Jr, Sawazaki R, et al. Surgical approaches and fixation patterns in zygomatic complex fractures. J Craniofac Surg 2010;21: 1213–7.
7. Kovács AF, Ghahremani M. Minimization of zygomatic complex fracture treatment. Int J Oral Maxillofac Surg 2001;30:380–3.
8. Kloss FR, Stigler RG, Brandstätter A, et al. Complications related to midfacial fractures: operative versus non-surgical treatment. Int J Oral Maxillofac Surg 2011;40:33–7.
9. Jamal BT, Pfahler SM, Lane KA, et al. Ophthalmic injuries in patients with zygomaticomaxillary complex fractures requiring surgical repair. J Oral Maxillofac Surg 2009;67:986–9.
10. Bogusiak K, Arkuszewski P. Characteristics and epidemiology of zygomaticomaxillary complex fractures. J Craniofac Surg 2010;21:1018–23.
11. Lee EI, Mohan K, Koshy JC, et al. Optimizing the surgical management of zygomaticomaxillary complex fractures. Semin Plast Surg 2010;24:389–97.
12. Knight JS, North JF. The classification of malar fractures: an analysis of displacement as a guide to treatment. Br J Plast Surg 1961;13:325–39.
13. Fujii N, Yamashiro M. Classification of malar complex fractures using computed tomography. J Oral Maxillofac Surg 1983;41:562–7.
14. Hwang K, Kim DH. Analysis of zygomatic fractures. J Craniofac Surg 2011;22:1416–21.
15. Andreasen JO, Jensen SS, Schwartz O, et al. A systematic review of prophylactic antibiotics in the surgical treatment of maxillofacial fractures. J Oral Maxillofac Surg 2006;64:1664–8.

16. Dorri M, Nasser M, Oliver R. Resorbable versus titanium plates for facial fractures. Cochrane Database Syst Rev 2009;(21):CD007158.

17. Adeyemo WL, Akadiri OA. A systematic review of the diagnostic role of ultrasonography in maxillofacial fractures. Int J Oral Maxillofac Surg 2011;40: 655–61.

18. Magarakis M, Mundinger GS, Kelamis JA, et al. Ocular injury, visual impairment, and blindness associated with facial fractures: a systematic literature review. Plast Reconstr Surg 2012;129:227–33.

19. Burnstine MA. Clinical recommendations for repair of orbital facial fractures. Curr Opin Ophthalmol 2003;14:236–40.

20. Hollier LH, Thornton J, Pazmino P, et al. The management of orbitozygomatic fractures. Plast Reconstr Surg 2003;111:2386–92 [quiz: 2393].

21. Evans BG, Evans GR. MOC-PSSM CME article: zygomatic fractures. Plast Reconstr Surg 2008; 121(Suppl 1):1–11.

22. Manson PN, Markowitz B, Mirvis S, et al. Toward CT-based facial fracture treatment. Plast Reconstr Surg 1990;85:202–12.

23. Kelley P, Hopper R, Gruss J. Evaluation and treatment of zygomatic fractures. Plast Reconstr Surg 2007;120(7 Suppl 2):5S–15S.

24. Xie L, Shao Y, Hu Y, et al. Modification of surgical technique in isolated zygomatic arch fracture repair: seven case studies. Int J Oral Maxillofac Surg 2009;38:1096–100.

25. Evans GR, Daniels M, Hewell L. An evidence-based approach to zygomatic fractures. Plast Reconstr Surg 2011;127:891–7.

26. Kim JH, Lee JH, Hong SM, et al. The effectiveness of 1-point fixation for zygomaticomaxillary complex fractures. Arch Otolaryngol Head Neck Surg 2012; 138:828–32.

27. Moreno EF, Vasconcelos BC, Carneiro SC, et al. Evaluation of fixation techniques with titanium plates and Kirschner wires for zygoma fractures: preliminary study. J Oral Maxillofac Surg 2012;70:2386–93.

28. Mueller CK, Zeiß F, Mtsariashvili M, et al. Correlation between clinical findings and CT-measured displacement in patients with fractures of the zygomaticomaxillary complex. J Craniomaxillofac Surg 2012;40:e93–8.

29. Ogunmuyiwa SA, Fatusi OA, Ugboko VI, et al. The validity of ultrasonography in the diagnosis of zygomaticomaxillary complex fractures. Int J Oral Maxillofac Surg 2012;41:500–5.

30. Kurita M, Okazaki M, Ozaki M, et al. Patient satisfaction after open reduction and internal fixation of zygomatic bone fractures. J Craniofac Surg 2010;21:45–9.

31. McLoughlin P, Gilhooly M, Wood G. The management of zygomatic complex fractures: results of a survey. Br J Oral Maxillofac Surg 1994;32:284–8.

32. Knepil GJ, Loukota RA. Outcomes of prophylactic antibiotics following surgery for zygomatic bone fractures. J Craniomaxillofac Surg 2010;38:131–3.

33. Chole RA, Yee J. Antibiotic prophylaxis for facial fractures. A prospective, randomized clinical trial. Arch Otolaryngol Head Neck Surg 1987;113: 1055–7.

34. Holmes KD, Matthews BL. Three-point alignment of zygoma fractures with miniplate fixation. Arch Otolaryngol Head Neck Surg 1989;115:961–3.

35. Manson PN, Hoopes JE, Su CT. Structural pillars of the facial skeleton: an approach to the management of Le Fort fractures. Plast Reconstr Surg 1980;66:54–62.

36. Jones GM, Speculand B. A splint for the unstable zygomatic arch fracture. Br J Oral Maxillofac Surg 1986;24:269–71.

37. Champy M, Lodde JP, Kahn JL, et al. Attempt at systematization in the treatment of isolated fractures of the zygomatic bone: techniques and results. J Otolaryngol 1986;15:39–43.

38. Eisele DW, Duckert LG. Single-point stabilization of zygomatic fractures with the minicompression plate. Arch Otolaryngol Head Neck Surg 1987; 113:267–70.

39. Ogden GR. The Gillies method for fractured zygomas: an analysis of 105 cases. J Oral Maxillofac Surg 1991;49:23–5.

40. Covington DS, Wainwright DJ, Teichgraeber JF, et al. Changing patterns in the epidemiology and treatment of zygoma fractures: 10-year review. J Trauma 1994;37:243–8.

41. Tarabichi M. Transsinus reduction and one-point fixation of malar fractures. Arch Otolaryngol Head Neck Surg 1994;120:620–5.

42. Makowski G, Van Sickels J. Evaluation of results with three-point visualization of zygomaticomaxillary complex fractures. Oral Surg Oral Med Oral Pathol Oral Radiol Endod 1995;80:624.

43. O'Sullivan ST, Panchal J, O'Donoghue JM, et al. Is there still a role for traditional methods in the management of fractures of the zygomatic complex? Injury 1998;29:413–5.

44. Fujioka M, Yamanoto T, Miyazato O, et al. Stability of one-plate fixation for zygomatic bone fracture. Plast Reconstr Surg 2002;109:817–8.

45. Enislidis G, Lagogiannis G, Wittwer G, et al. Fixation of zygomatic fractures with a biodegradable copolymer osteosynthesis system: short- and long-term results. Int J Oral Maxillofac Surg 2005; 34:19–26.

46. Hwang K. One-point fixation of tripod fractures of zygoma through a lateral brow incision. J Craniofac Surg 2010;21:1042–4.

47. Kharkar VR, Rudagi BM, Halli R, et al. Comparison of the modified lateral orbitotomy approach and modified hemicoronal approach in the treatment

of unstable malunions of zygomatic complex fractures. Oral Surg Oral Med Oral Pathol Oral Radiol Endod 2010;109:504–9.

48. Kim ST, Go DH, Jung JH, et al. Comparison of 1-point fixation with 2-point fixation in treating tripod fractures of the zygoma. J Oral Maxillofac Surg 2011;69:2848–52.

49. Gaziri DA, Omizollo G, Luchi GH, et al. Assessment for treatment of tripod fractures of the zygoma with microcompressive screws. J Oral Maxillofac Surg 2012;70:e378–88.

50. Rana M, Warraich R, Tahir S, et al. Surgical treatment of zygomatic bone fracture using two points fixation versus three point fixation—a randomised prospective clinical trial. Trials 2012;12:13–36.

51. Dal Santo F, Ellis E 3rd, Throckmorton GS. The effects of zygomatic complex fracture on masseteric muscle force. J Oral Maxillofac Surg 1992;50:791–9.

52. Davidson J, Nickerson D, Nickerson B. Zygomatic fractures: comparison of methods of internal fixation. Plast Reconstr Surg 1990;86:25–32.

53. Heiland M, Schulze D, Blake F, et al. Intraoperative imaging of zygomaticomaxillary complex fractures using a 3D C-arm system. Int J Oral Maxillofac Surg 2005;34:369–75.

54. Pohlenz P, Blake F, Blessmann M, et al. Intraoperative cone-beam computed tomography in oral and maxillofacial surgery using a C-arm prototype: first clinical experiences after treatment of zygomaticomaxillary complex fractures. J Oral Maxillofac Surg 2009;67:515–21.

55. Ibrahim AM, Rabie AN, Lee BT, et al. Intraoperative CT: a teaching tool for the management of complex facial fracture fixation in surgical training. J Surg Educ 2011;68:437–41.

56. Rabie A, Ibrahim AM, Lee BT, et al. Use of intraoperative computed tomography in complex facial fracture reduction and fixation. J Craniofac Surg 2011;22:1466–7.

57. Yu H, Shen G, Wang X, et al. Navigation-guided reduction and orbital floor reconstruction in the treatment of zygomatic-orbital-maxillary complex fractures. J Oral Maxillofac Surg 2010;68:28–34.

58. Buijs GJ, van Bakelen NB, Jansma J, et al. A randomized clinical trial of biodegradable and titanium fixation systems in maxillofacial surgery. J Dent Res 2012;91:299–304.

59. Hanemann M Jr, Simmons O, Jain S, et al. A comparison of combinations of titanium and resorbable plating systems for repair of isolated zygomatic fractures in the adult: a quantitative biomechanical study. Ann Plast Surg 2005;54:402–8.

60. Banks P. Outline of definitive treatment of fractures of the middle third of the facial skeleton. In: Banks P, editor. Kelley's fractures of the middle third of the facial skeleton. London: Wright; 1985. p. 59–104.

61. Ellis E, Zide MF. Periorbital approaches. In: Ellis E, Zide MF, editors. Surgical access to the facial skeleton. Baltimore (MD): Williams & Wilkins; 1995. p. 7–54.

62. Kushner GM. Surgical approaches to the infraorbital rim and orbital floor: the case for the transconjunctival approach. J Oral Maxillofac Surg 2006; 64:108–10.

63. Khan AM, Varvares MA. Traditional approaches to the orbit. Otolaryngol Clin North Am 2006;39: 895–909.

64. Ridgway EB, Chen C, Colakoglu S, et al. The incidence of lower eyelid malposition after facial fracture repair: a retrospective study and meta-analysis comparing subtarsal, subciliary, and transconjunctival incisions. Plast Reconstr Surg 2009;124:1578–86.

65. Wray RC, Holtmann B, Ribaudo JM, et al. A comparison of conjunctival and subciliary incisions for orbital fractures. Br J Plast Surg 1977; 30:142–5.

66. Appling WD, Patrinely JR, Salzer TA. Transconjunctival approach vs subciliary skin-muscle flap approach for orbital fracture repair. Arch Otolaryngol Head Neck Surg 1993;119:1000–7.

67. Mueller R. Endoscopic treatment of facial fractures. Facial Plast Surg 2008;24:78–91.

68. Santosh BS, Giraddi G. Transconjunctival preseptal approach for orbital floor and infraorbital rim fracture. J Maxillofac Oral Surg 2011;10: 301–5.

69. Baumann A, Ewers R. Use of the preseptal transconjunctival approach in orbit reconstruction surgery. J Oral Maxillofac Surg 2001;59:287–91.

70. Fernandes R, Fattahi T, Steinberg B, et al. Endoscopic repair of isolated orbital floor fracture with implant placement. J Oral Maxillofac Surg 2007; 65:1449–53.

71. Yan Z, Zhou Z, Song X. Nasal endoscopy-assisted reconstruction of orbital floor blowout fractures using temporal fascia grafting. J Oral Maxillofac Surg 2012;70:1119–22.

72. Bayat M, Momen-Heravi F, Khalilzadeh O, et al. Comparison of conchal cartilage graft with nasal septal cartilage graft for reconstruction of orbital floor blowout fractures. Br J Oral Maxillofac Surg 2010;48:617–20.

73. Enislidis G, Pichorner S, Kainberger F, et al. Lactosorb panel and screws for repair of large orbital floor defects. J Craniomaxillofac Surg 1997;25: 316–21.

Management of Fractures of the Nasofrontal Complex

Archibald D. Morrison, DDS, MS, FRCD(C)[a,b,*],
Curtis E. Gregoire, BSc, DDS, MS, MD, FRCD(C)[a,b]

KEYWORDS

- NOE (naso-orbital-ethmoidal) fractures • Frontal sinus fractures • Nasofrontal fractures

KEY POINTS

- Nasofrontal fractures are commonly encountered in everyday OMF surgery practice.
- Studies suggest that the incidence may be decreasing as a result of seat belt use and the introduction of air bags.
- Concomitant CNS injuries are commonly associated with nasofrontal injuries and these must be identified early and managed appropriately.
- Nasofrontal injuries must be properly diagnosed through a thorough clinical examination and ancillary maxillofacial injuries.
- Close long-term follow-up must be done to assess for the development of early and late complications.

INTRODUCTION

Fractures involving the nasofrontal region of the face can affect the root of the nose, the orbits, the naso-orbital-ethmoidal (NOE) complex, and the frontal bone including the frontal sinuses. These types of fractures are routinely encountered by practicing oral and maxillofacial (OMF) surgeons. Management of facial fractures and injuries remains a mainstay of the specialty. Fractures of the nasofrontal complex are unique in that the occlusion is not typically affected, thereby removing the element of precision required to restore a functional occlusion. The exception is a Lefort II fracture that traverses the face in an anterosuperior direction across the nasal bridge, thus involving the nasofrontal region by definition. However, there are unique characteristics in this region that require their own attention to detail in restoring the injured parts back to the premorbid state.

This includes the functional and cosmetic restoration of these structures. Fractures of this region can occur as part of a panfacial injury (**Fig. 1**) or as a localized injury (**Fig. 2**).

EPIDEMIOLOGY
Motor Vehicle Collisions

Two decades ago, facial trauma was the main injury resulting from motor vehicle collisions (MVC).[1] With the advent of seat belts and now air bags, injuries to this region of the face from MVC have decreased greatly. This is assuming seat belts are worn and vehicles are equipped with air bags. A retrospective review of US data collected by the National Automotive Sampling System Crashworthiness Data System between 1993 and 2005 has shown yearly decreases in facial injuries as a result of MVC.[2] Interestingly, the authors found that restraint was of paramount importance (ie, air

Disclosures: There are no funding sources or conflicts of interest to disclose by either author.
[a] Department of Oral and Maxillofacial Surgery, QEII Health Sciences Centre, Halifax, Nova Scotia B3H 2Y9, Canada; [b] Department of Oral and Maxillofacial Sciences, Faculty of Dentistry, Dalhousie University, 5981 University Avenue, Halifax, Nova Scotia B3H 4R2, Canada
* Corresponding author. Department of Oral and Maxillofacial Sciences, Faculty of Dentistry, Dalhousie University, 5981 University Avenue, Halifax, Nova Scotia, Canada B3H 4R2.
E-mail address: archie.morrison@dal.ca

Oral Maxillofacial Surg Clin N Am 25 (2013) 637–648
http://dx.doi.org/10.1016/j.coms.2013.08.001
1042-3699/13/$ – see front matter © 2013 Elsevier Inc. All rights reserved.

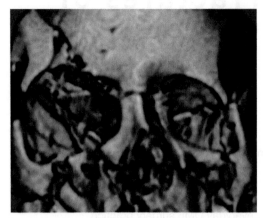

Fig. 1. A 23-year-old woman involved in a car crash with panfacial fractures involving in part the nasofrontal region.

bags alone do not always prevent facial injury). Fortunately, the prevalence of safety belt use in passenger vehicles on the road reached 85% in 2010 according to the US National Highway Transportation and Safety Administration.[3]

Frontal sinus fractures account for roughly 5% to 15% of maxillofacial fractures, and not surprisingly, the most common cause of frontal sinus fractures is MVC followed by sport-related injuries.[4] Significant force is required to fracture the anterior table of the frontal sinus. It has been estimated that a force of 800 to 2000 lb is required to fracture the anterior table of the frontal sinus.[5] As such, concomitant injuries are common and must be appropriately diagnosed and managed. In particular, cervical spine and intracranial injury must be identified as soon as possible after the injury. Frontal sinus fractures and concomitant

injuries are diagnosed by performing a thorough clinical examination in conjunction with radiographic imaging.

Interpersonal Violence and Sport

Unfortunately, interpersonal violence remains a common cause for NOE and frontal sinus fractures. These types of injuries tend to be lower-energy injuries compared with MVC. As a result, these types of injuries are generally less likely to have concomitant brain injuries. Frontal bone fractures may result from sports, such as soccer. However, aside from pure nasal fractures and frontal sinus fractures, nasofrontal fractures are relatively rare from sporting injuries.

PERTINENT ANATOMY OF THE NASOFRONTAL REGION AND ITS RELATION TO SURGERY

The nasofrontal region of the face is a complex area from an anatomic perspective. The nasofrontal region is composed of bones, muscles, nerves, and blood vessels. It also contains the eyelids, orbits, nasolacrimal apparatus, and frontal sinus with its outflow tract.

The nasofrontal region is composed of several bones (**Fig. 3**). These include the frontal, nasal, lacrimal, maxillary, and ethmoid bones. The frontal bone forms the upper portion of the face and contains the frontal sinus. Injuries to the nasofrontal region of the face typically do not affect the occlusion. However, there are important structures that require care in their reconstruction. Failing to do so can result in dysfunction of the affected area and cosmetic deformity. Because the eyes are often the first area of visual contact when one meets

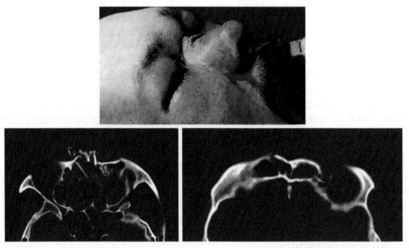

Fig. 2. A 28-year-old man with associated CT images who was struck across the bridge of the nose with a baseball bat with a resultant isolated nasofrontal injury.

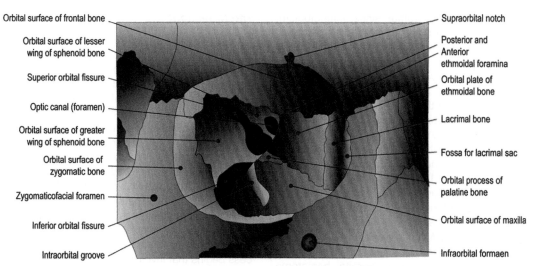

Fig. 3. The osseous anatomy of the nasofrontal complex. (*Data from* Hansen JT, Lambert DR. Netter's Clinical Anatomy. Philadelphia: Elsevier, 2006.)

another person, it is important to reconstruct the NOE complex properly so as to avoid the stigmata of previous trauma.

Frontal Sinus

The frontal sinus is absent at birth and only fully pneumatizes after puberty (**Fig. 4**). It is lined by a pseudostratified columnar respiratory epithelium that consists of four cell types: (1) ciliated, (2) intermediate, (3) basal, and (4) goblet cells. Goblet cells produce mucus, which drains through the nasofrontal outflow tract (NFOT).

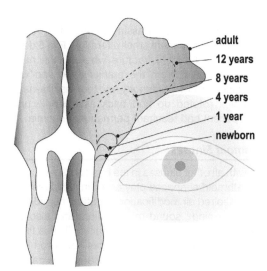

Fig. 4. Frontal sinus pneumatizes after birth. (*Adapted from* Manolidis S, Hollier LH Jr. Management of frontal sinus fractures. Plast Reconstr Surg 2007;120(Suppl 2):32S–48S; with permission.)

The frontal sinuses are paired and rarely symmetric. Ten percent to 12% of adults possess a rudimentary frontal sinus or may completely lack pneumatization of one or the other of the sinuses.[6] A further 4% of the population fails to develop both frontal sinuses.[6] The nasofrontal ducts drain the frontal sinuses and their course is highly variable. They are located in the posteromedial aspect of the floor of the sinuses and are the only drainage pathway for the sinuses. A true duct is absent in 85% of people, in which case drainage is through a foramen. From here they drain into their respective infundibulae, then into the ethmoid sinuses, and finally into the middle meati.[6]

The frontal bone has a vertical and a horizontal portion.[6] The vertical component forms the forehead and contains the frontal sinus, which lies between its anterior and posterior tables.[6] The thick anterior table contains cancellous bone between its cortical plates. The posterior table is much thinner and lies in direct contact with the dura. The horizontal portion of the frontal bone forms the roof of the orbit and articulates with the ethmoid bone to form the roof of the nasal cavity and the floor of the anterior cranial fossa.[6]

The paired typically asymmetric frontal sinuses are separated by a central intersinus septum. The average dimensions in adults are 24.3 mm in height, 29 mm in width, and 20.5 mm in depth.[6] In contrast with the thick anterior table of the vertical portion of the frontal bone, the horizontal orbital plate of the frontal bone forms the thinnest wall of the frontal sinus. The inferior portion of the frontal sinus cavity narrows toward the frontal ostium in an area known as the frontal infundibulum.[6] The frontal sinus infundibulum, frontal sinus ostium, and frontal recess comprise a functional unit for drainage that has loosely been referred to as the NFOT.[6]

The blood supply to the frontal sinus is from the anterior ethmoid artery and the supraorbital branch of the ophthalmic artery, which are both branches of the internal carotid artery.[6] The anterior ethmoid artery may be surrounded by dura along its entire ethmoidal extent or only at its passage through the ethmoidal sulcus.[6] In a small portion of cases the artery remains extradural along its entire course. This is important because injury to the anterior ethmoid artery poses two obvious risks: cerebrospinal fluid (CSF) leakage and hemorrhage. More importantly, if the artery is injured close to the orbit, the vessel can retract intraorbitally and lead to intraorbital hematoma and blindness.[6]

The supraorbital artery branches from the ophthalmic artery within the orbit where the ophthalmic artery crosses the optic nerve. The supraorbital artery then runs between the orbital plate periosteum and the superior levator palpebrae muscle to exit the orbit at the supraorbital notch or foramen. It then divides into superficial and deep branches, supplying the skin, muscles, and frontal periosteum, and anastomoses with the supratrochlear and frontal branch of the supratrochlear arteries.[6,7] At the superior orbital rim, the supraorbital artery sends a branch to the diploe of the frontal bone and, occasionally, the mucoperiosteum in the frontal sinus.[7]

Venous drainage of the frontal sinus mucosa occurs through small vascular pits that pockmark the cortical bone. These mucosa-lined pits mark the exit points of the diploic veins named after Gilbert Breschet, the French anatomist who extensively described venous drainage of the head and neck in the early nineteenth century.[6,8] The foramina through which the diploic veins of Breschet pass (Breschet canals) have been described in the anterior and posterior walls of the frontal sinus, although the diploe is minimal in the posterior wall.[6,8] They usually coalesce with larger frontal diploic veins and eventually drain to the ipsilateral frontal diploic vein, which is oriented vertically between the plates of cortical bone above the supraorbital notch. In the supraorbital notch, the frontal diploic and supraorbital veins join to form the superior ophthalmic vein, which then drains posteriorly to the cavernous sinus.[6,7] Lymphatics of the forehead and frontal scalp region terminate in the anterior auricular and parotid lymph nodes. The lymphatics drain the anterior parts of the nasal cavity and travel across the face to the submandibular lymph nodes.[6,7]

The Nasal Root

Injuries to the nasofrontal complex may result in a permanent change in the individual's appearance. The subtleties of the shape and contour of this area of the face are as varied as the facial characteristics that make us individual in appearance. We are well aware how a cosmetic rhinoplasty can have such a dramatic effect on one's appearance. In profile, the transition from the frontal bone to the nasal dorsum can be dramatically or subtly altered. From the frontal view, a perceived profile change can be apparent. This is especially true if there is comminution and obvious disruption of the medial orbital walls with subsequent loss of support for nasal projection. When comminuted injuries to the nasal root are reduced and fixated, a natural remodeling process begins that involves initial resorption of small bone fragments. This physiologic process may result in undercontouring of the nasal root after healing is complete. If this type of deformity does occur, it results in the appearance of a much wider nasal bridge even in the absence of telecanthus. It is for this reason that many surgeons perform nasal bone grafting at the time of initial fracture repair for severe injuries to the nasal root.[9]

Cribriform Plate

The cribriform plate represents a transition from the base of the skull to the face at the upper aspect of the nose. The cribriform plate plays a role in the passage of olfactory nerves and disruption of this can lead to partial or total anosmia. A review of the incidence and factors involved in this sensory loss caused by trauma has been summarized.[10] It is therefore intuitive to understand that disruption of the sensory fibers passing through this region can lead to permanent smell alteration. **Fig. 5** demonstrates a Lefort II fracture whereby the nasal bone separated from the cranial base and was displaced 1-cm posteriorly as the maxilla-nasal complex rotated up and back as a single unit. This patient had resultant permanent anosmia.

Ethmoid Sinuses

As with all other sinuses in the head and neck area, the ethmoid airspaces play a role in nasal respiration; inspired air modification (filtration, humidification, warming); sound modification; and also act to reduce the weight of the cranium. These finely arranged and septated spaces between the medial orbital walls and the nasal cavity can be easily disrupted from trauma to this region. Fractures involving the ethmoid sinuses are usually only grossly reduced and fortunately subsequent complications related to their damage are rare.

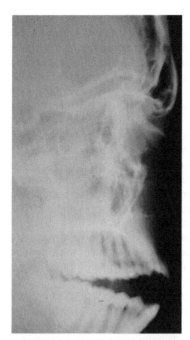

Fig. 5. A 24-year-old man with pure Lefort II fracture affecting the nasofrontal region by definition. Note the posteriorly displaced maxilla with upward rotation. Nasion can be seen about 1 cm from its usual location at the frontonasal suture.

Drainage usually remains patent and risk of mucocele formation is very low. One review of 47 mucoceles of the ethmoid and sphenoid sinuses shows none to be related to previous trauma.[11] However, there is an isolated report in the literature of a bilateral posttraumatic mucocele.[12]

Ethmoid Arteries

The anterior and posterior ethmoid arteries can be damaged as a result of nasofrontal trauma. The origin of these arteries has been discussed. They are commonly encountered during surgical repair of injuries to this region of the face. Cauterization of these vessels, when necessary, is associated with no long-term deleterious consequences. However, if the vessels are injured and begin to bleed during surgical exploration, they may retract causing a retrobulbar hemorrhage if bleeding persists.

Trochlea and Superior Oblique Muscle

The trochlea, which acts as the pulley for the superior oblique muscle, is found at the antero-supero-medial aspect of the medial orbital. Because the medial wall of the orbit is often involved in these injuries, the trochlea is at risk of avulsion or displacement. Pure avulsion is presumed to be rare because there is little in the literature describing this type of injury.[13] Displacement as part

of a larger piece of medial orbital wall is likely more common. Although palsy or paresis of this muscle secondary to cranial nerve injury from head trauma is more likely, there are reports of trauma to the muscular tendon leading to superior oblique muscle dysfunction either from the trauma itself or the surgical repair.[14–16] Again, these are relatively rare. In our experience we do not routinely consider this specific structure as a potential area of injury because it is uncommon to find dysfunction of the superior oblique muscle in patients with facial trauma. Nevertheless, the eye function including cranial nerves, eye movement, and visual acuity needs to be carefully assessed in patients with nasofrontal injuries.

Nasolacrimal Duct

The nasolacrimal apparatus may be disrupted in the setting of traumatic injury to the nasofrontal region of the face. This ductal system drains the lacrimal sac that is precariously located between the anterior and posterior lacrimal crests. A recent review of the patterns of injury and subsequent outcomes was done by Ali and colleagues.[17] Unless the OMF surgeon has particular experience in operating on the nasolacrimal apparatus, attention to this type of injury is best left in the hands of an oculoplastic surgeon or trauma ophthalmologist, both of whom manage these types of injuries on a regular basis.

The early identification of this type of injury is important because it may not be readily apparent if other more obvious and serious injuries are present. However, careful assessment of the nasolacrimal system is mandatory to prevent late complications related to obstruction of the canal. This complication is much more difficult to manage than repairing the duct at the time of initial injury.[18]

Medial Canthal Tendon

The medial canthal tendon (or ligament) is a complex and important structure often involved in trauma to this region. Traumatic telecanthus (widening of the intercanthal distance) is a common sequella of fractures of the NOE complex or medial orbital walls. The medial canthal tendon plays a role in providing attachment of the medial aspect of the eyelid to the medial orbital wall. It also provides a pumping action to the lacrimal sac, which it surrounds. Disruption of this structure can lead to a significant cosmetic deformity that normally supersedes any noticeable functional deficit.

For the most part, the medial canthal tendon has been described as having an anterior and a posterior limb that attach to the anterior and posterior lacrimal crests, respectively, and the adjacent medial orbital wall.[19] Recent investigation[20] questions this and as with anatomic study of many structures, it is often necessary to look at the detailed histology of the part to understand the gross anatomic relationships and hence its function. Poh and colleagues[20] remind us that the anterior limb is by far the more robust piece of this tendon and question the existence of a true posterior limb of the medial canthal tendon. Rather, it seems as though the presumed posterior limb may in fact be the tendon of Horner muscle that arises from the periosteum of the posterior lacrimal crest and the anterior aspect of the medial orbital wall. It then inserts into the medial tarsal plate. The connective tissue covering of the lacrimal sac seems to be confluent with the fascia of Horner muscle. This suggests that the posterior limb is therefore Horner muscle and its tendon and not a part of the canthal tendon proper.

Despite a better appreciation of this detailed anatomy, the surgical management of the disruption of soft tissue attachments in this area remains the same. The classic paper by Markowitz and colleagues[21] stands as an accurate descriptor of the three types of fracture patterns involving this tendon and its attachments. In a type 1 NOE fracture, the tendon is attached to the bony fragment that is disrupted from the medial orbital wall. This type of fracture is amenable to open reduction and internal fixation with microplates, thereby relocating the tendon in its correct anatomic relation. A type 2 NOE fracture involves more comminution of the medial orbital wall. However, the tendon is still attached to a bony fragment and is usually still amenable to reduction and fixation. Type 3 is the most difficult to treat because it involves severe comminution and avulsion of the tendon from its bony attachment.

DIAGNOSIS AND IMAGING

It is important to have a systematic approach to the examination of these types of patients. Although some patients may have an isolated fracture of the nasofrontal region, others may have life-threatening concomitant injuries. After a patient is stabilized and life-threatening injuries managed appropriately, a careful inventory of facial fractures needs to be attained as part of the secondary survey. After this inventory of injuries is established and a treatment plan is formulated, the plan should be to definitively repair these fractures rather than delay treatment as long as the patient is suitable for surgery. There is no evidence to support delaying repair or partial reduction of these fractures with more definitive repair to follow.

Features on clinical examination suggestive of a frontal sinus fracture are variable. The signs may be subtle, such as bruising or edema of the skin overlying the frontal bone. An obvious cosmetic deformity may be present if the fracture is grossly displaced and lacerations of the forehead skin may be present. The patient may also present with V1 anesthesia and periorbital ecchymosis. CSF rhinorrhea may be present if the posterior table is involved. Other signs and symptoms may be present if concomitant injuries are present.

The main goals of treatment of frontal sinus fractures are the protection of intracranial structures, elimination of CSF leak, maintenance of patent sinus drainage, prevention of complications, and preservation of esthetics.[22] Various classifications of frontal sinus fractures have been proposed; however, the type and extent of surgery is generally based on involvement of the anterior and posterior tables, the integrity of the NFOT, and dural integrity.[4,23,24]

Computed tomography (CT) is considered the gold standard for diagnosing fractures of the nasofrontal region. Newer-generation scanners allow for submillimeter slices in axial, coronal, and sagittal planes. These fine slices allow for accurate evaluation of the integrity of the hard and soft tissues of the region.

Not only is it important for detailing the specifics of the anatomic structures traumatized in the nasofrontal region but including the head in the CT scan helps identify concomitant injuries if present. Examples include the ability to assess the integrity of the posterior table of the frontal sinus, the NFOT, and intracranial structures. The details of the anatomy of NOE fractures may help to avoid surprises at the time of exposure, reduction, and fixation. These fractures can be challenging to manage and high-quality CT imaging is of paramount importance.

Three-dimensional reformatting of the CT data can be extremely useful for diagnosis and treatment planning of fractures involving the nasofrontal region as highlighted in **Fig. 6**. These reformatted images can also be used as a very

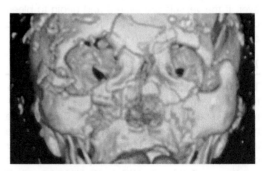

Fig. 6. Standard three-dimensional reformatted image of midfacial fractures.

effective teaching tool for OMF surgery residents. It is important to remember that images in two opposing planes of space are useful in revealing fractures that otherwise may go unappreciated. The patient in **Fig. 7** sustained an injury to the nasofrontal region and as part of the work-up an axial CT scan was obtained by the neurosurgery department. At the time of assessment by OMF surgeons (before modern reformatting technology), a further coronal scan was requested that revealed multiple large bony fragments rotated into the anterior cranial fossa. Obviously, this was important to identify before manipulating and reducing these fractures.

Neurologic Injuries

A significant portion of patients with frontal sinus fractures have concomitant neurologic injuries because of the significant forces involved with this type of injury. Radiographic evidence of neurologic injury, such as epidural and subdural hematomas and depressed skull fractures, are commonly seen on CT imaging. It is imperative that these types of injuries be appropriately identified and managed. Management should involve neurosurgical consultation, because a team approach to treatment can often be accomplished.[23,25] Depressed skull fractures other than those of the frontal bone are also a common feature in severe motor vehicle–associated frontal sinus fractures. If a CSF leak is present, the source must be identified. The two most common causes of a CSF leak are the result of disruption of the posterior table resulting in a tear of the dura or disruption of the anterior cranial fossa.[23,25]

SURGICAL MANAGEMENT
Access

Most nasofrontal fractures are accessed by a coronal (bicoronal) incision. Pre-existing lacerations may be used for isolated fractures directly in the underlying area. However, the best view and appreciation of the bony anatomy and subsequent repair is by a well-extended, properly dissected coronal flap. Using an existing laceration often affords poor surgical access, which results in poor surgical outcomes. Other approaches to the nasofrontal region have been described and include the Lynch incision (**Fig. 8**), brow incision, and butterfly incision. However, these incisions often offer poor access to the fracture and result in poor cosmesis. With preauricular extension, the complete upper facial skeleton can be accessed including the zygomatic root and arches, upper lateral orbital rims including the frontozygomatic sutures, supraorbital rims, orbital roofs, frontal bone, nasal bone, and the anterior aspect of the upper medial orbital walls. One exception is the classic Lefort II fracture that involves the frontonasal suture without telecanthus or NOE injury. The radiographic image in **Fig. 5** depicts such an injury. This can be reduced and plated intraorally, securing the maxilla to stable zygomatic bones bilaterally. However, when the medial orbital walls are disrupted, a coronal flap allows for proper access to repair the fractures.

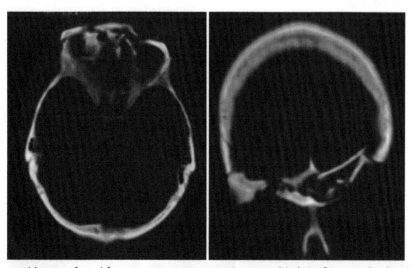

Fig. 7. A 30-year-old man referred from neurosurgery to repair supraorbital rim fractures (in the absence of any neurologic deficit). The initial axial scan was provided. The coronal scan was requested to have a two-plane view of the injury (in the time before three-dimensional reconstructions were readily available). Note the obvious involvement of the anterior cranial fossa, which prepared us for possible CSF leak during manipulation and to have the neurosurgery department on standby if needed. Fortunately, they were not required.

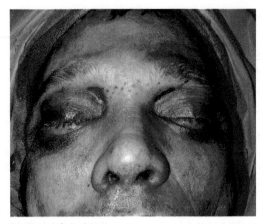

Fig. 8. Lynch incision.

near to anatomic reduction as possible. Microplates (1 or 1.3 mm) are most commonly used and offer acceptable rigidity in this area of the face. Less than anatomic reduction may be acceptable in such areas as the frontal bone where a scaffold of comminuted bone pieces reduced well may be adequate enough to prevent a postoperative cosmetic defect.

For NOE fractures, particularly type 3, osseosynthesis with plates may not be possible. Transnasal wiring is often used to reduce and fixate the medial canthal tendons. Sometimes a heavy nonresorbable or slowly resorbable suture is sufficient to maintain orientation of the medial canthal tendons until mature fibrosis ensues.

Some authors have suggested that baldness is a relative contraindication to using this approach. However, in our experience, the coronal incision can be used on patients with alopecia with little to no effect on cosmesis. The decision to do so is always a weighing of the pros of access and subsequent ideal reparative results versus the cons of a coronal scar and the possibility of poor esthetics secondary to an inadequately visualized repair.

Although there are those that suggest that NOE fractures that require surgical repair can on occasion be accessed from a midline dorsal nasal incision or intraorally or from an infraorbital incision,[26] we almost always access these from the coronal approach.

Reduction and Fixation

As with most facial fractures treated in this era, plate and screw fixation is used to perform as

Bone Grafting

Fractures of the nasal dorsum as it transitions from the forehead to the nose can lead to the classic saddle nose deformity if not properly managed. Even when anatomically repositioned, if there is comminution, this can lead to a noticeable defect later. Although personal family photographs are of limited use in repairing these injuries, a profile picture may be beneficial in appreciating the frontonasal angle and the general contour of the area when combined with a frontal photograph.

If there is a question of whether or not to graft, the authors err on the side of grafting because a more defined nasal bridge of the nose tends to have a favorable effect of cosmesis and prevents a saddle deformity. For these cases, a split-thickness calvarial graft is used and can be readily harvested as an appropriately shaped strip while the coronal flap is elevated (**Fig. 9**). This is harvested from the parietal bone away from the

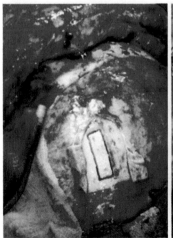
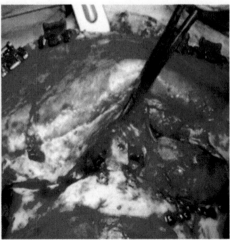

Fig. 9. Harvesting of a split-thickness calvarial bone graft for nasal root reconstruction followed by its placement and securing with one fixation screw.

midline in the event of an aberrant sagittal sinus or absent diploe.

Fig. 10 is an example of presurgical nasofrontal trauma with significant saddle deformity and post-treatment several months later.

FRONTAL SINUS FRACTURES
Anterior Table Fractures

Nondisplaced or minimally displaced anterior table fractures generally do not require surgical treatment unless the NFOT is involved. These types of fractures are generally low-energy injuries and concomitant injuries are less common but must not be overlooked if present.[5,27] Appropriate antibiotics should be considered and long-term follow-up planned to evaluate for late complications. Decongestants are also commonly prescribed in the setting of minimally displaced frontal sinus fractures involving the anterior table.[27]

Isolated anterior table fractures that are displaced often require open reduction and internal fixation. After this type of fracture has been accessed, the fragments should be removed and a careful assessment of the posterior table and NFOT completed. If either of these structures is disrupted they must be treated appropriately. Any damaged sinus lining should be removed by vigorous curettage to reduce the likelihood of

subsequent mucocele formation.[5] Sinus obliteration is generally not indicated with this type of fracture especially if the posterior table and NFOT are intact. The displaced fragments are repositioned and fixated with titanium micro plates. This type of fixation plate has minimal risk of complications and generally is difficult to palpate.

If an isolated anterior table fracture involves the NFOT, it must be addressed at the time of surgery. Preoperative CT is extremely helpful in identifying fractures that involve the NFOT but occasionally they may not be identified on CT. Thus, the NFOT should be explored at the time of surgery in all cases. If the NFOT is involved, the sinus may be obliterated.[12] This involves removing all of the sinus mucosa with the use of sharp curettes. To avoid leaving remnants of mucosa behind, a bur may be used on the walls of the sinus. The NFOT mucosa must also be inverted into the nasal cavity. After this step is complete, the NFOT must be occluded. There are several materials that have been used for this purpose. Pericranium is the authors' choice because it can easily be harvested during the approach to the sinus. However, fibrin glue, fat, muscle plugs, and bone graft have also been described for this purpose.[25]

After the NFOT is plugged, the sinus should be obliterated. Several materials have been used for this purpose including autogenous fat, muscle, cartilage, pericranium, silicone, hydroxyapatite, and methyl methacrylate.[4] Autogenous fat (**Fig. 11**) is the most commonly described material used for the purpose of obliterating the frontal sinus; however, a vascularized pericranial flap is becoming more popular and is the authors' choice for this procedure. The procedure for harvesting a pericranial flap is simple. The pericranium is left attached to the cranium at the time of coronal flap elevation (**Fig. 12**A). After the coronal flap is elevated, an inferiorly based pericranial flap is elevated based off the supratrochlear vessels. The pericranium can be rotated into the frontal sinus to plug the NFOT and to obliterate the sinus (see **Fig. 12**B). The outer table is then repositioned and fixated with micro plates (see **Fig. 12**C).

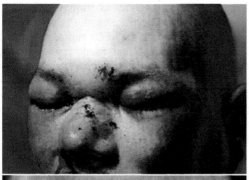
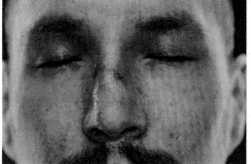

Fig. 10. Same patient in **Fig. 2** demonstrating presurgical nasofrontal deformity and 3 months postsurgical repair with cranial bone graft to the nasofrontal region.

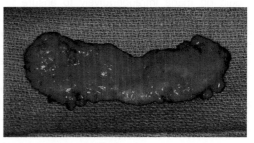

Fig. 11. Autogenous fat harvest.

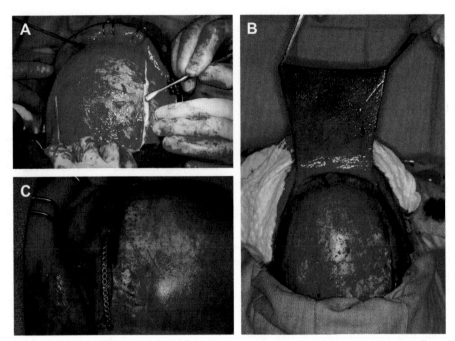

Fig. 12. (*A*) The coronal flap is elevated above the pericranium. (*B*) Inferiorly based pericranial flap after elevation. (*C*) Sinus obliterated with pericranial flap and fracture reduced with micro plates.

Posterior Table Fractures

Posterior table fractures almost always occur in conjunction with anterior table fractures and require a different treatment approach. If the posterior table fracture is nondisplaced or minimally displaced and no CSF leak is present, observation is the treatment of choice.[25] If a CSF leak is present in a nondisplaced posterior table fracture it is generally treated conservatively with observation. The patient should be placed on bed rest with the head of the bed elevated 30 degrees. If the leak persists beyond 4 days, a spinal drain is recommended.[25] A significant proportion of these cases respond favorably to this type of conservative therapy. However, if there is no resolution within 7 to 14 days, the sinus must be surgically explored by a coronal approach and craniotomy. This allows access to the dura that must be repaired with sutures or a dural patch. An attempt should be made intraoperatively to ensure the repair is water tight.[25] After the repair is complete, the sinus lining should be removed as previously described, the NFOT plugged, and the sinus obliterated. In this instance, the posterior table can be removed to allow cranialization of the sinus.[5] Cranialization involves removal of the entire posterior wall of the sinus and separating the intracranial cavity from the aerodigestive tract using a temporoparietal or pericranial flap. This allows room for the frontal lobe to expand and fill the frontal sinus.[4]

This procedure is typically used when concomitant neurosurgical intervention is required and should not be used routinely for purposes of frontal sinus obliteration in the absence of surgical neurologic injuries.[4]

If no involvement of the NFOT is present and no CSF leak is present, the fracture is generally treated with either preservation of the sinus or obliteration depending on the type of fracture.[25] If the posterior table fracture is significantly displaced or comminuted, the sinus is generally obliterated after the lining is completely removed and the NFOT plugged.[25]

FOLLOW-UP AND COMPLICATIONS

Patients who sustain injuries to the nasofrontal region must be closely followed for the development of complications. Because the occlusion is not generally a concern with most nasofrontal fractures, there does not exist a critical time period so as to manage a malocclusion. For potential occlusal disturbances, following a Lefort II fracture for example, these need to be intercepted within the first week or two ideally if surgical repair is required. With respect to NOE fractures, complications include the following: stability of medial canthal tendon repair; function of the lacrimal drainage system; and eye function, both extraoccular movements and visual acuity.

Any surgery involving the orbits can result in a postoperative, retrobulbar hemorrhage, which can threaten the visual acuity of the eye. Therefore, it is important to have the patient's eyes tested for visual acuity, pupillary light reflex, pain, and proptosis according to the following schedule: every 15 minutes for the first postoperative hour, every 30 minutes for the next hour, then every hour for the next 4 hours, and then every 4 hours until 24 hours postoperative.

One of the primary goals of treating frontal sinus fractures, as with any facial fracture, is avoiding complications. There are early and late complications that may occur. Early complications are those that occur during the first few weeks after treatment of the fracture. The most common early complication is CSF leak. If the decision is made to manage a CSF leak conservatively, a lumbar drain is placed and the patient is put on bed rest. The use of antibiotics is controversial in this setting.[28,29] Antibiotics are usually administered prophylactically if a lumbar drain is in place and there are other independent reasons for their administration.[25]

Meningitis is another early complication related to nasofrontal injuries.[25] Patients with these types of injuries often have concomitant neurologic injuries that result in decreased levels of consciousness. This can be problematic in the setting of meningitis because the early manifestations of meningitis are often changes in mental status. Thus, a suspected case of meningitis must be recognized early and patients who develop signs or symptoms suggestive of meningitis should undergo immediate lumbar puncture to ensure a prompt diagnosis is made and appropriate antibiotics initiated. If meningitis is not recognized, the outcome can be fatal.

Other minor early complications include diplopia and anesthesia of the skin overlying the frontal sinus. These are usually related to surgical access and are transient.

Late complications may present at any point after treatment of a frontal sinus fracture. These include mucoceles, mucopyoceles, brain abscesses, frontal bone osteomyelitis, chronic frontal headaches, and cosmetic deformities.[25]

A mucocele is an expansile lesion of the sinus that becomes filled with fluid being produced from remnants of the respiratory epithelial lining of the sinus. They enlarge progressively as a result of blockage of the NFOT and may cause significant local bone expansion and resorption. If a mucocele becomes secondarily infected it is termed a mucopyocele. These may develop several years after the injury and as such, patients should be placed on close long-term follow-up. The signs and symptoms of a mucocele or mucopyocele include frontal headaches, fullness in the forehead and upper eyelid region, diplopia, proptosis, nasal discharge, and obstruction.[24] If the posterior table is resorbed by a mucocele or mucopyocele, they may develop direct communication with the epidural and intracerebral space. If they result in resorption of the floor of the sinus they often cause ocular symptoms. Both are treated surgically. Depending on their size, this may be done endoscopically if they are small or by an open approach if they become large.

Osteomyelitis of the frontal bone is another uncommon late complication of frontal sinus fractures. This normally results because of direct extension of infection from the frontal sinus into the surrounding marrow space, or even by way of the valveless diploic venous system.[24] Finally, a pericranial abscess, or Pott puffy tumor, is often associated with frontal bone obliteration or cranialization of the frontal sinus.[24]

Other articles in this issue discuss management of several other late complications of fractures in this area. It is important to remember that, as with most facial fractures, complications, be they malpositions (ie, malreductions) or otherwise, are easier to deal with sooner rather than later. With this in mind, regular follow-up every week or two for the first 6 weeks is appropriate so as to intercept any problems early.

REFERENCES

1. Nakhgevany KB, LiBassi M, Esposito B. Facial trauma in motor vehicle accidents: etiological factors. Am J Emerg Med 1994;12:160–3.
2. McMullin BT, Rhee JS, Pintar FA, et al. Facial fractures in motor vehicle collisions: epidemiological trends and risk factors. Arch Facial Plast Surg 2009;11:165–70.
3. Dept of Transportation (US), National Highway Traffic Safety Administration (NHTSA). Traffic safety facts: seat belt use in 2010—Overall results. Washington, DC: NHTSA; 2010. Available at: http://www-nrd.nhtsa.dot.gov/Pubs/811378.pdf. Accessed August, 2012.
4. Yavuzer R, Sari A, Kelly C, et al. Management of frontal sinus fractures. Plast Reconstr Surg 2005; 115:79e–93e.
5. Doonquah L, Brown P, Mullings W. Management of frontal sinus fractures. Oral Maxillofac Surg Clin North Am 2012;24:265–74.
6. McLaughlin RB Jr, Rehl RM, Lanza DC. Clinically relevant frontal sinus anatomy and physiology. Otolaryngol Clin North Am 2001;34:1–22.
7. Williams PL, Warwick R, Dyson M, et al, editors. Gray's anatomy. 37th edition. New York: Churchill Livingstone; 1989.

8. Miller AJ, Amedee RG. Functional anatomy of the paranasal sinuses. J La State Med Soc 1997;149: 85–90.

9. Potter JK, Muzaffar AR, Ellis E, et al. Aesthetic management of the nasal component of naso-orbital ethmoid fractures. Plast Reconstr Surg 2006;117: 10e–8e.

10. Jiminez DF, Sundrani S, Barone CM. Posttraumatic anosmia in craniofacial trauma. J Craniomaxillofac Trauma 1997;3:8–15.

11. Moriyama H, Nakajima T, Honda Y. Studies on mucoceles of the ethmoid and sphenoid sinuses: analysis of 47 cases. J Laryngol Otol 1992;106:23–7.

12. Grigoriu V, Stefaniu A. Post-traumatic bilateral naso-ethmoidal mucocele. Rev Chir Oncol Radiol O R L Oftalmol Stomatol Otorinolaringol 1981;26: 309–12.

13. Laure B, Arsene S, Santallier M, et al. Post-traumatic disinsertion of the superior oblique muscle trochlea. Rev Stomatol Chir Maxillofac 2007;108:551–4.

14. Harish AY, Ganesh SC, Narendran K. Traumatic superior oblique tendon rupture. J AAPOS 2009; 13:485–7.

15. Seo IH, Rhim JW, Suh YW, et al. A case of acquired Brown syndrome after surgical repair of a medial orbital wall fracture. Korean J Ophthalmol 2010;24: 53–6.

16. Sydnor CF, Seaber JH, Buckley EG. Traumatic superior oblique palsies. Ophthalmology 1982;89: 134–8.

17. Ali MJ, Gupta H, Honavar SG, et al. Acquired nasolacrimal duct obstructions secondary to naso-orbital-ethmoidal fractures: patterns and outcomes. Ophthal Plast Reconstr Surg 2012;28:242–5.

18. Becelli R, Renzi G, Mannino G, et al. Posttraumatic obstruction of lacrimal pathways: a retrospective analysis of 58 consecutive naso-orbito-ethmoid fractures. J Craniofac Surg 2004;15:29–33.

19. Ritleng P, Bourgeon A, Richelme H. New concepts of the anatomy of the lacrimal apparatus. Anat Clin 1983;5:29–34.

20. Poh E, Kakizaki H, Selva D, et al. Anatomy of the medial canthal tendon in caucasians. Clin Experiment Ophthalmol 2012;40:170–3.

21. Markowitz BL, Manson PN, Sargent L, et al. Management of the medial canthal tendon in nasoethmoid orbital fractures: the importance of the central fragment in classification and treatment. Plast Reconstr Surg 1991;87:843–53.

22. Winkler A, Smith T, Meyer T, et al. The management of frontal sinus fractures. In: Rhinologic and sleep apnea surgical techniques. New York: Springer; p. 149–58.

23. Gerbino G, Roccia F, Benech A, et al. Analysis of 158 frontal sinus fractures: current surgical management and complications. J Craniomaxillofac Surg 2000;28:133–9.

24. Lee TT, Ratzker PA, Galarza M, et al. Early combined management of frontal sinus and orbital and facial fractures. J Trauma 1998;44:665–9.

25. Manolidis S, Hollier LH Jr. Management of frontal sinus fractures. Plast Reconstr Surg 2007; 120(Suppl 2):32S–48S.

26. Sargent L. Nasoethmoid orbital fractures: diagnosis and management. Plast Reconstr Surg 2007; 120(Suppl 2):16S–31S.

27. Sawatari Y, Caceres J. Frontal sinus fractures. In: Bagheri SC, Bell RB, Khan HA, editors. Current therapy in oral and maxillofacial surgery. Chicago: Elsevier Saunders; 2012. p. 346–53.

28. Kaufman BA, Tunkel AR, Pryor JC, et al. Meningitis in the neurosurgical patient. Infect Dis Clin North Am 1990;4:677–701.

29. Mollman HD, Haines SJ. Risk factors for postoperative neurosurgical wound infection: a case-control study. J Neurosurg 1986;64:902–6.

Panfacial Fractures
An Approach to Management

William Curtis, MD, DMD, Bruce B. Horswell, MD, DDS, MS*

KEYWORDS

- Panfacial fracture • Injury • Reconstruction • Treatment

KEY POINTS

- Reestablishing proper vertical columns and anterior facial projections at skeletal supports through anatomic reduction and rigid fixation with possible grafts are essential to optimal treatment.
- The approach to facial fracture reconstruction should focus on reestablishing proper occlusal, vertical, and horizontal relationships in the facial frame as well as restoration of orbital, oral, and nasal cavities/volume.
- Time and detail should be devoted to nasal projection and patency, as well as facial soft tissue support and resuspension.

INTRODUCTION

Panfacial fractures are defined as fractures involving the lower, middle, and upper face. Treatment can be challenging and requires an individualized treatment plan. A firm understanding of the treatment principles of each individual fracture is necessary before attempting to tackle the patient with panfacial fractures. Historically, these fractures were treated conservatively, which led to significant postoperative problems, including crippling malocclusion, significant increase in facial width, and decreased facial projection.[1] Secondary deformities that were surgically addressed were and still remain extremely difficult to correct. Advances in rigid fixation, wide exposure, primary bone grafting, and attention to soft tissue reattachment have significantly improved the treatment of the patient with panfacial fractures.

EPIDEMIOLOGY

Panfacial fractures are caused by impact from high-energy mechanisms and have characteristics beyond that seen in more common isolated facial fractures.[2,3] Such high-energy forces directed at the craniofacial region result in secondary vectors of injury or contre-coup forces, which necessitate a high degree of suspicion for other injuries. Features of panfacial fractures include the following[2–5]:

- Most frequently caused by motor vehicle collisions and gunshot wounds
- Approximately 4% to 10% of all facial fractures
- 80% have condylar neck or intracapsular fractures
- More likely to involve comminuted and avulsed segments
- Lower Glasgow Coma Scale score (average GCS 10)
- Higher hospital complication rate (18%)
- 20% chance of cervical spine injuries

SUPPORT STRUCTURE OF THE FACIAL SKELETON

The face is made up of vertical and horizontal buttresses (**Fig. 1**) where bone is thicker to neutralize

Disclosures: The authors have nothing to disclose.
FACES, Women and Children's Hospital, 830 Pennsylvania, Charleston, WV 25302, USA
* Corresponding author.
E-mail address: bruce.horswell@camc.org

Oral Maxillofacial Surg Clin N Am 25 (2013) 649–660
http://dx.doi.org/10.1016/j.coms.2013.07.010
1042-3699/13/$ – see front matter © 2013 Elsevier Inc. All rights reserved.

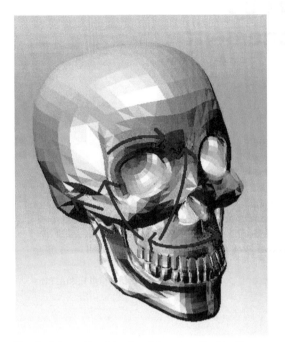

Fig. 1. Schematic of horizontal and vertical buttresses and the vectors (*arrows*) of support and resistance of the skeletal frame. (*From* Herford AS. Pan-facial trauma. In: Bagheri SC, Bell RB, Khan HA, editors. Current therapy in oral and maxillofacial surgery. Philadelphia: Saunders; 2012. p. 355; with permission.)

forces applied to it.[6,7] Reduction and fixation of these key areas are the basis of maxillofacial reconstruction. Key features or purposes of these buttresses include the following[6–9]:

- Maintain projection and protection of the airway
- Provide for anchoring suspension of the muscular-aponeurotic system, which is under constant function
- House and protect key functional units
  - Anterior brain
  - Eye and visual pathways
  - Neurovascular passages
  - Oral-pharyngeal mechanisms for speech, chewing, and swallowing
- Facial buttresses must be adequately reduced to restore height, width, and projection
- Vertical buttresses include the nasomaxillary, zygomaticomaxillary, pterygomaxillary, and the condyle and posterior mandible.
  - The pterygomaxillary buttress is not usually repaired due to difficulty of access
- Horizontal buttresses include the frontal, zygomatic, maxillary, and mandibular
- The central mid face is weak in horizontal buttress support and especially prone to decreased projection after injury (**Fig. 2**).

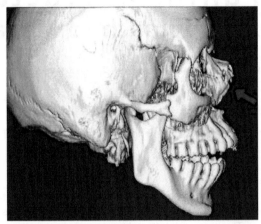

Fig. 2. CT 3D of panfacial fractures demonstrating the force of injury resulting in midfacial impaction in a superoposterior vector (*arrow*).

INITIAL EVALUATION

A thorough evaluation of the patient with panfacial fractures is invaluable. It is easy for the novice clinician to be overwhelmed by distracting injuries and neglect the basics of a physical examination. The examination should focus on stabilizing the patient by securing the airway if necessary, management of bleeding, and prompt consultation with other specialists. Many times a thorough examination is not possible because of intubation, cervical collar, or patient cooperation. Sequential examinations may be necessary as the patient progresses to avoid missed injuries. Refer to **Figs. 3–5** for examples of panfacial injuries with extensive soft tissue disruption over open fractures, airway, and bleeding considerations. Each case requires prompt attention to the following critical points in assessment and early management.

- Airway

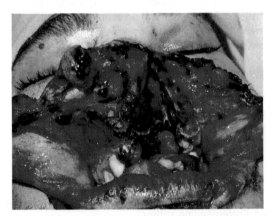

Fig. 3. Blast injury with extensive soft tissue loss and open midfacial fractures and attendant posterior hemorrhage requiring interventional embolotherapy.

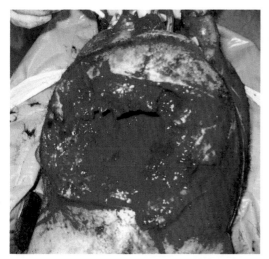

Fig. 4. Gunshot wound with avulsion of the submental tissues and tongue with exposed, comminuted bone and loss of airway support and patency.

Many times a patient may be brought to the trauma bay with an unsecured airway. Factors that should be considered for airway placement involve severe comminution of the mandible, neurologic compromise, and significant mid-face bleeding. In severe cases an emergent surgical airway may be necessary; however, an oral intubation can typically be performed without complication. In most cases an oral tube will have to be exchanged at the time of surgery to facilitate the management of panfacial fractures (see **Fig. 5**). The submental pull-through technique can be used to facilitate fixation while avoiding the

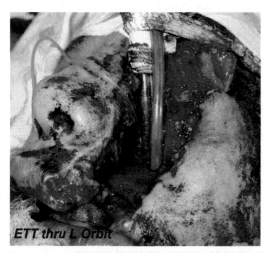

ETT thru L Orbit

Fig. 5. An avulsive panfacial injury with endotracheal tube exiting through the shattered orbit, which should be secured inferiorly and a more stable airway provided with tracheotomy.

placement of a tracheotomy.[10] An algorithm to help decide airway management is provided in **Fig. 6**.

- Bleeding

Common sites of troublesome bleeding include tongue, scalp, and mid face/nose. Arterial bleeders need to be identified and controlled. Temporary tacking sutures can be placed to aid with hemostasis, especially in large scalp wounds. Nasal passages may need to be packed with bilateral Foley catheters and intranasal gauze to tamponade the area of hemorrhage (**Fig. 7**).

- Specialist consultation

Prompt recognition of injuries that may require emergent treatment is essential. Depending on the comfort level of the surgeon, various consultations may be obtained. A list of important structures to focus on during the initial evaluation as well as related consultations is shown in **Fig. 8**.

RECONSTRUCTION—PRINCIPLES

- Prioritize function and preservation of brain, vision, hearing
- Open mandible fractures should be stabilized as soon as possible for osseous health
- Support framework until final reconstruction can take place
- Preserve integrity and health of overlying soft tissue and subunits
  - Neurovascular and ductal elements
  - Cranial nerves
  - Lacrimal system
- Fracture planning
- Grafting (augment support system)
- Final soft tissue reconstruction

SEQUENCING—PRINCIPLES

Historically and traditionally oral and maxillofacial surgeons have been comfortable starting with the occlusal unit, this owing to their base in dentistry. As a starting point, establishing occlusal integrity and stability provides for some initial horizontal and vertical relationship from which other related units may be established. Many oral and maxillofacial surgeons can recall past interactions with surgical colleagues in other disciplines who ask for help in this area of dental expertise or fabrication of dental casts and splints that the oral and maxillofacial surgeon would then apply under curious gaze. For many who treat panfacial fractures, starting "low" at the maxillary-mandibular unit is one of experience and comfort from which treatment progresses superiorly.[11]

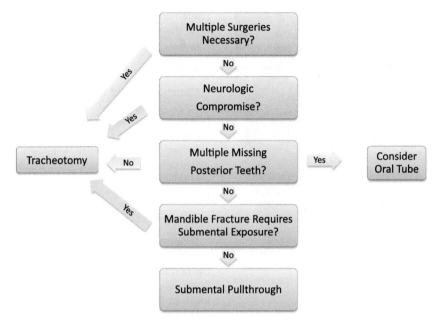

Fig. 6. Airway decision-making in panfacial fractures.

Although a "bottom-up" approach may be preferred, many surgeons prefer a "top-down" approach and achieve very satisfactory results with this alternative algorithm, provided the occlusion has been restored (please refer to **Figs. 9–12** for a representation of this systematic approach).

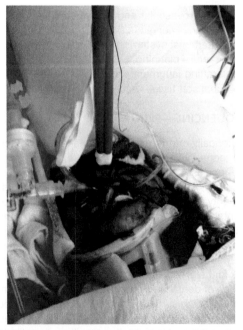

Fig. 7. Placement of Foley catheters in nasal passageways with intranasal gauze packing to control severe posterior midfacial hemorrhaging.

This latter approach uses a stable fronto-orbital frame from which to proceed inferiorly and outside-in. The vertical pillars at the naso-frontal region and the lateral orbital rims further provide for proper horizontal projection and stability of the orbital frame and other related mid-facial units. The main argument in favor of a "top-down" approach is the ability to avoid opening and fixating condylar fractures.[12,13] When addressing the mid and upper face (whether it is done before or after the mandible), the prudent surgeon is able to adjust to the individual variances of each fracture rather than stick dogmatically to one treatment algorithm. Working from a "known" or stable area (less displacement or comminution) and proceeding to an "unknown" area can make proper reduction more manageable and achievable.

In areas of comminution that involve important structures and buttresses, primary bone grafting has been shown to help with osseous union, re-establishment of buttresses, and preservation of the soft tissue drape.[6,7,14] Orbital volume compromise from comminution of the thin walls and loss of support frames at the rims and lateral wall require focused reduction and fixation or augmentation with bone grafts.[15] Similarly, comminution at the zygomatic-maxillary buttress and fronto-nasal-maxillary column requires restoration, often with grafting if bony fragments are too small or avulsed to achieve structural integrity.

The authors' preferred approach for treatment of panfacial fractures is presented in **Fig. 13**. The reader is referred to the other articles in this *Oral*

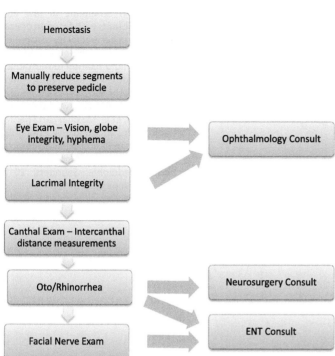

Fig. 8. Order of priority evaluations and attendant consultations for panfacial injuries.

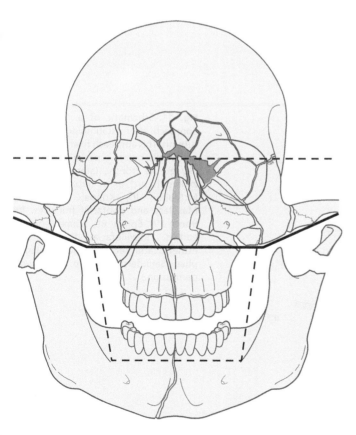

Fig. 9. Schematic of panfacial fractures with separation into units and subunits of focus and reconstruction. (*From* Holland IS, McMahon JD, Koppel DA, et al. Maxillary and panfacial fractures. In: Booth PW, Eppley BL, Schmelzeisen R, editors. Maxillofacial trauma and esthetic facial reconstruction. Philadelphia: Saunders; 2012. p. 237; with permission.)

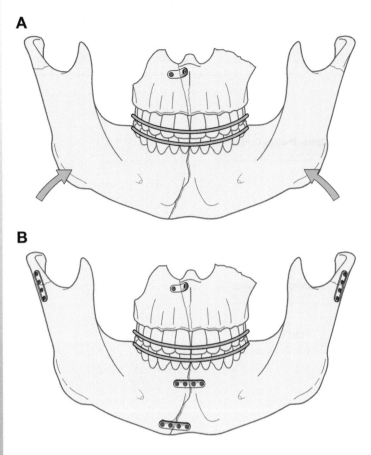

Fig. 10. (*A*) Schematic of jaw and occlusal subunits with focus on diastasis reduction via medial forces applied at the mandibular angle and body (*arrows*). (*B*) Rigid fixation to reestablish proper width and arch relationships and vertical (condylar-ramal) height. (*From* Holland IS, McMahon JD, Koppel DA, et al. Maxillary and panfacial fractures. In: Booth PW, Eppley BL, Schmelzeisen R, editors. Maxillofacial trauma and esthetic facial reconstruction. Philadelphia: Saunders; 2012. p. 237; with permission.)

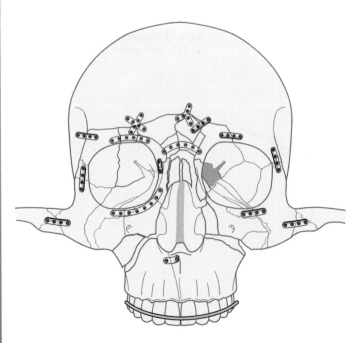

Fig. 11. Schematic of a "top-down" approach after establishing the lower subunit. This approach fixates to known and stable points superiorly and laterally at the frontal, lateral orbit, and zygomatic arch areas. (*From* Holland IS, McMahon JD, Koppel DA, et al. Maxillary and panfacial fractures. In: Booth PW, Eppley BL, Schmelzeisen R, editors. Maxillofacial trauma and esthetic facial reconstruction. Philadelphia: Saunders; 2012. p. 238; with permission.)

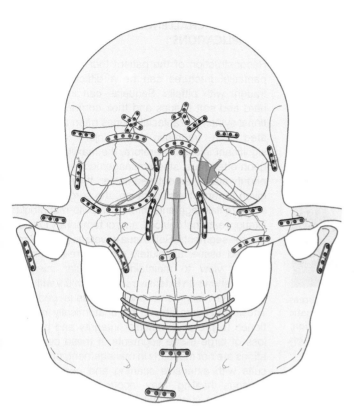

Fig. 12. Schematic of final panfacial fracture fixation with orbital volume and nasal projection restored with grafts. (*From* Holland IS, McMahon JD, Koppel DA, et al. Maxillary and panfacial fractures. In: Booth PW, Eppley BL, Schmelzeisen R, editors. Maxillofacial trauma and esthetic facial reconstruction. Philadelphia: Saunders; 2012. p. 239; with permission.)

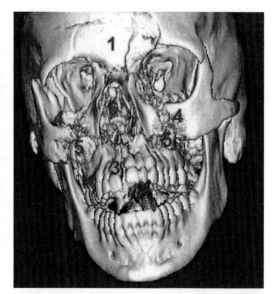

Fig. 13. CT 3D of panfacial fractures showing stepwise planning for reduction, fixation, and reconstruction in a "top-down" manner. 1, frontal-supraorbital rim; 2, lateral orbit and zygoma; 3, maxillary diastasis and establish occlusion; 4, orbital rims and walls; 5, zygomatic buttress and grafts; 6, nasal projection.

and Maxillofacial Surgery Clinics of North America for details on treatment of isolated facial fractures. To summarize, the approach to sequencing fracture reduction and fixation is to establish support from known to unknown, and to accomplish stability with rigidity and grafts. Any questionable or "insufficient" fracture reduction and stability, including correct occlusion, will invite discrepancy and error elsewhere in the adjacent skeleton with subsequent late deformity and dysfunction. **Fig. 14** identifies those key areas of injury that need to be addressed to obtain a predictable, stable, and satisfactory result. What follows is a systematic outline to panfacial fracture reconstruction.

A. Panfacial fractures—all or most levels of the facial skeleton
B. Mandible
    a. Placement in maxillo-mandibular fixation (fixate midline fracture in maxilla or model surgery and splints)
    b. Fixation of condylar region
       • Unilateral if significant displacement
       • Bilateral fractures and need for vertical reference
    c. Fixation of symphysis and body fractures
       • Splayed fractures require firm medialized reduction

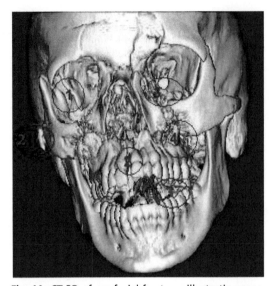

Fig. 14. CT 3D of panfacial fractures illustrating areas of priority focus for stabilization. 1, sphenozygomatic suture diastasis; 2, maxillary diastasis with separation; 3, orbital frame and volume disruption; 4, buttress comminution and disruption.

C. Zygomas and maxilla
   a. May require bone grafting to re-create buttresses
   b. Confirm correct vertical and horizontal restoration
D. Reconstruction of upper mid face (see **Fig. 2**, which illustrates superior-posterior impaction of the mid face requiring complete disimpaction for reduction)
   a. Orbital rim fixation (critical focus on inferior and lateral rim reduction and form)
     • Vertical supports and horizontal frames
     • Volume restoration with attendant wall reconstruction
   b. Nasal-orbital-ethmoid complex
     • Must have firm anterior support at the frontal region
     • Medial reduction if telecanthus is present (overcorrection?)
     • Often requires grafts
   c. Establishment and maintenance of nasal patency particularly if concomitant soft tissue and cartilaginous disruption
E. Implants and augmentation
   a. Orbital floor/wall implants
     • Porous polyethylene
     • Split calvarial grafts
   b. Nasal dorsal onlay grafting
     • Graft sources—calvarium, rib, alloplasts
   c. Other onlay grafts (malar eminence, frontal bar)
F. Soft tissue supports

COMMON CHALLENGES AND COMPLICATIONS

Reconstruction of the patient that has sustained panfacial fractures can be a difficult endeavor fraught with pitfalls. Sequelae can involve both hard and soft tissues and their component functional systems. Panfacial injuries often are associated with traumatic brain injury and other significant injuries; therefore, the maxillofacial surgeon often must stage management according to priority status, as outlined earlier. If limitations are given for anesthetic duration, the surgeon should stabilize flail segments through maxillo-mandibular fixation, external devices, and/or temporary fixation of large segments. Soft tissue envelope (particularly avulsed tissue) absolutely requires re-placement with a view to maintaining vascular integrity. **Fig. 15** shows an extensive panfacial injury with displaced jaw segments and soft tissue pedicles. These segments should be anatomically repositioned to preserve vascular integrity and prevent loss of large tissue segments. If these considerations are not met early in management, poorer results with extensive scarring and compromised osseous healing may occur. Furthermore, a cascade of suboptimal healing events in bone, cartilage, skin, and other specialized tissues (nerves, eyelids, ears, nose) can make future attempts at restoration very difficult, if not achievable. Bedside procedures in the surgical intensive care unit/trauma ward can be undertaken to optimize tissue health while patient stabilization is underway.

HARD TISSUE CONSIDERATIONS

Superoposteriorly rotated and impacted mid-facial fractures (see **Fig. 2**) can be difficult to mobilize, which requires firm and controlled disimpaction with forceps. During disimpaction, profuse

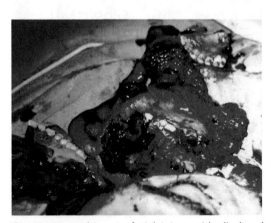

Fig. 15. An avulsive panfacial injury with displaced segments.

bleeding can be encountered by the surgeon from posterior areas of the internal maxillary artery distribution and venous plexus. Impaction may have temporarily achieved occlusion of these vascular entities but during mobilization they may be opened or further torn, resulting in brisk hemorrhage. For this reason it is important to correct any coagulopathies before surgery.

Inadequate reduction and fixation can lead to problems with facial width, height, and projection.[16,17] Common problematic sites and techniques to avoid or address them are presented in **Tables 1** and **2**. Functional cavities also need to be addressed and restored to their preoperative volume. The 3 functional areas potentially altered in panfacial injury are the orbit, oral, and nasal cavities.

Orbit

Orbital volume, if not properly restored early in reconstructive management, can be a very difficult problem to manage after healing. Some surgeons think that late enophthalmos is a nearly impossible condition to treat successfully.[15] Volumetric analysis through computed tomographic (CT) planning is possible if there is unilateral injury and a mirror image established through stereotactic means.[18] Bilateral volume loss will necessitate critical focus on orbital frame reduction and reestablishing the superolateral orbital walls if involved. From these stable points, one can proceed more reliably to the inferior and medial orbital walls. Calvarial bone grafts, as shown in **Fig. 16**, are an excellent choice for restoring orbital wall integrity if the contour can be managed. It is important to be aware of ocular pressure during and after volume restoration.

Oral

The oral cavity is often neglected as a functional unit in panfacial injury. Both vertical loss of the posterior mandible and maxilla and anterior underprojection of the maxillary-mandibular complex can adversely impact speech and swallowing. The posteriorly displaced complex can also push the tongue retrograde with resultant altered breathing. Significant or avulsive injuries to the tongue, lips, cheeks, and palate contribute to hurdles in achieving pretraumatic speech and swallowing mechanisms, in turn decreasing patient quality of life.[19]

Nasal

Nasal patency goes hand in hand with nasal projection. Nasal passage patency depends on properly positioned vertical and horizontal supports at the nasofrontal unit and septal stability. Cartilaginous resuspension, if disrupted, requires direct suturing to stable nasal bones and/or support via dorsal bolsters and splints. Frequently, dorsal grafting is necessary to preserve projection and attendant patency (**Fig. 17**). Inward displacement of comminuted piriform and nasal bones can reduce patency and also interfere with physiologic nasal airflow. If the septum is displaced, then rigid stents should be placed for 2 weeks to provide vertical support, prevent hematoma formation, and provide support to shredded mucosa.

SOFT TISSUE CONSIDERATIONS

Although the importance of a stable base in facial reconstruction cannot be understated, the soft tissue envelope must be given adequate attention to avoid disappointing results. Whenever wide

Table 1
Problems and solutions in panfacial fractures: projection and height issues

Bone	Problem Encountered	Approach or Solution
Frontal	Supraorbital comminution and postoperative flattening	May need primary bone grafting
Nasal-orbital-ethmoid	Comminution due to lack of buttressing	Primary bone graft with nasal strut of calvarium or rib
Zygomatic arch	Postoperative lateral displacement ("bowing") under function after fixation	Heavier plating to support and withstand the forces of mastication
Zygomatic-maxillary	Buttress collapse	Primary bone grafting
Maxilla/mandible	Malocclusion (anterior open bite) due to posterior mandibular foreshortening and elongation of posterior maxilla	• Ensure condylar-ramal proportions and stability • Adequate maxillary disimpaction before fixation

Table 2
Problems and solutions in panfacial fractures: facial width issues

Bone	Problem Encountered	Approach or Solution
Mandible	Splaying of the lingual cortex at the symphysis and ramal region	Exposure of inferior border to visualize lingual cortex with medializing force applied at the angles
Maxilla	Comminuted maxilla or multiple dento-alveolar segments	• Plating the palate or diastasis directly • Model surgery and fabrication of a surgical splint
Zygoma	Improper reduction (medial or lateral displacement)	Visualization and fixation at fronto-zygomatic and/or spheno-zygomatic sutures
Nasal-orbital-ethmoid	Telecanthus or widened nasal roof	Transnasal wiring and medial canthopexy or fixation of canthal-bearing fragments if large enough

exposure is obtained, as is frequently necessary in panfacial fracture treatment, soft tissue sagging is possible and will result if resuspension is not performed.[9,20] If possible, limiting exposure and extent of dissection to fractured elements can help prevent some soft tissue sagging. **Fig. 18** demonstrates wide dissection of a comminuted left zygomatic-maxillary complex and orbital floor for access to fractures. Suspension of the lower eyelid with canthopexy and the malar fat pad is important to avoid lid laxity/incompetence and cheek sagging. This is more easily achieved in the recently fractured patient when reduction is easier. Reapproximation of periosteum and resuspension of the musculo-aponeurotic envelope are critical to restoration of form and function after injury. Some areas of the face are more prone to inadequate soft tissue resuspension—these are the lower eyelids and the malar soft tissue pad and to a lesser extent the oral musculature.[21]

It has been shown that suspensory fascial ligaments exist in the face (zygomatic, masseteric, and mandibular slings) that add significant support to the superficial muscular aponeurotic system.[8] Following are important areas at which to obtain deep closure and resuspension.

- Orbital rim
  - Every effort should be made to reapproximate the periosteum
  - Resuspension is indicated if periosteum cannot be closed
- Lateral canthus
  - Downslanting palpebral fissures with incompetence and epiphora can occur without resuspension after wide periorbital dissection

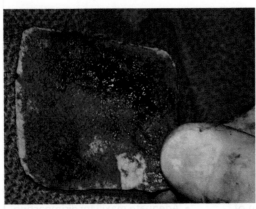

Fig. 16. A calvarial graft to restore an entire orbital floor.

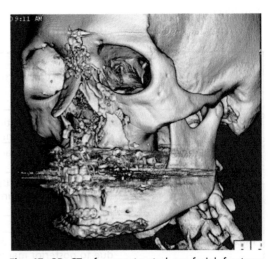

Fig. 17. 3D CT of reconstructed panfacial fractures with calvarial graft to restore the nasal profile and projection.

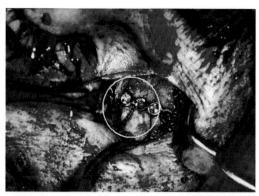

Fig. 18. Left zygomatic-maxillary complex with rigid fixation after wide dissection to the orbital floor, lateral rim, and zygoma. Resuspension of the eyelid and malar fat pad (white circle, with attendant musculo-aponeurosis) is necessary to prevent ptosis and sagging.

- If canthotomy is performed, the lower tarsus should be dissected and attached directly to the lateral orbital rim in a slightly superior position
- Malar eminence
  - Point of attachment of the zygomatic ligament
  - If not fractured, should avoid stripping
  - If stripped, it can be resuspended to the deep temporal fascia lateral to the fronto-zygomatic suture or to the bone directly
- Mentalis
  - The mentalis periosteal-muscle margin must be reattached
  - Chin support dressings can be used in the perioperative period
- Deep temporal fascia
  - Temporal hollowing can occur if the temporal fat pad is violated or the muscle is not repositioned properly resulting in muscle prolapse
  - Every effort should be made to resuspend (even overcorrect) the deep temporal fascia with direct suturing or suspension slings

SOFT TISSUE AUGMENTATION

Soft tissue augmentation is often necessary to lend support to either extensively stripped or avulsed soft tissue, or where loss of bulk may be anticipated. Depending on the nature of the initial injury, contracture and unsightly scarring, prolapsed tissue, asymmetry, and poor function of soft tissue subunits may be anticipated. After the facial skeleton, which serves as an important foundation to overlying and housed soft tissue, precise attention must be turned to the accompanying soft tissue. These areas are outlined above in the text

in terms of criticality for repositioning and resuspension of the soft tissue. If there has been true loss of tissue or resuspension is suspect, there are several tissue sources available to assist in contour and support measures.

- Acellular dermis
- Fascia
- Fat

Acellular dermis (human skin allograft) is available in various thicknesses and sizes and affords a good way to provide temporary dermal coverage or augment the subcutaneous tissues in the event of tissue loss. By so doing, the surgeon may achieve a more normal postoperative contour and avoid excessive scarring of the overlying skin to deeper tissues or bone. Acellular dermis or fascial strips harvested from the temporalis or lateral thigh can also be used as suspensory ligament bolsters in the oral commissure or malar area in the event of avulsion or shredding of the attendant musculo-aponeurosis. Placement at the time of injury provides a key support to these tissues and may avoid late cicatrization and accompanying dysfunction.

Harvested fat can be placed as an injectable or dermal-fat graft to achieve facial form and contour where tissue has been lost, particularly over the malar eminence. Pericranial pedicled flaps can be placed over comminuted nasofrontal bone or grafted defects to provide vascularity and improved contour. These free grafts cannot be expected to replace missing hard tissue and they should not be placed over bone with questionable viability as such osseous tissue requires an established viable tissue envelope to ensure survival. Finally, for intraoral defects the buccal fat graft is an excellent local source for augmentation and protection of exposed palatal bone or defects.

SUMMARY

Panfacial fractures are challenging because of the association of concomitant injuries, increased patient morbidity, and functional impairment often accompanying these injuries. Management must focus on prompt and thorough evaluation, prioritizing treatment (often staged) to preserve function and tissue viability, and providing for support to fractures if reduction and fixation cannot be achieved quickly. A systematic approach to planning and carrying out that plan for facial fracture reconstruction will involve focus on reestablishing proper occlusal, vertical and horizontal relationships in the facial frame, as well as restoration of orbital, oral, and nasal cavities/volume. Last, detail and time given to soft tissue resuspension and augmentation will help achieve a lasting and satisfying result after a devastating facial injury.

REFERENCES

1. He D, Zhang Y, Ellis E. Panfacial fractures: analysis of 33 cases treated late. J Oral Maxillofac Surg 2007;65:2459–65.
2. Follmar KE, Debruijn M, Baccarani A, et al. Concomitant injuries in patients with panfacial fractures. J Trauma 2007;63(4):831–5.
3. Erdmann D, Follmar KE, Debruijn M, et al. A retrospective analysis of facial fracture etiologies. Ann Plast Surg 2008;60(4):398–403.
4. Stacey D, Doyle J, Gutowski K. Safety device use affects the incidence patterns of facial trauma in motor vehicle collisions: an analysis of the national trauma database from 2000 to 2004. Plast Reconstr Surg 2008;121(6):2057–64.
5. Yang R, Zhang C, Liu Y, et al. Why should we start from mandibular fractures in the treatment of panfacial fractures? J Oral Maxillofac Surg 2012;70:1386–92.
6. Gruss J, Mackinnon S. Complex maxillary fractures: role of buttress reconstruction and immediate bone grafts. Plast Reconstr Surg 1986;78:9.
7. Gruss J, Phillips J. Complex facial trauma: the evolving role of rigid fixation and immediate bone graft reconstruction. Clin Plast Surg 1989;16:93.
8. Moss C, Mendelson B, Taylor G. Surgical anatomy of the ligamentous attachments in the temple and periorbital regions. Plast Reconstr Surg 2000;105(4): 1475–90.
9. Manson P, Clark N, Robertson B, et al. Subunit principles in midface fractures: the importance of sagittal buttresses, soft-tissue reductions, and sequencing treatment of segmental fractures. Plast Reconstr Surg 1999;103:1287–307.
10. Altemir F. The submental route for endotracheal intubation: a new technique. J Maxillofac Surg 1986;14:64.
11. Tullio A, Sesenna E. Role of surgical reduction of condylar fractures in the management of panfacial fractures. Br J Oral Maxillofac Surg 2000;38:472.
12. Markowitz B, Manson P. Panfacial fractures: organization of treatment. Clin Plast Surg 1989;16:105.
13. Kelly K, Manson P, Van der Kolk C, et al. Sequencing Le Fort fracture treatment. J Craniofac Surg 1990;1:168.
14. Manson P, Crawley W. Midface fractures: advantages of immediate extended open reduction and bone grafting. Plast Reconstr Surg 1985;76(1):1–12.
15. Grant M, Iliff N, Manson P. Strategies for the treatment of enophthalmos. Clin Plast Surg 1997;24(3): 539–50.
16. Ellis E, Tharanon W. Facial width problems associated with rigid fixation of mandibular fractures: case reports. J Oral Maxillofac Surg 1992;50:87.
17. Gruss J, Wyck L, Phillips J, et al. The importance of the zygomatic arch in complex midfacial fracture repair and correction of posttraumatic orbitozygomatic deformities. Plast Reconstr Surg 1990;85:878.
18. Collyer J. Stereotactic navigation in oral and maxillofacial surgery. Br J Oral Maxillofac Surg 2010;48(2): 79–83.
19. Niezen E, Bos R, de Bont L, et al. Complaints related to mandibular fuction impairment after closed treatment of fractures of the mandibular condyle. Int J Oral Maxillofac Surg 2010;39(7):660–5.
20. Gruss J, Antonyshyn O, Phillips J. Early definitive bone and soft-tissue reconstruction of major gunshot wounds of the face. Plast Reconstr Surg 1991;87(3):436–50.
21. Phillips J, Gruss J, Wells M, et al. Periosteal suspension of the lower eyelid and cheek following subciliary exposure of facial fractures. Plast Reconstr Surg 1991;88(1):145–8.

Late Reconstruction of Condylar Neck and Head Fractures

Ben Davis, DDS, Dip OMFS and Anesthesia, FRCD

KEYWORDS

- Condyle fracture • Complication • Reconstruction • Costochondral graft • Total joint prosthesis

KEY POINTS

- Condyle fractures are a common injury, but only a few of these injuries require immediate or late reconstruction.
- The complications that most frequently necessitate condylar reconstruction include proximal segment degeneration, malunion, and ankylosis.
- Costochondral grafts and total joint prostheses, both stock and custom, remain the most common methods of reconstruction.
- Reconstruction plates with condylar extensions should only be used temporarily as an unacceptable number cause serious complications.
- Distraction osteogenesis may have an occasional role in reconstructing the posttraumatic condyle.

INTRODUCTION

Because of their location and comparatively small cross-sectional volume, fractures of the mandibular condyle are among the most common maxillofacial injuries, and their management still elicits passionate debate. This debate is largely the result of the complex anatomy of the area, making access challenging and because different treatment options provide seemingly similar results. Nevertheless, it is important to continually scrutinize our outcomes to ensure that we are providing a high standard of care and minimizing complications. When discussing the outcomes of condylar fracture management, many areas need to be assessed (**Box 1**). Although the list is not exhaustive, it does show the need for careful, long-term clinical and radiographic follow-up in order to be able to assess outcomes.

Complications after condyle fractures (**Box 2**) can be the result of misdiagnosis or inadequate management. However, they can occur even when appropriate treatment has been rendered. Although uncommon, these complications can result in the loss of the condyle and damage to the glenoid fossa. The need to partially or completely reconstruct the temporomandibular joint (TMJ) after trauma represents significant morbidity to the patient and cost to the health care system and every attempt should be made to minimize this occurrence.

INCIDENCE OF RECONSTRUCTION AFTER CONDYLE FRACTURES

At our quaternary-care, level-I trauma center, approximately 30% of patients presenting with facial fractures have at least 1 condyle fracture, with the most common cause being interpersonal violence. Isolated and bilateral condyle fractures are less common than a single condyle fracture in combination with a second fracture of the mandible. Although controversy still exists regarding the appropriate management of condyle

Disclosures: The author has nothing to disclose.
Department of Oral and Maxillofacial Sciences, Dalhousie University, Halifax, NS B3H 1W2, Canada
E-mail address: bdavis@dal.ca

Oral Maxillofacial Surg Clin N Am 25 (2013) 661–681
http://dx.doi.org/10.1016/j.coms.2013.07.006
1042-3699/13/$ – see front matter © 2013 Elsevier Inc. All rights reserved.

ability to remodel and regenerate usually results in a complete return to normal function and occlusion with conservative management alone (**Fig. 1**). Adult patients who suffer nondisplaced to minimally displaced fractures, particularly in which the occlusion is unchanged, are also appropriately managed conservatively with close follow-up.

The incidence of complications after either conservative or surgical management of condyle fractures is low. Nonetheless, complications such as infection, ankylosis, malunion, and degeneration of the proximal segment do occur. These complications are often managed by reconstructing the mandibular condyle and occasionally the fossa. Although the frequency is unknown, of 364 condyle fractures managed by our service between 2002 and 2011, only 5 required late reconstruction for an incidence of 1.4%. Five other patients initially treated elsewhere for condylar trauma were referred to our service for reconstruction during the same period. Six of the 10 patients had initially undergone no treatment or had a period of maxillomandibular fixation (MMF) to manage their condyle fracture. The remaining 4 patients had undergone primary ORIF of their condyle fracture.

Young children frequently present with more significant condylar disruption, but it is the adult population, likely because of their diminished capacity for regeneration and remodeling, who present with more frequent and significant dysfunction after the management of condyle fractures, particularly when the fractured proximal segment is dislocated.[3,4] It is also the adult population who more frequently require posttraumatic condylar reconstruction. Other factors that increase the probability that a condyle fracture will require reconstruction are listed in **Box 3**.

MINIMIZING THE INCIDENCE OF RECONSTRUCTION AFTER TRAUMA

Some cases of reconstruction after condylar fracture are likely preventable. This observation is particularly true in circumstances in which reconstruction has been secondary to inadequate initial management or misdiagnosis (see case 5). This situation can be prevented by ensuring that a thorough clinical and radiographic examination is performed on all individuals with suspected facial trauma. During the clinical examination, the health care provider should look for the signs and symptoms of a mandibular condyle fracture (**Box 4**).

Plain film examination alone, particularly when interpreted by someone who is not an oral and maxillofacial surgeon (OMS), can result in numerous mandible fractures being missed (**Fig. 2**).[5,6] This

fractures, in our experience most patients not only prefer but are better managed by open reduction and internal fixation (ORIF). Consequently more than 70% of these fractures are treated in this manner by our department. The incidence of permanent neurologic injury is uncommon when ORIF is performed by experienced surgeons, but a few individuals have a perceptible scar.[1,2] We do not advocate ORIF for every condylar fracture; fractures in young, growing patients are usually best treated by conservative management. Their

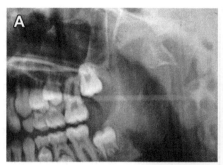
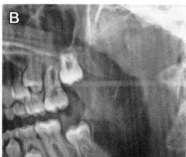
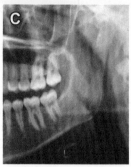

Fig. 1. (*A*) Initial radiographic presentation of an 8.5-year-old patient with a displaced condylar neck fracture. (*B*) Radiographic appearance of the condyle 4 months later. Notice the significant morphologic changes that have occurred to the proximal segment. The patient had been managed with MMF and physiotherapy. (*C*) By age 16 years, a normal-appearing condyle is noted, showing the regenerative ability of young patients.

situation has certainly resulted in condylar fractures being misdiagnosed and underscores the importance of reviewing the patient's history and performing a thorough clinical examination. Computed tomography has been helpful in not only diagnosing but also planning the surgical management of maxillofacial trauma. It has become overused and represents a real lifetime radiation exposure risk. Cone-beam imaging likely has a role in diagnosing maxillofacial injuries and does decrease the radiation exposure.[7] However, neither of these modalities images the important soft tissue anatomy of the TMJ. Although less frequently used for maxillofacial trauma, magnetic

resonance imaging (MRI) of the TMJ in patients with known or suspected condyle fractures has a role in determining the extent of soft tissue trauma.[8] This may affect management and help assess the potential for future complications such as ankylosis.[9,10]

COMPLICATIONS OF CONDYLE FRACTURES AND INDICATIONS FOR RECONSTRUCTION

When condyle fractures are correctly diagnosed and appropriately managed complications should occur infrequently. However, complications do occasionally compromise the form and function

Box 3
Factors that increase the probability of a condyle fracture requiring reconstruction

Patient Factors	Injury Factors	Treatment Factors	Posttreatment Factors
• Preexisting malocclusions	• Avulsive injuries	• Misdiagnosis	• Postoperative infection
• Arthritides	• Penetrating injuries	• Inadequate reduction	• Ankylosis
• Poor/inadequate dentition	• Intracapsular fractures	• Inadequate fixation	• Condylar degeneration
	• Sagittal fractures	• Free grafting	• Dysfunction
	• Disk disruption	• Inadequate MMF	• Loss of posterior facial height
		• Prolonged MMF	

of the TMJ, with the most common indications for late reconstruction after condylar trauma being:

- Development of ankylosis
- Significant proximal segment degeneration with functional impairment or pain
- Malunion with unacceptable function or pain

The development of these complications, and thus the need to reconstruct the TMJ, is often multifactorial. Apart from avulsive injuries and ankylosis, most of the factors listed in **Box 3** do not usually individually result in the need to reconstruct the condyle. The patient and injury factors are difficult to modify, but the clinician should

appreciate that these factors increase the possibility of developing posttraumatic ankylosis or condylar degeneration and consequently close long-term follow-up is warranted. Every attempt should be made to minimize those treatment factors that increase the risk of developing complications that require late condylar reconstruction.

Although ankylosis or degeneration are the most obvious reasons that require reconstructing the TMJ after trauma, any one of the following complications has the potential to necessitate reconstruction.

Malocclusion

One of the primary goals in managing patients with fractures of the maxillomandibular complex is to return their occlusion to its preinjury state. With only an estimated 40% of the US population having an ideal preinjury occlusion, this goal is often challenging.[11] Returning the occlusion to its preinjury state requires an appreciation of both normal and abnormal occlusal anatomy, as well as careful monitoring during and after treatment to ensure that this goal has been obtained and maintained.

Malocclusions are not uncommon after condylar fractures. ORIF seems to result in fewer patients developing a posttraumatic malocclusion than closed management with MMF.[12] Neuromuscular adaptation and occlusal wear often allow most patients to accept a minor change in their occlusion after management. However, there is variation in a patient's ability to adapt, and consequently some individuals require management. Large and

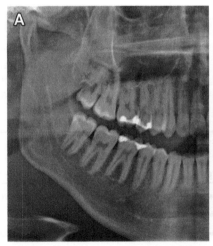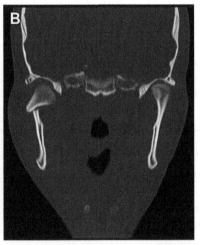

Fig. 2. A patient was seen in the emergency room after a fall. (*A*) Clinical signs and symptoms of a condyle fracture were noted in the hospital record, but the treating service detected no injury on the orthopantomograph and discharged the patient home. The patient was seen by our department, and clinical examination and subtle findings on the radiograph suggested a condyle fracture. (*B*) This was confirmed by computed tomography.

early changes in the occlusion are usually the result of a malposition of the proximal segment and are best managed by correctly reducing and fixating it. Once bone healing has occurred, or when it is impossible to reduce and fixate the proximal segment, then management is dependent on condylar function. Condylar reconstruction usually has little role when good, pain-free range of motion is present. When a malocclusion occurs in light of good condylar function, the management strategies include occlusal equilibration, orthodontic correction, and/or osteotomies (**Fig. 3**).[13,14] When a malocclusion occurs in the presence of diminished or unacceptable TMJ function, consideration needs to be given to reconstructing the TMJ. The ability to correct a malocclusion at the same time the TMJ is reconstructed is dependent on the magnitude/type of the malocclusion, the reconstruction technique/material, and the relationship of the ramus to the fossa once the occlusion has been corrected. Custom-made total joint prostheses simplify the simultaneous correction of malocclusions and reconstruction of the TMJ.[15]

Hypomobility

Range of mandibular motion, which includes maximum interincisal opening (MIO), lateral excursive jaw movements, and protrusion, is frequently adversely affected by mandibular condyle trauma. This situation seems to be more common after the management of these injuries with a period of MMF.[16] Management of diminished range of motion must first involve determining the cause. If the loss of function is secondary to ankylosis, proximal segment malposition or degeneration, then surgery is required. In the absence of these problems, a return to a preinjury, or at least acceptable, level of stomatognathic function can often be obtained by physiotherapy. Physiotherapy needs to be overseen by a clinician who appreciates and understands normal stomatognathic function.

Facial Pain

The development of the subcondylar osteotomy for managing certain intra-articular pain conditions resulted from Terence Ward noticing that many patients with preexisting TMJ symptoms had an improvement in their symptoms after condyle fractures.[17] Consequently the development of facial pain after condyle fractures is not common but also seems to occur with a slightly higher frequency in patients managed with MMF.[2] As with any patient presenting with facial pain, correct diagnosis is vital before initiating management, particularly nonreversible treatment modalities. Most patients presenting with posttraumatic facial pain suffer from myofascial pain, but when clinical examination suggests an intra-articular source of the pain, then imaging of the soft and hard tissue of the TMJ is necessary before recommending surgical intervention. Pain can be the result of posttraumatic condylar degeneration, which sometimes necessitates reconstruction (**Fig. 4**).

Alteration of Facial Growth

Condyle fractures in the growing child can alter future facial growth, causing facial asymmetries.[18] The decision as to how and when to manage this complication is challenging, because many children who develop this problem show acceptable TMJ function.[19] Furthermore, reconstruction of the condyle with a costochondral graft (CCG) does not guarantee that future growth will be predictable or equal to the contralateral side. Consequently, when acceptable function exists, consideration should be given to managing these secondary dentofacial deformities with predictable, and less morbid, orthognathic surgery procedures. These procedures can be undertaken in the growing child or delayed until growth is complete. CCG reconstruction should be contemplated only for these patients when TMJ function is also impaired.

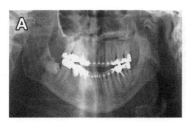
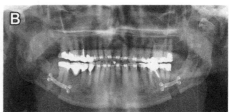

Fig. 3. (*A*) A patient presented with a chief complaint of a significant malocclusion after bilateral condyle fracture. The patient's stomatognathic function was within normal limits and pain free. Clinical and radiographic examination noted a malunion of both condyle fractures, causing a posttraumatic anterior open-bite deformity. (*B*) Because good, pain-free range of mandibular motion was possible it was decided to not perform reconstruction of the TMJs and correct the malocclusion with orthognathic surgery alone.

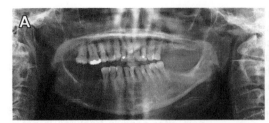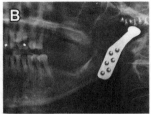

Fig. 4. (*A*) A patient was referred with severe pain, a malocclusion, and limited opening approximately 2 years after a left high condylar neck fracture. The orthopantomograph shows complete degeneration of the previously fractured condyle. (*B*) The TMJ was reconstructed with a Biomet stock total joint prosthesis.

Infection

The development of a postoperative infection remains one of the most common complications after management of mandibular fracture.[20] This complication is uncommon after ORIF of condyle fractures. **Box 5** lists those factors that predispose a condyle fracture to becoming infected. In a 2012 article, Mercuri[21] outlined several recommendations to minimize surgical site infections when performing total joint replacement, with several of these recommendations also being appropriate for management of open condyle fracture. Infection can cause the rapid resorption of the proximal segment, thus requiring reconstruction (see case 4).

Fixation Failure

Fixation failure can increase the likelihood of condylar degeneration, malunion, or infection. **Box 6** lists the factors that increase the probability of fixation failure. When this complication is noted, the surgeon must first assess whether adequate

bone exists to reduce and refixate the proximal segment. If inadequate bone exists, then the proximal segment likely requires removal and the site immediately reconstructed with either a CCG or total joint prosthesis (TJP).

Malunion

Malunion, either because of misdiagnosis, inadequate initial reduction, or movement of the proximal segment after treatment, results in the healing of the proximal segment in an anatomically incorrect position (see case 2). Malunion frequently causes a malocclusion or dysfunction. Condylar reconstruction is required when the malunion causes TMJ dysfunction. Malunion causing a malocclusion but with acceptable stomatognathic function can usually be managed with orthodontics or orthognathic surgery (see **Fig. 3**).[22] Malunion or nonunion can occasionally be managed by proper positioning and fixation of the proximal segment. However, this option is often impractical if a significant delay has occurred, because the proximal segment is either resorbed or healed in an incorrect position.

Degeneration

Proximal segment degeneration (**Fig. 5**) can occur secondary to infection, fixation failure, or if there is a decrease in vascularity to the proximal segment. The third reason may explain why some condylar

---

Box 5
Factors that increase the risk of a condyle fracture managed with ORIF becoming infected

- Communication with the oral cavity
- Contamination of the site with cutaneous flora
- Contamination of the site with oral flora
- Contamination of the site with otologic flora
- Fixation failure with loose hardware
- Immunocompromised host
- Inadequate fracture stability
- Multiple operations
- Poor vascularity
- Presence of a foreign body
- Smoker/ethanol abuse/illicit drug use

Box 6
Factors that increase the likelihood for fixation failure

- Early, excessive, loading
- Inadequate bone stock
- Inadequate plate strength
- Infection
- Poor initial reduction
- Reinjury

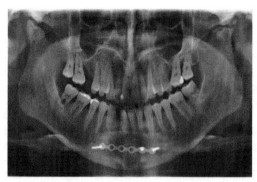

Fig. 5. This patient had their facial injuries managed with ORIF of their symphyseal fracture and MMF for their bilateral condyle fractures. The patient was referred to our department 18 months after their injury because of radiographic evidence of significant condylar degeneration.

free grafts undergo rapid and significant resorption (see case 1).[23] The location of the fracture is also related to the likelihood of developing condylar resorption. Condylar head fractures, particularly when comminuted, predictably undergo more resorption then less significant injuries.[24] However, the role that trauma plays in the development of future condylar resorption is unknown. Preexisting malocclusions and arthritides likely increase a patient's risk for this complication after condylar trauma. Nevertheless, degeneration of the proximal segment requires reconstruction only when it results in pain and dysfunction. Malocclusions secondary to degeneration but with pain-free acceptable function can often be corrected without the need for TMJ reconstruction.

Ankylosis

Posttraumatic ankylosis is uncommon and is suggested to occur in approximately 0.2% to 0.4% of condyle fractures (see case 6).[25] Even though the overall incidence is low, condylar fractures remain the most common cause of pediatric TMJ ankylosis in developed countries.[26] This complication usually results from comminuted intracapsular injuries, particularly when the articular disk is disrupted. It has also been suggested that concomitant anterior mandibular fractures, which allow posterior facial widening and consequent lateral displacement of sagittally fractured condyles, are also a risk factor for this complication.[27]

As mentioned earlier, a correctly positioned intact articular disk likely minimizes the risk of ankylosis. Dislocated high condylar neck fractures and condylar head fractures are frequently associated with disk displacement and capsular and retrodiskal soft tissue damage.[28,29] MRI imaging of

the TMJ is helpful in identifying those patients who may benefit from disk repair, which may minimize the risk of future ankylosis. When ankylosis does occur, the surgeon must first release the ankylosis and then reconstruct the defect.

Most of these complications, apart from ankylosis, only occasionally necessitate late reconstruction of the mandibular condyle or TMJ. Reconstruction should be contemplated only when these complications are causing TMJ dysfunction that is affecting the patient's quality of life. When reconstruction of the TMJ following condylar trauma is required, the patient needs to understand their operative options.

MATERIAL OPTIONS WHEN RECONSTRUCTING THE MANDIBULAR CONDYLE

The surgeon has 2 principal options when reconstruction is required after condylar trauma. Autogenous options can either be nonvascularized or vascularized grafts, with the latter being used rarely for late reconstruction of the mandibular condyle after trauma. The most commonly used autogenous product for reconstructing the TMJ is the CCG. The CCG does not reconstruct the entire TMJ, because an intact or reconstructed fossa is a requirement for its use. The advantages and disadvantages of CCGs are listed in **Box 7**.

Historically, the CCG has been considered the workhorse for reconstruction of the condyle but it does have limitations. One of the principal shortcomings of this technique is the inability to initiate aggressive physiotherapy immediately after surgery, which is important in cases of ankylosis or

Box 7		
The advantages and disadvantages of CCG reconstruction of the TMJ		
Advantages		**Disadvantages**
• Autogenous		• Donor site morbidity (pain, scar, risk of pneumothorax)
• Cartilage cap		
• Cost		• Increased operating time
• Growth potential		• Period of MMF usually required
• Modifiable		• Risk of resorption
		• Unpredictable growth
		• Requires relatively normal fossa and ramus anatomy

hypomobility. Even when rigid fixation is used to stabilize the rib graft, the bone quality rarely allows for immediate, aggressive, postoperative physiotherapy. Although the incidence of pneumothorax is low in experienced hands, it is still a possible complication of the procedure.

More recently, distraction osteogenesis (DO) for reconstructing the TMJ has gained popularity among some surgeons. The principal advantages of creating a neocondyle with this method are the avoidance of the morbidity associated with CCG harvesting and decreased cost compared with an alloplast. Disadvantages include a lack of growth, occasional difficulty in controlling the direction of the neocondyle, cost of the distraction device, and the need for strict compliance with activating the device. In the animal model, DO has been shown to be as effective as CCGs for reconstructing an ankylosed TMJ.[30]

The most basic type of alloplast is a reconstruction plate with a condylar extension. This treatment option is frequently used when ablative surgery for disease necessitates the removal of the mandibular condyle. No fossa component exists, and the condylar extension rests against the glenoid fossa or, preferably, the meniscus. There is a long history of their successful use.[31] However, manufacturers warn that these devices are intended to be only temporary and should be removed within 2 years of placement.[32] Complications such as fracture, loosening of the fixation hardware, heterotopic bone formation, perforation though skin, and erosion through the glenoid fossa, mastoid process,

or tympanic plate are all possible (**Fig. 6**).[33] We have seen 4 metal condyles erode into the middle cranial fossa, with 1 case occurring in as little as 5 months after placement. However, numerous patients have had the device placed and because of good, pain-free function, have refused to have the device removed.

The history of total joint (fossa/condyle) alloplast use for reconstruction of the TMJ is checkered primarily because of significant complications associated with prostheses containing Proplast-Teflon, because it tended to fragment under prolonged cyclical loading. This situation often resulted in a locally destructive foreign body giant cell reaction (**Fig. 7**). Improvements in materials and designs have occurred, with devices now being fabricated out of materials that have been successfully used in orthopedic prostheses for many decades. The advantages and disadvantages of their use are listed in **Box 8**.

In North America, 3 companies produce total joint prostheses. TMJ Concepts (Ventura, CA, USA) produces a patient-specific device only, whereas Biomet Microfixation (Warsaw, IN, USA) and TMJ Medical Inc (Salt Lake City, UT, USA) produce both stock and patient-specific devices. Both the fossa and condyle of the TMJ Medical device are constructed of surgical grade cobalt-chromium-molybdenum alloy. The fossa component of the Biomet Microfixation device is made of ultra–high-molecular-weight polyethylene (UHMWPE), whereas the ramus-condyle unit is constructed of cobalt-chromium alloy with the

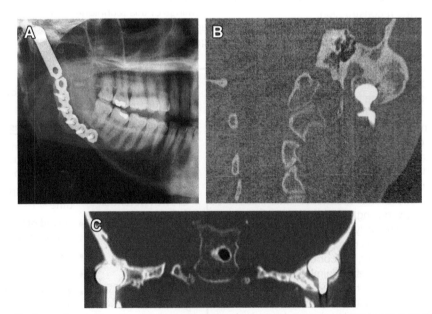

Fig. 6. Complications of reconstruction plates with condylar extension: (*A*) fracture, (*B*) heterotopic bone formation, and (*C*) erosion through the cranial base into the middle cranial fossa.

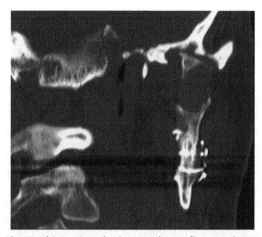

Fig. 7. This patient had a Proplast-Teflon total TMJ prosthesis removed 15 years earlier because of pain and a locally destructive foreign body giant cell reaction. The site was immediately reconstructed with a CCG. In 2007, the patient had increasing pain and a decreasing mouth opening. Imaging showed a destructive process involving the CCG. The CCG was removed and the site was immediately reconstructed with a stock TJP (Biomet). Histopathology demonstrated a foreign body giant cell reaction.

undersurface of the ramus portion, which lies adjacent to bone, being titanium plasma sprayed. The fossa portion of the TMJ Concept device has an articulating surface of UHMWPE attached to a commercially pure titanium body, which lies against the cranial base and zygomatic arch. The mandibular component of this device is made from medical grade titanium, except for the condylar head, which is made of cobalt-chromium-molybdenum alloy.

Box 8
The advantages and disadvantages of alloplastic reconstruction of the TMJ

Advantages	Disadvantages
• Decreased operating time	• Cost
• Immediate function/ no need for postoperative MMF	• Possible need for replacement
	• No growth potential
• No donor site	• Plain film imaging of contralateral side often difficult
• Patient-specific devices available	
• Simultaneous correction of malocclusions possible	• Possible displacement
	• Possible fixation failure
	• Wear

Stock alloplastic options are available in various sizes and styles, with the position of the inferior alveolar nerve and the anatomy of the ramus/fossa dictating which condyle and fossa prosthesis to use. The Biomet Microfixation device has a right and left condylar prosthesis, which is available in 3 lengths (45 mm, 50 mm, and 55 mm) and 3 styles (regular, narrow, and offset). The fossa prosthesis also comes in small, medium, and large, with the difference being in the length of the flange that allows for fixation of the device to the zygomatic arch. The condylar head and fossa size/morphology are consistent. Both components are fixed to underlying bone with titanium screws. The stock TMJ Medical devices come with a series of sizers that are used to select the correct fossa and ramus/condyle given the patient's anatomy. Both are secured with cobalt-chromium-molybdenum alloy screws.

Custom-made prostheses are fabricated using stereolithographic modeling of the patient's craniomaxillofacial region. This technique requires a company-specific computed tomogram protocol. The clinician is provided with a detailed model of the patient's maxillomandibular complex. TMJ Medical provides the surgeon with a wax-up of the proposed device before fabricating a definitive device (**Fig. 8**). TMJ Concept provides the clinician with the model, allowing the surgeon to confirm the occlusion and note or address any areas that may interfere with the fabrication or placement of the definitive prosthesis. At our center, because of the increased cost associated with these patient-specific devices, they are typically reserved for cases in which the associated anatomy is too complex for either autogenous options or stock alloplastic devices.

An ongoing concern surrounding alloplastic devices is their longevity, with the expectation that, like in orthopedics, many devices will require

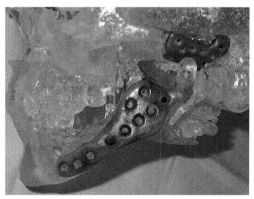

Fig. 8. A stereolithic model showing a wax-up of a patient-specific TJP.

replacement. Metal-on-metal prostheses are of particular concern in the orthopedic community.[34] Revision surgery, as in orthopedics, tends to be more complicated than the initial surgery and often requires patient-specific devices to replace them. In 2011, the US Food and Drug Administration ordered a postmarket surveillance of the 3 US manufacturers of TMJ implants to determine the length of time before removal or replacement of the devices because of pain or other reasons.[35]

There is a lack of well-designed prospective studies comparing the outcomes of alloplastic versus autogenous reconstruction of the TMJ. Most case series suggest that both CCG and newer-generation alloplasts have good success. Failures do occur with either technique.

MANAGEMENT GUIDELINES

Patients with a history of a condyle fracture who present with TMJ dysfunction must have the position and morphology of their proximal segment evaluated (**Fig. 9**). Plain films alone are often insufficient in detailing the morphology and three-dimensional position of the condyle. TMJ dysfunction with radiographic corroboration of a proximal segment abnormality supports the need for reconstruction. However, when comfortable and acceptable TMJ function exists, radiographic evidence of a proximal segment problem alone does not indicate a need for reconstruction. Most posttraumatic complications not causing TMJ dysfunction can be managed without reconstruction. Furthermore, TMJ dysfunction in the absence of a proximal segment abnormality rarely requires reconstruction. In these situations, clinical and MRI findings guide appropriate management.

In patients who require reconstruction, the clinician must assess the anatomy of the ramus and fossa. When it is determined to be abnormal, the most predictable option is the use of a custom TJP. When normal ramus and fossa anatomy exists, the clinician can use a CCG or stock TJP. In our experience, a custom-made prosthesis is rarely required when normal anatomy is present. Preexisting ankylosis or inflammatory arthritides likely decrease the success of CCGs. Furthermore, relatively normal fossa and ramus anatomy must exist for CCGs. CCG survival is dependent on the vascularity of the recipient bed, so multiple previous operations or irradiation decrease graft success.

In a growing child, a CCG still represents the best option. Undergrowth and overgrowth do occur, so close, long-term follow-up is mandatory. Either of these CCG outcomes requires secondary osteotomies to be corrected. Although a case report of using an alloplastic total joint in a growing child has been reported,[36] this is not considered the standard of care.

Reconstruction is indicated when proximal segment degeneration is accompanied by TMJ dysfunction. Comminuted, small, unstable, poorly vascularized, and infected proximal segments are all at risk for resorption. When infection is present, initial management includes the use of empiric broad-spectrum antibiotics and radiographic assessment of the proximal segment. If fixation appears intact and the proximal segment is normal in terms of position and morphology, then the usual protocols for managing an infection of a fracture or TMJ apply.[37,38] Infection is difficult to eliminate in the presence of mobile fracture segments, and failure to remove loose hardware and stabilize the segments results in rapid degeneration of the proximal segment.

When resorption of the proximal segment prevents correct anatomic reduction or if the articulating surface has undergone degeneration, then the segment should be removed and the area reconstructed. Noninfected sites can be reconstructed immediately with a CCG or TJP. Infected sites can be temporarily reconstructed with a reconstruction plate with condylar extension. As mentioned, these devices can fail catastrophically, and it is therefore critical that once the infection has resolved, that the site be definitively managed with either a CCG or TJP.

When a malposition or malunion of the condyle is noted the clinician must first determine if dysfunction is present. Occasionally, patients function well with a malunited condyle, in which case TMJ reconstruction is likely not indicated. When dysfunction is noted, the clinician must determine if the remaining proximal segment can be properly repositioned. Repositioning is often impractical, because the segment often undergoes some degree of resorption or becomes fused to the ramus. In this circumstance, removal of the segment and reconstruction is usually indicated.

When ankylosis occurs, the surgeon must first release the entire ankylosis and then reconstruct the defect. Kaban and colleagues[39] described a rational approach to managing ankylosis in the pediatric population. However, Nitzan and colleagues[40] suggested that in some cases, this approach is overly aggressive and that simply removing the lateral ankylotic mass and preserving the medial displaced disk/condyle provides good results, if aggressive physiotherapy is provided postoperatively. In the adult population, autogenous options such as CCGs likely increase the risk for reankylosis, and consequently, TJPs are usually recommended.[41]

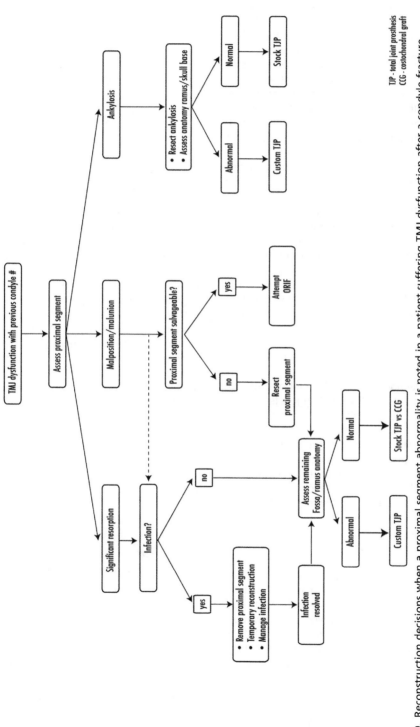

Fig. 9. Reconstruction decisions when a proximal segment abnormality is noted in a patient suffering TMJ dysfunction after a condyle fracture.

Regardless of the reconstruction technique and material used, close, long-term follow-up is mandatory. We typically see these patients back for follow-up at 1, 2, and 4 weeks and then at 3, 6, and 12 months. More regular follow-up is scheduled if complications ensue or the patient's progress is slower than expected. Patients are typically seen on a twice-yearly basis thereafter, but eventually progress to annual follow-up.

Aggressive physiotherapy is typically initiated the day after the placement of an alloplastic prosthesis and is continued for at least 6 months postoperatively. If the patient's range of mandibular function is not progressing as quickly as expected, they are referred to a physiotherapist for oversight of their rehabilitation.

Perioperative use of antibiotics is the standard of care, but the issue of long-term prophylactic coverage of patients with TMJ TJP before invasive dental, genitourinary, or gastrointestinal procedures is controversial.[42] The 2009 American Academy of Orthopedic Surgeons (AAOS) information statement was contentious, so applying these recommendations to temporomandibular TJPs is inappropriate.[43] In December, 2012, the AAOS and American Dental Association jointly published a clinical practice guideline (CPG), which states, "While evidence supports a strong association between certain dental procedures and bacteremias, there is no evidence to demonstrate a direct link between dental-procedure-associated bacteremia and infection of prosthetic joint or other orthopedic implants."[44] The CPG suggests that the clinician may consider discontinuing the practice of routinely prescribing prophylactic antibiotics for patients with hip and knee prosthetic joint implants undergoing dental procedures.[44] There seems to be even less evidence to support the routine use of prophylactic antibiotics before invasive dental procedures in patients with TMJ TJPs.

PROCEDURE

Once the patient has undergone nasoendotracheal intubation, arch bars or MMF screws are placed before preparing or draping the patient. This procedure is performed using a separate surgical tray and before scrubbing and gowning. MMF screws are typically used when the TMJ is reconstructed using an alloplast, and arch bars are used when a CCG is used. The patient is not initially placed into MMF, because recipient site preparation is easier if the mandible can be manipulated.

When a CCG is required, a right fifth or sixth rib is harvested, as it is thought that an adult right rib can be used to reconstruct either condyle. This

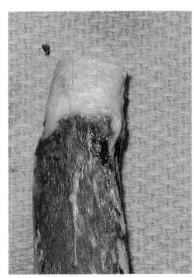

Fig. 10. A CCG showing the irregular bone/cartilage junction present in adolescents and adults. Maintenance of a cuff of soft tissue at the costochondral junction is not required in these age groups, because separation of the cartilage from the bone is unlikely.

strategy avoids postoperative confusion between surgical site and cardiogenic pain. For midadolescent and older patients, maintaining a cuff of perichondrial/periosteal tissue at the costochondral junction is not only unnecessary but likely increases the risk of pleural tears. By this age, the bone-cartilage junction is not a butt joint but is irregular, which prevents separation of the bone and cartilage (**Fig. 10**). With careful dissection, pleural tears should be uncommon. Typically 5 cm of bone is harvested, with 5 mm of cartilage being sufficient (**Fig. 11**). The graft is stored in a clearly identified separate basin and is wrapped in a saline-soaked sponge. Skin-to-skin operating time is normally 45 minutes.

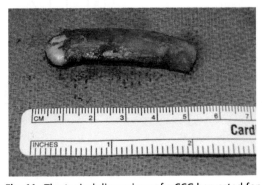

Fig. 11. The typical dimensions of a CCG harvested for reconstructing a mandibular condyle. Typically, 5 mm of cartilage is adequate, with this being modified with a blade to create a rounded, smooth articulating surface.

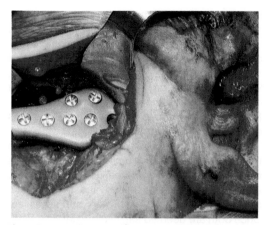

Fig. 12. A patient-specific custom TJP with a long anterior extension, which required modification of the previously made retromandibular incision.

The head and neck area is prepared and draped in a typical fashion for TMJ surgery. A recent study offered[21] several recommendations regarding preparation of the surgical site so as to minimize the risk of infection. We isolate the oral cavity with a clear adhesive drape (D1010, Medical Concepts Development), which can be reflected in a manner so as to not contaminate the surgical field while MMF is applied or released.

Access to the ramus is by a de novo or preexisting submandibular or retromandibular incision line. Previous surgery can alter the typical location of cranial nerve VII branches, so the use of a nerve stimulator is recommended during the dissection down to the ramus. Consequently, the patient should not be paralyzed during this portion of the surgery. Retromandibular incisions often provide limited access to the mandibular body and

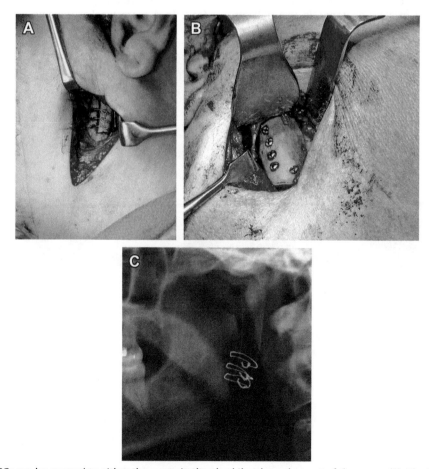

Fig. 13. CCGs can be secured to either the posterior border (*A*) or lateral aspect of the ramus (*B*). The fossa/ramus anatomy and morphology of the CCG determine the most suitable location for the graft. When placing the graft at the posterior border, a ramus osteotomy creates a butt joint, which helps prevent vertical displacement of the graft (*C*).

have to be modified, particularly when a custom-made prosthesis has a large anterior extension (**Fig. 12**).

A standard preauricular incision is used with a slight hockey-stick extension to facilitate anterior access to the arch. If a CCG is to be placed, removal of the proximal fragment is performed, but the disk, if healthy, is maintained (see case 5). Alloplasts require a meniscectomy and modification of the ramus and cranial base. Once the condylectomy and bone reduction have been performed, the patient's range of mandibular motion is assessed and if adequate, the patient is placed into MMF. If inadequate, unilateral or bilateral coronoidectomies are undertaken and the mandibular range of motion is reassessed. Once range of motion is deemed adequate, the patient is placed into MMF.

When using a CCG to reconstruct the condyle, the graft is either placed at the posterior border or on the lateral aspect of the mandibular ramus (**Fig. 13**). The decision regarding placement is based on the existing anatomy. In thin patients,

lateral placement of the graft often results in a noticeable asymmetry between the operated and unoperated sides. However, rigid fixation of laterally positioned grafts is often technically simple if the quality of the CCG is sufficient to hold screws. When placing the graft at the posterior border, a careful vertical osteotomy of the ramus is first performed to create a slot in which the graft is secured, typically with 3 stainless steel wires.

The alloplastic prosthesis is placed according to the manufacturer's recommendations and is initially secured with a minimal number of screws, after which MMF is released and the patient's range of motion and occlusion are assessed. Once both are deemed satisfactory, MMF is reapplied and the remaining fixation screws are placed in the fossa and condyle components. After either an alloplast or CCG is secured, the range of motion and the occlusion are confirmed one last time before closure. Patients with CCGs are typically placed in tight MMF using elastics for 2 to 4 weeks followed by progressively lighter elastics for 2 to 4 more weeks. Patients with alloplasts

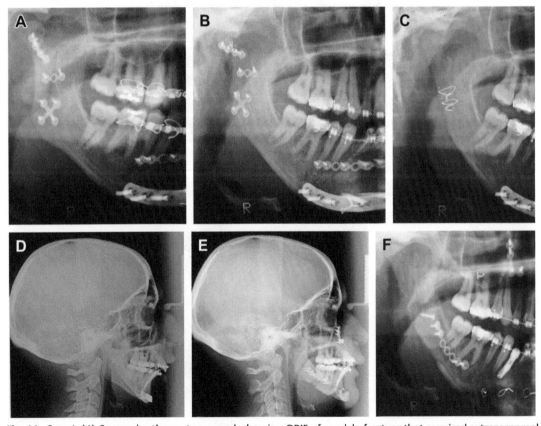

Fig. 14. Case 1. (*A*) Cropped orthopantomograph showing ORIF of condyle fracture that required extracorporeal reduction and fixation. (*B*) Rapid degeneration of the proximal segment was noted. (*C*) A CCG was used to reconstruct the condyle. (*D*) Lateral cephalogram before the patient's preexisting dentofacial deformity was corrected. (*E*) Postoperative lateral cephalogram. (*F*) Postoperative orthopantomograph.

have no postoperative MMF so that physiotherapy can be initiated immediately.

CASE PRESENTATIONS
Case 1

An 18-year-old woman with a preexisting dentofacial deformity consisting of mandibular retrognathia and vertical maxillary excess was involved in a motor vehicle collision (**Fig. 14**). She sustained a right displaced high condylar neck fracture and a symphyseal fracture. The significant preexisting malocclusion necessitated ORIF of both fractures. Because of difficulty in reducing the dislocated high condylar neck fracture it was rigidly reduced and fixated extracorporeally (see **Fig. 14**A). MMF was used postoperatively for 2 weeks. At the 3-month follow-up, the patient was experiencing pain and limited mouth opening. Radiographic examination noted proximal segment degeneration (see **Fig. 14**B). The patient was returned to the operating room and the proximal segment and hardware were removed and the site immediately reconstructed with a CCG (see **Fig. 14**C). A 4-week period of MMF was used. Follow-up noted

good function, and the preexisting dentofacial deformity was corrected with orthodontics and LeFort 1 and bilateral sagittal split osteotomies (see **Fig. 14**D–F). No problem was encountered when the sagittal split osteotomy was performed on the side of the CCG.

Case 2

A 58-year-old man fell and suffered a condylar neck fracture. Reduction of the fracture was attempted 3 times (**Fig. 15**). The patient was referred to our service complaining of pain and a malocclusion. Radiographic examination noted a malunion, with the proximal segment lying anterior in the infratemporal fossa (see **Fig. 15**A). Repositioning of the malpositioned proximal segment proved impossible, and the site was temporarily reconstructed using a reconstruction plate with condylar extension. A stable occlusion and good range of mandibular opening were obtained, and the patient refused definitive reconstruction of his TMJ. Three years after placement, the patient presented back complaining of decreasing mouth opening and a recent onset of discomfort and

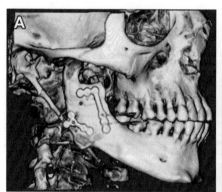
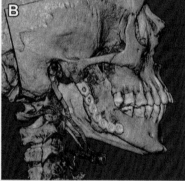
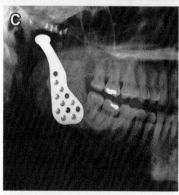

Fig. 15. Case 2. (A) Three-dimensional computed tomography showing that the fractured condyle, which has undergone 3 attempts at ORIF, is still lying well anterior to the glenoid fossa. (B) Heterotopic bone formation and fracture of the reconstruction plate with condylar extension, which had been used to temporarily manage the site once the malunited proximal segment had been removed. (C) Stock Biomet TJP placed immediately after removal of the fractured reconstruction plate with condylar extension.

malocclusion. Radiographic examination noticed the presence of heterotopic bone and a plate fracture (see **Fig. 15**B). The patient was returned to the operating room and had a stock TJP placed (see **Fig. 15**C). He has been followed for 8 years and still shows a stable preinjury occlusion and an MIO of 42 mm.

Case 3

A 53-year-old woman was involved in a motor vehicle collision and suffered a condylar neck fracture, which was managed initially with MMF (**Fig. 16**). She was referred to our service when a malocclusion was noted after the release of the MMF. Radiographic examination noted resorption and malunion of a small proximal fragment (see **Fig. 16**A). The patient elected to undergo CCG grafting of the site. The CCG

completely resorbed within 12 months (see **Fig. 16**B). Because of the small size of her ramus, it was believed that a custom prosthesis was the patient's best option. Stereolithographic modeling allowed for the production of a custom glenoid fossa and condyle, which was placed without injuring the inferior alveolar nerve (see **Fig. 16**C). The patient continues to function well and has an MIO of 44 mm.

Case 4

A 24-year-old man with a preinjury malocclusion suffered a symphyseal and bilateral condylar neck fractures (**Fig. 17**A–H). ORIF was performed for all 3 fractures (see **Fig. 17**A). One week after discharge, he presented back with a left-sided wound infection (see **Fig. 17**B). Despite appropriate management, the infection persisted, and

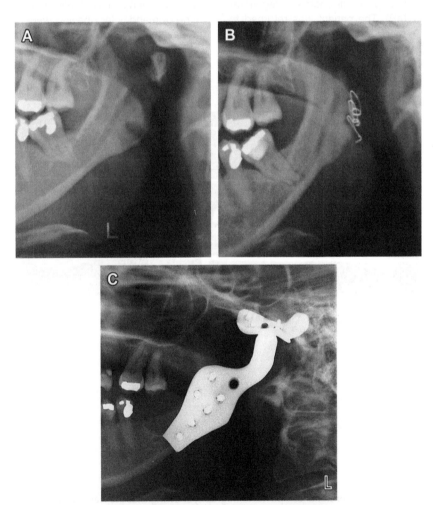

Fig. 16. Case 3. (*A*) A radiograph showing significant resorption of the proximal segment after a condyle fracture. (*B*) Reconstruction of the condyle was attempted with a CCG. This failed. (*C*) Because of a small ramus and an atypical fossa/ramus relationship, a patient-specific (custom) TJP was used to definitively reconstruct this patient's TMJ.

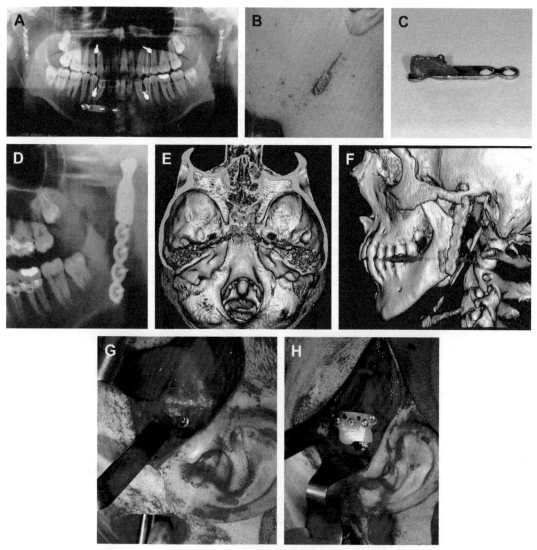

Fig. 17. Case 4. (*A*) ORIF of all 3 fractures. (*B*) Postoperative infection involving the left condyle fracture site. (*C, D*) Rapid resorption of the proximal segment necessitated removing the condylar remnants and, because of persistent infection, the temporary management of the site with a reconstruction plate with condylar extension. (*E, F*) Erosion of the condylar portion of the reconstruction plate into the middle cranial fossa. (*G, H*) Removal of the reconstruction plate and immediate reconstruction using a stock Biomet TJP.

fixation failure with rapid proximal segment degeneration was seen radiographically. The fixation hardware and remnants of the left condyle were removed, and a temporary reconstruction plate with condylar extension was placed (see **Fig. 17**C, D). The patient was continued on appropriate antibiotics and told that definitive TMJ reconstruction would be undertaken once the infection had been eliminated.

Five months after placement of the reconstruction plate, the patient began complaining of increasing pain and progressive limitation in mouth opening. Radiographic examination noted superior migration of the condylar portion of the reconstruction plate into the middle cranial fossa (see **Fig. 17**E, F). Of interest is that this situation occurred rapidly and without a noticeable clinical change in the patient's occlusion. The patient was returned to the operating room and had the reconstruction plate removed and the site immediately reconstructed with stock TJP (see **Fig. 17**G, H). He has maintained a reproducible occlusion and a mouth opening of greater than 37 mm for close to 5 years.

Case 5

A 45-year-old woman was seen in an emergency department after an assault (**Fig. 18**). No facial fracture was detected. The patient consulted an OMS because of persistent pain, dysfunction, and a malocclusion. A left condyle fracture was diagnosed. The patient was referred to our center 3 months after the injury, because of a persistent malocclusion. The proximal segment (see **Fig. 18**A) was determined not to be useable, and the patient elected to have a CCG to reconstruct her condyle. After the proximal segment was resected, the disk was examined and deemed to be intact, so it was maintained (see **Fig. 18**B). A ramus osteotomy was performed, which allowed for the secure positioning of the CCG at the posterior border (see **Fig. 18**C). Postoperatively, she was maintained in tight MMF for 3 weeks and then had guiding elastics used for another 3 weeks. She is functioning well with a mouth opening of 39 mm.

Case 6

A 33-year-old patient presented with a history of a condyle fracture as a youngster, which was managed with a period of MMF (**Fig. 19**). The patient underwent multiple operations for hypomobility, with the site being reconstructed with a CCG. Examination in 2007 noted a mouth opening limited to 7 mm. Radiographic examination noted a large ankylosis (see **Fig. 19**A). The patient underwent resection of the ankylosis, bilateral coronoidectomies, and immediate reconstruction using a stock TJP (see **Fig. 19**B, C). Aggressive physiotherapy was prescribed for more than 6 months and the patient has been able to maintain a maximum mouth opening of 35 mm for more than 6 years.

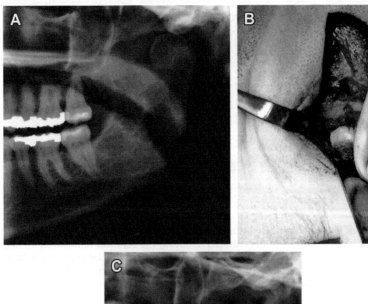

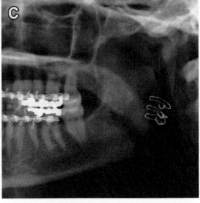

Fig. 18. Case 5. (*A*) Cropped orthopantomograph showing the displaced condyle fracture. (*B*) After the proximal segment was resected, the disk was examined and deemed to be intact, so it was maintained. (*C*) An osteotomy at the posterior border of the ramus allows the CCG to be more adequately secured and provides resistance to vertical displacement of the graft.

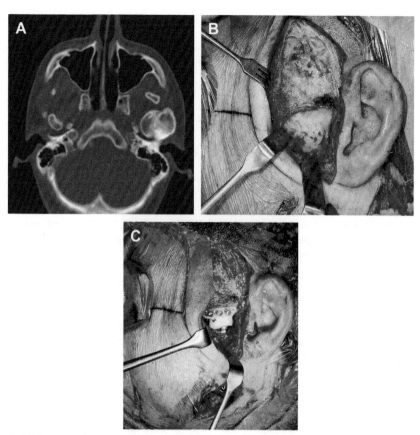

Fig. 19. Case 6. (*A*) Computed tomography and (*B*) clinical photograph showing a large ankylotic mass. (*C*) The management included resection of the ankylosis, bilateral coronoidectomies, and immediate reconstruction using a stock Biomet TJP.

SUMMARY

The need to reconstruct the TMJ after a condyle fracture is uncommon. Some instances of this complication can be prevented by the correct and early diagnosis of these injuries and by adherence to accepted management strategies. Nevertheless, reconstruction of the mandibular condyle is occasionally necessary when TMJ dysfunction is significant. This situation is usually a result of proximal segment degeneration, malunion, or ankylosis. Apart from instances of ankylosis, reconstruction is rarely needed after condyle fractures in the young child, because of their tremendous regenerative and adaptive capacity. When reconstruction is necessary in children, then CCG is likely the most acceptable option, with the patient and clinician understanding that further surgery may be necessary to correct asymmetrical facial growth. In the adult population, the development of alloplastic prostheses with similar properties to those used successfully in orthopedics for several decades suggests that these TJPs likely provide good long-term success.[45] In our experience, the stock TJP is suitable for most patients who require alloplastic reconstruction of their TMJ after trauma. Nevertheless, there remain advantages and disadvantages for all reconstructive options, so the decision to use one material versus another should be made in conjunction with the patient.

REFERENCES

1. Ellis E III, McFadden D, Simon P, et al. Surgical complications with open treatment of mandibular condylar process fractures. J Oral Maxillofac Surg 2000;58:950–8.
2. Haug RH, Assael LA. Outcomes of open versus closed treatment of mandibular subcondylar fractures. J Oral Maxillofac Surg 2001;59:370–5.
3. Dahlstrom L, Kahnberg KE, Lindahl L. 15 years follow-up on condylar fractures. Int J Oral Maxillofac Surg 1989;18:18–23.
4. Takenoshita Y, Ishibashi H, Oka M. Comparison of functional recovery after nonsurgical and surgical treatment of condylar fractures. J Oral Maxillofac Surg 1990;48:1191–5.

5. Wilson IF, Lokeh A, Benjamin CI, et al. Prospective comparison of panoramic tomography (zonography) and helical computed tomography in the diagnosis and operative management of mandibular fractures. Plast Reconstr Surg 2001;107:1369–75.

6. Roth FS, Kokoska MS, Awwad EE, et al. The identification of mandible fractures by helical computed tomography and panorex tomography. J Craniofac Surg 2005;16:394–9.

7. Shintaku WH, Venturi JS, Azevedo B, et al. Applications of cone-beam computed tomography in fractures of the maxillofacial complex. Dent Traumatol 2009;25:358–66.

8. Oezmen Y, Mischkowski R, Lenzen J, et al. MRI examination of the TMJ and functional results after conservative and surgical treatment of mandibular condyle fractures. Int J Oral Maxillofac Surg 1998;27:33–7.

9. Li Z, Zhang W, Li ZB. Induction of traumatic temporomandibular joint ankylosis in growing rats: a preliminary experimental study. Dent Traumatol 2009;25:136–41.

10. Zhang Y, He DM. Clinical investigation of early posttraumatic temporomandibular joint ankylosis and the role of repositioning discs in treatment. Int J Oral Maxillofac Surg 2006;35:1096–101.

11. Proffit WR, Fields HW Jr, Moray LJ. Prevalence of malocclusion and orthodontic treatment need in the United States: estimate from NHANES III survey. Int J Adult Orthodon Orthognath Surg 1988;13:97–106.

12. Ellis E, Simon P, Throckmorton GS. Occlusal results after open or closed treatment of fractures of the mandibular condylar process. J Oral Maxillofac Surg 2000;58:260–8.

13. Ishihara Y, Kuroda S, Nishiyama A, et al. Functional improvements after orthodontic-surgical reconstruction in a patient with multiple maxillofacial fractures. Am J Orthod Dentofacial Orthop 2012;142:534–45.

14. Laine P, Konito R, Salo A, et al. Secondary correction of malocclusion after treatment of maxillofacial trauma. J Oral Maxillofac Surg 2004;62:1312–20.

15. Wolford LM, Bourland TC, Rodrigues D, et al. Successful reconstruction of nongrowing hemifacial microsomia patients with unilateral temporomandibular joint total joint prosthesis and orthognathic surgery. J Oral Maxillofac Surg 2012;70:2835–53.

16. Schneider M, Erasmus F, Gerlach KL, et al. Open reduction and internal fixation versus closed treatment and mandibulomaxillary fixation of fractures of the mandibular condylar process: a randomized, prospective, multicentre study with special evaluation of fracture level. J Oral Maxillofac Surg 2008;66:2537–44.

17. Ward TG. Surgery of the mandibular joint. Ann R Coll Surg Engl 1961;28:139–52.

18. Choi J, Oh N, Kim IK. A follow-up study of condyle fractures in children. Int J Oral Maxillofac Surg 2005;34:851–8.

19. Hovinga J, Boering G, Stegenga B. Long-term results of nonsurgical management of condylar fractures in children. Int J Oral Maxillofac Surg 1999;28:429–40.

20. Lovato C, Wagner JD. Infection rates following perioperative prophylactic antibiotics versus postoperative extended regimen prophylactic antibiotics in surgical management of mandibular fractures. J Oral Maxillofac Surg 2009;67:827–32.

21. Mercuri LG. Avoiding and managing temporomandibular joint total joint replacement surgical site infections. J Oral Maxillofac Surg 2012;70:2280–9.

22. Rubens BC, Stoelinga PJ, Weaver TJ, et al. Management of malunited mandibular condylar fractures. Int J Oral Maxillofac Surg 1990;19:22–5.

23. Davis BR, Powell JE, Morrison AD. Free-grafting of mandibular condyle fractures: clinical outcomes in 10 consecutive patients. Int J Oral Maxillofac Surg 2005;34:871–6.

24. Park JM, Jang YW, Kim SG, et al. Comparative study of the prognosis of an extracorporeal reduction and a closed treatment in mandibular condyle head and/or neck fractures. J Oral Maxillofac Surg 2010;68:2986–93.

25. Ellis E. Complications of mandibular condyle fractures. Int J Oral Maxillofac Surg 1998;27:255–7.

26. Zimmermann CE, Troulis MJ, Kaban LB. Pediatric facial fractures: recent advances in prevention, diagnosis and management. Int J Oral Maxillofac Surg 2006;35:2–13.

27. He D, Ellis E, Zhang Y. Etiology of temporomandibular joint ankylosis secondary to condylar fractures: the role of concomitant mandibular fractures. J Oral Maxillofac Surg 2008;66:77–84.

28. Emshoff R, Rudisch A, Ennemoser T, et al. Magnetic resonance imaging findings of temporomandibular joint soft tissue changes in type V and VI condylar injuries. J Oral Maxillofac Surg 2007;65:1550–4.

29. Chen M, Yang C, He D, et al. Soft tissue reduction during open treatment of intracapsular condylar fracture of the temporomandibular joint: our institution's experience. J Oral Maxillofac Surg 2010;68:2189–95.

30. Cheung LK, Zheng LW, Ma L, et al. Transport distraction versus costochondral graft for reconstruction of temporomandibular joint ankylosis: which is better? Oral Surg Oral Med Oral Pathol Oral Radiol Endod 2009;108:32–40.

31. Marx RE, Cillo JE Jr, Broumard V, et al. Outcome analysis of mandibular condylar replacements in tumor and trauma reconstruction: a prospective analysis of 131 cases with long-term follow-up. J Oral Maxillofac Surg 2008;66:2515–23.

32. DePuySynthes. Condylar head add-on system product monograph. Available at: http://www.synthes.com/sites/NA/Products/CMF/Mandible/Pages/Condylar_Head_Add-On_System.aspx. Accessed January 6, 2013.

33. Carlson ER. Disarticulation resections of the mandible: a prospective review of 16 cases. J Oral Maxillofac Surg 2002;60:176–81.

34. Smith AJ, Dieppe P, Vernon K, et al. Failure rates of stemmed metal-on-metal hip replacements: analysis of data from the National Joint Registry of England and Wales. Lancet 2012;379:1199–204.

35. US Food and Drug Administration. FDA orders postmarket surveillance of certain TMJ implants. Available at: http://www.fda.gov/NewsEvents/Newsroom/PressAnnouncements/ucm242421.htm. Accessed January 23, 2013.

36. Mercuri LG, Swift JQ. Considerations for the use of alloplastic temporomandibular joint replacement in the growing patient. J Oral Maxillofac Surg 2009;67:1979–90.

37. Mehra P, Van Heukelom E, Cottrell DA. Rigid internal fixation of infected mandibular fractures. J Oral Maxillofac Surg 2009;67:1046–51.

38. Cai XY, Yang C, Zhang ZY, et al. Septic arthritis of the temporomandibular joint: a retrospective review of 40 cases. J Oral Maxillofac Surg 2010;68:731–8.

39. Kaban LB, Bouchard C, Troulis MJ. A protocol for management of temporomandibular joint ankylosis in children. J Oral Maxillofac Surg 2009;67:1966–78.

40. Nitzan DW, Tair JA, Lehman H. Is entire removal of a post-traumatic temporomandibular joint ankylotic site necessary for an optimal outcome? J Oral Maxillofac Surg 2012;70:e683–99.

41. Mercuri LG. Total joint reconstruction–autologous or alloplastic. Oral Maxillofac Surg Clin North Am 2006;18:399–410.

42. Mercuri LG, Psutka D. Perioperative, postoperative, and prophylactic use of antibiotics in alloplastic total temporomandibular joint replacement surgery: a survey and preliminary guidelines. J Oral Maxillofac Surg 2011;69:2106–11.

43. Antibiotic Prophylaxis for bacteremia in patients with joint replacements. Information statement from the AAOS Board of Directors. Released February 2009. Available at: http://www.aaos.org/news/aaos-now/may09/cover2.asp. Accessed January 24, 2013.

44. Prevention of orthopedic implant infection in patients undergoing dental procedures. Executive summary on the AAOS/ADA Clinical Practice Guideline. Released December, 2012. Available at: http://www.aaos.org/news/aaosnow/jan13/cover1.asp. Accessed January 24, 2013.

45. Mercuri LG, Edibam NR, Giobbie-Hurder A. Fourteen-year follow up of a patient-fitted total temporomandibular joint reconstruction system. J Oral Maxillofac Surg 2007;65:1140–8.

Late Reconstruction of Orbital and Naso-orbital Deformities

Jan Wolff, DDS, PhD[a,b],
George K.B. Sándor, MD, DDS, PhD, Dr Habil[c,d,*],
Mikko Pyysalo, DDS[b], Aimo Miettinen, DDS[b],
Antti-Veikko Koivumäki, DDS[b],
Vesa T. Kainulainen, DDS, PhD[e]

KEYWORDS

- Orbital fracture • Acute injury • Deformity • Treatment • Reconstruction

KEY POINTS

- Acute orbital fractures and naso-orbital ethmoid fractures can result in chronic orbital and naso-orbital deformities.
- Understanding the acute injury is the first step in reconstructing the established late deformity.
- New technologies from computer-guided surgical planning and additive manufacturing technology produce passive fitting implants tailored for patient-specific needs.
- Secondary late corrections, including intracranial osteotomies in severe cases of orbital hypertelorism, are extremely difficult to perform, less predictable, and associated with increased postoperative morbidity.
- The best management strategy for reconstruction of orbital hypertelorism is to avoid late complications by repairing these deformities early near the time of the original fractures.

INTRODUCTION

Acute orbital fractures and naso-orbital ethmoid (NOE) fractures can result in extremely difficult to manage chronic orbital and naso-orbital deformities. Understanding the acute injury is the first step in reconstructing the established late deformity. Acute and chronic orbital fractures are commonly classified on the basis of anatomic considerations[1] including fractures of the orbital floor, orbital walls, supraorbital and infraorbital rims, and the NOE complex.

Isolated fractures of the orbital floor, medial wall, and roof only involving the internal orbital skeleton are often described as blow-out and blow-in fractures.[2] Orbital blow-out fractures are divided into the following fractures: trapdoor fractures, medial blow-out fractures and lateral blow-out fractures, and orbital fractures involving the orbital rim.

THE BLOW-OUT FRACTURE

The blow-out fracture is the most common fracture of the orbit often caused by motor vehicle accidents, interpersonal violence, or sports injuries.[3] Such fractures occur when external forces strike the orbital rim causing a sudden increase in intra-orbital pressure.[4] This force is transmitted in a

Disclosures: The authors have nothing to disclose.
[a] Tissue Engineering, Regea-BioMediTech, University of Tampere, Biokatu 12 Krs 6, Tampere FIN-33520, Finland; [b] Oral and Maxillofacial Unit, Department of Otorhinolaryngology, Tampere University Hospital, PO Box 2000, Tampere FIN-33521, Finland; [c] Regea-BioMediTech, University of Tampere, Biokatu 12 Krs 6, Tampere FIN-33520, Finland; [d] Institute of Dentistry, University of Oulu, Oulu FIN-90014, Finland; [e] Institute of Dentistry, Oulu University Hospital, University of Oulu, Box 5281, Oulu FIN-90014, Finland
* Corresponding author. Regea-BioMediTech, University of Tampere, Biokatu 12 Krs 6, Tampere 33520, Finland.
E-mail address: george.sandor@uta.fi

posterior direction to the thinnest walls of the orbit causing them to fracture while the more resistant rim structure of the orbit usually remains intact.[1,5]

Fractures involving the orbital floor tend to produce greater functional problems.[3] Diplopia and enophthalmos are symptoms of an acute orbital injury. Diplopia and enophthalmos are also the most common late sequelae of the blow-out fractures of the orbit and represent the greatest reason for patients to seek late reconstruction of their orbital deformities (**Figs. 1–8**).

Binocular diplopia is caused by direct entrapment of the inferior rectus muscle. It may also be secondary to injury to the innervation of the extraoccular muscles and hemorrhage or contusion of the inferior rectus and inferior oblique muscle. In contradistinction, monocular diplopia may be caused by ocular trauma, for example, due to the luxation of the lens or retinal detachment.

In later stages, enophthalmos may be caused by fat atrophy or contracture of damaged extraoccular muscles. The most common cause of the enophthalmos is the increase in intraobital volume due to a combination of malposition of the bones surrounding the globe and orbital fat atrophy.[3]

Although a large variety of treatment approaches have been described for the management of orbital blow-out fractures, its treatment still remains a controversial topic. One school of thought recommends surgical intervention using

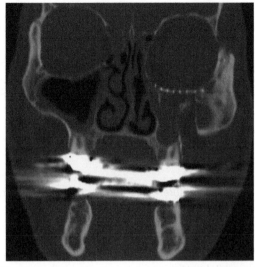

Fig. 2. Preoperative CT scan in coronal plane showing attempt to reconstruct orbital floor with a stock orbital floor plate. Note the discrepancy in the relative heights of the right and left orbital floors and the increased volume of the left orbit.

balloons, whereas others suggest titanium[6] or resorbable meshes.[7] Nevertheless, it is generally accepted that the presence of the clinical symptoms including diplopia, enophthalmos, motility disturbances of the globe, and fractures resulting in orbital floor or wall defects larger than 10 mm in diameter indicate the need for surgical treatment hence open reduction.[2,3]

Transcutaneous and transconjunctival approaches are the most commonly used approaches in both early and late open reductions of orbital floor fractures, because they allow good access and visualization of the fracture site. The transcutaneous incision can be made at subciliary or subtarsal levels.[8] Subciliary incisions are made immediately below the lower eyelashes, and when correctly executed, this approach is associated with no appreciable scar. According to the meta-analysis by Ridgway and colleagues,[8] the risk for lower lid ectropion associated with the subciliary approach was 14%.[8] The same meta-analysis showed that a 1.5% risk of ectropion was associated with transconjunctival approaches. Transconjunctival incision is made through the conjunctiva near the fornix. Transconjunctival incision can be extended medially to expose the medial orbit as well. This incision leaves no visible scar and the ectropion risk is minimal. Subtarsal or infraorbital incision is made through the first or second natural skin fold of the lower eyelid. It may result in a visible scar, which has been reported in 3.4% of cases, but the

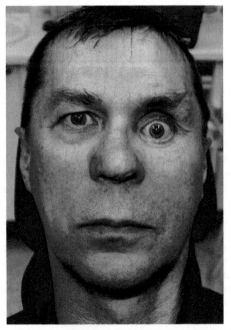

Fig. 1. Case 1. Preoperative frontal appearance of a 57-year-old man with severe left enophthalmos following 2 previous failed attempts at repair.

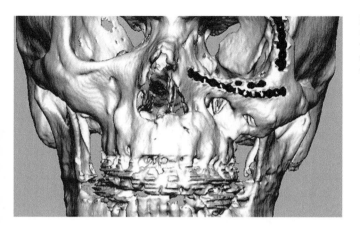

Fig. 3. Using the DICOM files from the CT scan, the files are converted to STL files with the existing periorbital hardware in blue. These STL files are useful for reconstruction hardware planning.

ectropion risk was found to be minimal, being only 3.8%.[8]

During the past decades, autogenous bone grafts have in general been considered to be ideal for the treatment of orbital floor fractures.[9] However, when using autogenous bone it is important to consider the following factors: the quantity of bone required at the recipient site, the biologic qualities of the donor bone, the unpredictable resorption of the bone graft, and the considerable donor site morbidity.[9] The above-listed shortcomings associated with autogenous bone grafting have led to the development of 4 basic types of implant materials for orbital wall reconstruction: allogeneic grafts, xenografts, nonresorbable synthetic alloplastic materials, and resorbable synthetic alloplastic materials.

Titanium meshes and high-density porous polyethylene implants are presently the most commonly used nonresorbable synthetic alloplastic materials for orbital floor reconstructions.[3] Titanium meshes are commonly used for larger defect sizes exceeding 2 cm[2].[3] Smaller defects are often treated using different commercially available resorbable materials such as PDS and Medpor (Stryker, Kalamazoo, MI, USA). Silastics, however, have fallen into disfavor due to frequent reports of

post-operative infections often leading to foreign material extrusion.[2,10] The major complications faced with orbital floor reduction are enophthalmos, lower lid ectropion, and ocular motility defects.[2] It is therefore very important to accurately restore the orbital volume preferably at the acute fracture stage to avoid chronic problems and patient dissatisfaction.

ADDITIVE MANUFACTURED ORBITAL FLOOR IMPLANTS

A major challenge when performing complex orbital surgery using commercially available stock materials is the need for tedious manual adaptation of the implants to the complex contours of the damaged orbital floor or walls. Most commercially available implants are supplied in generic sizes and shapes, which are designed on the basis of the "average" patient, not the "average" defect.

One novel way to circumvent this problem is by using new technologies from computer-guided surgical planning and additive manufacturing (AM) technology to produce passive fitting implants tailored for patient-specific needs.[11] Because the reconstruction of late orbital deformities is based on already existing chronic

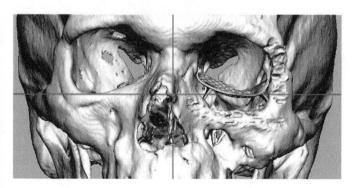

Fig. 4. Frontal view of the virtual planning of the orbital floor reconstruction in gold.

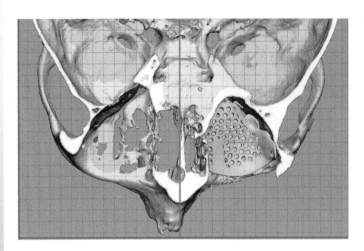

Fig. 5. Superior view of the virtual planning of the orbital floor reconstruction in gold.

defects, there is time to assess, plan, and custom manufacture highly precise implants. AM technology offers the possibility of physically replicating the morphology of damaged anatomic structures[12] and has proved to be highly advantageous within the field of craniofacial surgery (see **Figs. 4–7**; **Figs. 9–17**) where explaining, planning, and performing an operation is extremely difficult due to complex and highly variable anatomy.[13–16]

The combination of AM technology with electron beam, laser melting technology, and the development of the titanium materials have resulted in a new fabrication method for computer-aided design (CAD) or more specifically custom-designed titanium orbital implants.[6] Orbital implants fabricated from titanium are by their physical nature thin and stiff. They are easily stabilized, maintain their shape, and have the unique ability to compensate for volume without resorbing.[6]

Before planning an orbital operation, a 3-dimensional (3D) stereolithographic model of the patient's skull is fabricated using the patient's preoperative computed tomography (CT) DICOM voxel-based data set (see **Figs. 3–6** and **13–16**). In the future, as cone-beam CT (CBCT) scans become more available, the CBCT scanning protocol may offer a less invasive way to acquire DICOM data sets.[17] Planning with a DICOM data set allows a much better assessment and understanding of the shape, dimensions, and volume of the orbital defect area. After visual assessment of the defect site, the patient's DICOM data set is then imported into a virtual surgical planning software program of choice (Romexis Planmeca, Helsinki, Finland, Materialise Belgium) after which patient-specific 3D planning of the orbital floor area can be performed (see **Figs. 15** and **16**).

Most commercially available software programs are capable of manipulating bony segments and mirror the anatomy of the unaffected orbital site

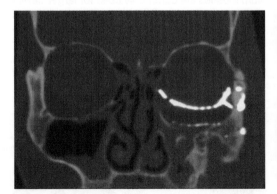

Fig. 7. Postoperative CT scan in coronal plane showing orbital floor rapid prototype in place. There are no screws securing the plate to the orbit. The device is kept in place by the weight of the orbital contents from above pushing the device against the inferior orbital rim and floor below.

Fig. 6. The rapid prototype metal orbital floor reconstruction in the orbit of the stereolithic skull reconstructed from the original CT scans.

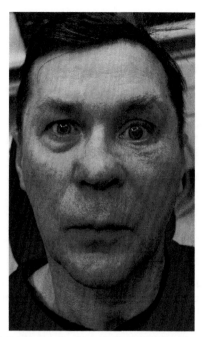

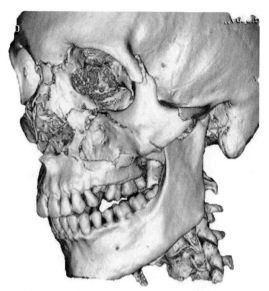

Fig. 10. Preoperative 3D CT scan, left lateral oblique view of a 22-year-old with NOE fracture, LeFort II fracture on right, and LeFort III fracture on left.

Fig. 8. Postoperative frontal view of patient 3 months following reconstruction of the left orbit to treat severe enophthalmos.

(see **Fig. 5**). After the planning phase is complete, the virtual reconstructions are drawn and converted into a stereolithography software file format (STL) to generate information needed to fabricate individual orbital floor implants using powder-based processes such as Selective Laser Sintering, Direct Metal Laser Sintering, or Three-Dimensional Printing.

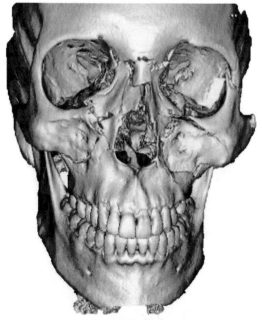

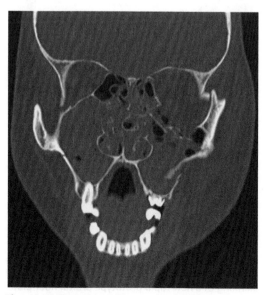

Fig. 9. Case 2. Preoperative 3D CT scan, frontal view of a 22-year-old man with NOE fracture, LeFort II fracture on right, and LeFort III fracture on left following an assault.

Fig. 11. Preoperative CT scan in the coronal plane showing severely comminuted NOE fracture and inferior displacement of the left orbital floor.

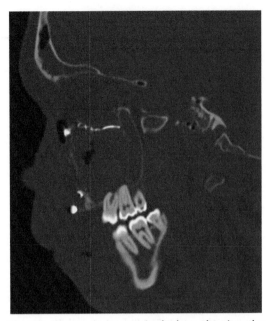

Fig. 12. CT scan in parasagittal plane showing the initial reconstruction of the orbital floor using a stock orbital floor plate secured with 2 screws in the inferior orbital rim. The orbital floor plate has become displaced inferiorly into the maxillary sinus.

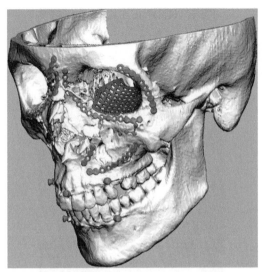

Fig. 14. Lateral oblique view of the STL skull reconstruction with the newly planed rapid prototype orbital floor plate.

STL is the most widely used format in rapid prototyping.[15] The STL model is formed by tessellation of the original model. Tessellation is the process of creating a 2D plane using the repetition of a geometric shape with no overlaps or gaps. Tessellation allows generalizations to higher dimensions, which helps to produce 3D constructs.

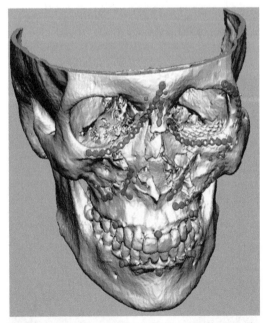

Fig. 13. This 3D model made by converting the DICOM CT scan files to STL files is useful for the virtual planning of a new rapid prototype orbital floor plate. The preexisting hardware is colored blue and there is a mesh on the left orbital floor represented by the serrated surface.

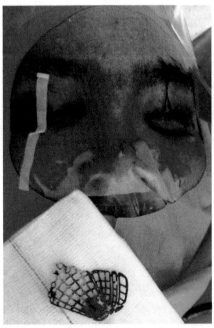

Fig. 15. Displaced stock manufactured orbital floor plate removed 8 weeks after insertion.

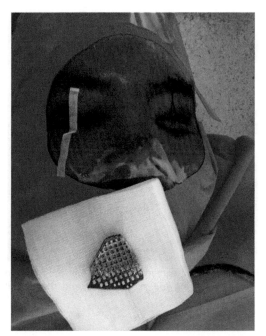

Fig. 16. Replacement rapid prototype orbital floor plate at the time of insertion.

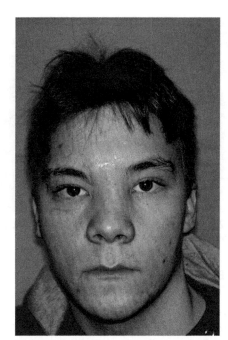

Fig. 18. Case 3. Preoperative frontal appearance of a 19-year-old man with traumatic telecanthus 6 months following reduction of NOE fracture.

The accuracy of CAD reconstruction hardware has been determined.[11,18–21] Once inserted, the fit of the construct is predictably stable and in terms of the wound and surrounding soft tissues, the device is well-tolerated. One major advantage of CAD and planned orbital hardware is that the construct can be precisely designed and fitted to cover only the defect and immediately adjacent tissue. By doing so, the minimum-sized implant and the minimum volume of material required to treat the defect is used. The construct can be designed to avoid the sensitive vital structures of the posterior orbit. This minimization of implanted hardware can be a significant issue when considering the post-operative edema that occurs following major orbital reconstruction of significant enophthalmos.

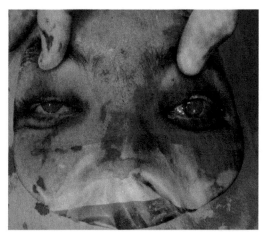

Fig. 17. Globe position checked after insertion of rapid prototype orbital floor plate.

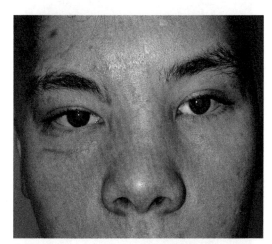

Fig. 19. Close-up of nasofrontal region showing widened interpupillary distance and lack of projection of nasal dorsum. In this case, the widening is asymmetric with greater widening on the right.

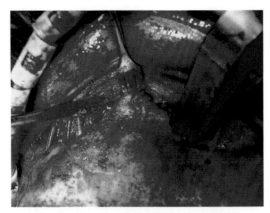

Fig. 20. Intraoperative view through coronal incision exposing the frontonasal suture.

LATE MANAGEMENT OF ORBITAL HYPERTELORISM AND NOE FRACTURES

One cause of orbital hypertelorism or increased interorbital width is traumatic telecanthus. Such traumatic telecanthus commonly occurs because of the displacement or detachment of the medial canthal tendon due to the fracture of the medial orbit, especially in combination with NOE fractures (see **Fig. 11**).[22] NOE fractures are to date most commonly classified according to the findings and recommendations published by Markowitz BL and colleagues[23] in 1991.

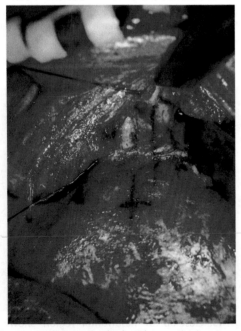

Fig. 21. Midline is marked with a scribed cross and then 2 incremental lines of 5 mm each is marked on the right side.

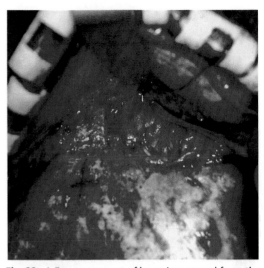

Fig. 22. A 5-mm segment of bone is removed from the right side leaving the midline bone and the medial orbital wall intact.

The NOE fractures are classified according to the pattern of the fracture and have been divided into the 3 groups. Type I fractures consist of a single-segment central fragment bearing the intact medial canthal tendon. Type II fractures comprise a comminuted central fragment with fractures remaining external to the medial canthal tendon. Type III fractures include a comminuted central fragment with fractures extending into bone bearing the medial canthal tendon insertion. There is often comminution of the NOE area and a detachment of the medial canthal tendon from the bone.

When the medial canthal tendon becomes detached, traumatic telecanthus results. However, if the medial canthal tendon is displaced laterally

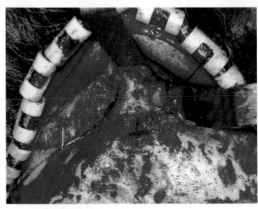

Fig. 23. The right medial orbital wall is moved 5 mm toward the midline.

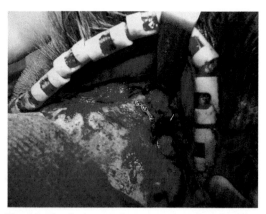

Fig. 24. The frontonasal segment is reduced with a plate.

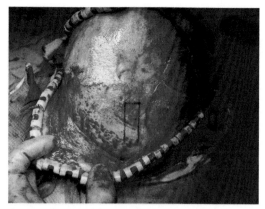

Fig. 26. Planning of calvarial bone graft harvest from right parietal bone.

with the bony medial orbital wall, the correct term should be medial orbital wall hypertelorism.[24] Traumatic displacement of the entire orbit is extremely rare but the incidence of increased distance between medial walls of the orbits due to the NOE injury is estimated to be 12% to 20% of cases.[25]

The severity of the orbital hypertelorism can be assessed using the Tessier score. In the mild type (type I) the interorbital distance is 30 to 34 mm, whereas in the moderate type (type II) the interorbital distance is 35 to 39 mm. Hypertelorism is classified as severe if the interorbital distance is more than 40 mm (type III).[26] Even in severe cases of hypertelorism the optic canals often lie in their normal positions. The diagnosis, hence scoring, (type I-III) can be made both by clinical assessment or using CT scans.

Traumatic orbital hypertelorism due to the NOE injury should be corrected at the first-stage operation. The surgical treatment is based on medial orbital wall and medial canthal tendon repositioning and fixation with miniplates. The detached medial canthal tendon can be repositioned by transnasal wiring methods. The aim of NOE injury treatment is to symmetrically restore the normal medial canthal anatomy, maintain the physiologic function of the lacrimal system, and to prevent complications particularly related to the frontal sinus. The frontal sinus must be evaluated especially if there are accompanying fractures of the supraorbital rim or the frontal bone.[27,28] Globe position must be restored by fixing the position of the orbital floor and finally restoring the orbital volume.

Frontonasal angle and nasal projection are essential for an aesthetic post-operative result.[29] Poor frontonasal angle and poor nasal projection combined with orbital hypertelorism compound the severity of the apparent deformity making the patient look worse.[22]

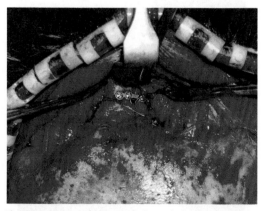

Fig. 25. Wiring of the medial canthal tendon on the right with a wire directly to the plate reducing the frontonasal bony segment. On the left side the medial canthal tendon wire is fixated to a screw diagonally to a screw in the right supraorbital region.

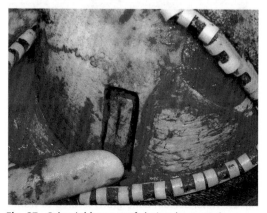

Fig. 27. Calvarial bone graft being harvested.

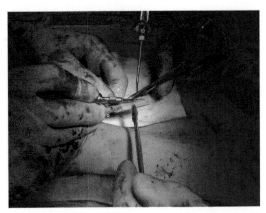

Fig. 28. Calvarial plate with plates applied being split on back table in preparation for grafting to right and left sides of nasal dorsum.

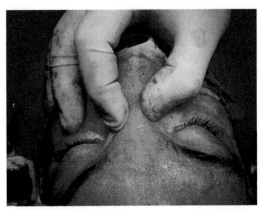

Fig. 30. Contour of nasal dorsum checked intraoperatively.

It is essential that during NOE surgery the surgeon be able to visualize and have access to the entire area of interest. The most predictable access is via the coronal approach. The order of treatment should be to first reconstruct the cranial base, frontal region, and the outer orbital frame.[30] The management of the frontal sinus should be done at this stage. Second, the frontonasal buttresses and orbital rims are fixed. Third, the nasal dorsum and nasal projection are restored by plating or using bone grafts. Fourth, the medial orbits and medial canthal tendons are repositioned and fixed by miniplates, meshes, and transnasal wires. The last stage is to repair the lacrimal canaliculi if necessary. Acute repair is preferred to dealing with the late complications associated with attempts to repair chronic long-standing deformities.

Secondary late corrections including intracranial osteotomies in severe cases of orbital hypertelorism are extremely difficult to perform, have less predictable results, and are associated with increased post-operative morbidity.[22] In milder cases, the subcranial osteotomies can be chosen. The principle is to restore the normal interorbital distance (**Figs. 18–35**). The improvement associated with late reconstruction of long-standing orbital hypertelorism may be disappointing. It is for this reason that the best management strategy is to avoid late complications by repairing these deformities early near the time of the original fractures.

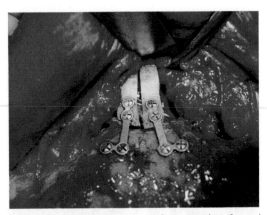

Fig. 29. Nasal dorsum bone grafts secured to frontal nasal area by bone plates.

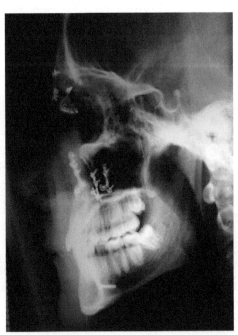

Fig. 31. Postoperative lateral skull film showing reduction of the nasofrontal region.

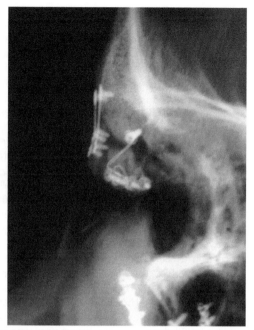

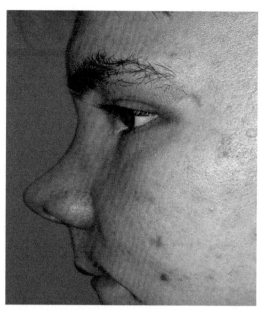

Fig. 34. Postoperative left lateral view of Case 3 with decreased interpupillary distance and improved projection of the dorsum of the nose.

Fig. 32. Magnified lateral skull view showing bone grafts to nasal dorsum secured by plates and screws and canthal tendon wiring.

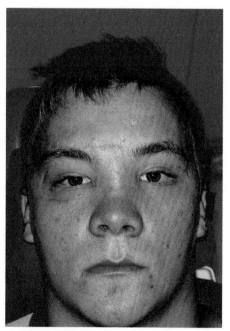

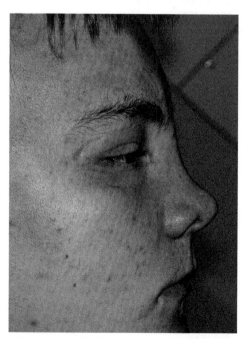

Fig. 33. Postoperative frontal view of Case 3 with decreased interpupillary distance and improved projection of the dorsum of the nose.

Fig. 35. Postoperative right lateral view of Case 3 with decreased interpupillary distance and improved projection of the dorsum of the nose.

REFERENCES

1. Kontio R, Lindqvist C. Management of orbital fractures. Oral Maxillofac Surg Clin North Am 2009; 21(2):209–20.
2. Cole P, Kaufman Y, Hollier L. Principles of facial trauma: orbital fracture management. J Craniofac Surg 2009;20(1):101–4.
3. Tabrizi R, Ozkan TB, Mohammadinejad C, et al. Orbital floor reconstruction. J Craniofac Surg 2010; 21(4):1142–6.
4. Al-Sukhun J, Lindqvist C, Kontio R. Modelling of orbital deformation using finite-element analysis. J R Soc Interface 2006;3(7):255–62.
5. Al-Sukhun J, Kontio R, Lindqvist C. Orbital stress analysis–part I: simulation of orbital deformation following blunt injury by finite element analysis method. J Oral Maxillofac Surg 2006;64(3):434–42.
6. Al-Sukhun J, Kontio R, Lindqvist C, et al. Use of a prefabricated titanium plate for accurate reconstruction of secondary orbital blow-out fracture. Plast Reconstr Surg 2006;117(5):1648–51.
7. Al-Sukhun J, Törnwall J, Lindqvist C, et al. Bioresorbable poly-L/DL-lactide (P[L/DL]LA 70/30) plates are reliable for repairing large inferior orbital wall bony defects: a pilot study. J Oral Maxillofac Surg 2006;64(1):47–55.
8. Ridgway EB, Chen C, Colakoglu S, et al. The incidence of lower eyelid malposition after facial fracture repair: a retrospective study and meta-analysis comparing subtarsal, subciliary, and transconjunctival incisions. Plast Reconstr Surg 2009; 124(5):1578–86.
9. Kontio RK, Laine P, Salo A, et al. Reconstruction of internal orbital wall fracture with iliac crest free bone graft: clinical, computed tomography, and magnetic resonance imaging follow-up study. Plast Reconstr Surg 2006;118(6):1365–74.
10. Morrison AD, Sanderson RC, Moos KF. The use of silastic as an orbital implant for reconstruction of orbital wall defects: review of 311 cases treated over 20 years. J Oral Maxillofac Surg 1995;53(4):412–7.
11. Abou-ElFetouh A, Barakat A, Abdel-Ghany K. Computer-guided rapid-prototyped templates for segmental mandibular osteotomies: a preliminary report. Int J Med Robot 2011;7(2):187–92.
12. Ibrahim D, Broilo TL, Heitz C, et al. Dimensional error of selective laser sintering, three-dimensional printing and PolyJet models in the reproduction of mandibular anatomy. J Craniomaxillofac Surg 2009;37(3):167–73.
13. Chang PS, Parker TH, Patrick CW Jr, et al. The accuracy of stereolithography in planning craniofacial bone replacement. J Craniofac Surg 2003;14(2): 164–70.
14. Campbell RI, de Beer DJ, Pei E. Additive manufacturing in South Africa: building on the foundations. Rapid Prototyping J 2011;17(2): 156–62.
15. Silva DN, Gerhardt de Oliveira M, Meurer E, et al. Dimensional error in selective laser sintering and 3D-printing of models for craniomaxillary anatomy reconstruction. J Craniomaxillofac Surg 2008;36(8): 443–9.
16. Laoui T, Shaik SK. Rapid prototyping techniques used to produce medical models/implants. Proceedings of the 4th national conference on rapid and virtual prototyping and applications, pp. 23–32, ISBN 1-86058-411-X, Centre for rapid design and manufacture, Buckinghamshire Chilterns University College. Buckinghamshire, United Kingdom, June 20, 2003.
17. Lukáts O, Bujtár P, Sándor GK, et al. Porous hydroxyapatite orbital implant evaluation using CBCT scanning: a method for in vivo porous structure evaluation. Int J Biomater 2012;2012:764749. http://dx.doi.org/10.1155/2012/764749 Article ID 764749.
18. Foley BD, Thayer WP, Honeybrook A, et al. Mandibular reconstruction using computer-aided design and computer-aided manufacturing: an analysis of surgical results. J Oral Maxillofac Surg 2013;71(2):111–9.
19. Arias-Gallo J, Maremonti P, González-Otero T, et al. Long term results of reconstruction plates in lateral mandibular defects. Revision of nine cases. Auris Nasus Larynx 2004;31(1):57–63.
20. Christensen AM, Humphries SM. Role of rapid digital manufacture in planning and implementation of complex medical treatments. In: Gibson I, editor. Advanced manufacturing technology for medical applications. Sussex (United Kingdom): John Wiley & Sons Ltd; 2006. p. 16.
21. McDonald JA, Ryall CJ, Wimpenny DI. Rapid prototyping casebook. London: Professional Engineering Publishing Stratasys; 2001. p. 260.
22. Sàndor GK, Clokie CM. Hypertelorism. In: Fonseca RJ, editor. Oral and maxillofacial surgery, vol. 6. Philadelphia: W.B. Saunders Company; 2000. p. 221–38 ISBN# 0-7216-9631-7.
23. Markowitz BL, Manson PN, Sargent L, et al. Management of the medial canthal tendon in nasoethmoid orbital fractures: the importance of the central fragment in classification and treatment. Plast Reconstr Surg 1991;87(5):843–53.
24. Yaremchuk MJ, Whitaker LA, Grossmann R, et al. An objective assessment of treatment for orbital hypertelorism. Ann Plast Surg 1993;30:27–34.
25. Sargent LA. Nasoethmoid orbital fractures: diagnosis and treatment. Plast Reconstr Surg 2007; 120(7 Suppl 2):16S–31S.
26. Tessier P. Anatomical classification of facial, craniofacial, and latero-facial clefts. J Maxillofac Surg 1976;4:69–89.
27. Lanigan DT, Stoelinga PJ. Fractures of the supraorbital rim. J Oral Surg 1980;38(10):764–70.

28. McGuire TP, Gomes PP, Clokie CM, et al. Fractures of the supraorbital rim: principles and management. J Can Dent Assoc 2006;72(6):537–40.

29. Biller JA, Kim DW. A contemporary assessment of facial aesthetic preferences. Arch Facial Plast Surg 2009;11(2):91–7.

30. Rodriguez ED, Bluebond-Langner R, Park JE, et al. Preservation of contour in periorbital and midfacial craniofacial microsurgery: reconstruction of the soft-tissue elements and skeletal buttresses. Plast Reconstr Surg 2008;121(5):1738–47.

Late Revision or Correction of Facial Trauma–Related Soft-Tissue Deformities

Kevin L. Rieck, DDS, MD*, W. Jonathan Fillmore, DMD, MD, Kyle S. Ettinger, DDS

KEYWORDS

- Facial trauma • Maxillofacial surgery • Soft-tissue injury • Wound healing • Treatment

KEY POINTS

- Facial soft-tissue deformities can arise that require specific evaluation and management for correction.
- The contemporary maxillofacial surgeon has continued to expand on the historical management of facial fractures established by pioneers in the specialty.
- Advances in understanding the biological aspects of wound healing and surgical options to rectify acute and delayed facial soft-tissue deformities, combined with current technology, facilitate improved outcomes.

INTRODUCTION

Facial trauma is the foundation underlying contemporary oral and maxillofacial surgery. We have a long history of managing these patients and providing excellent care for their complex injuries. As specialists we owe a great deal to those who pioneered various treatments for facial fracture repair and paved the way for oral and maxillofacial surgeons to further expand their scope to include all aspects of facial trauma. The surgical approaches used in accessing the facial skeleton for fracture repair are often the same as or similar to those used for cosmetic enhancement of the face, an aspect that has contributed to the expansion of cosmetic procedures performed by maxillofacial surgeons. Rarely does facial trauma result in injuries that do not in some way affect the facial soft-tissue envelope either directly or as sequelae of the surgical repair. Knowledge of both skeletal and facial soft-tissue anatomy is paramount to successful clinical outcomes. Facial soft-tissue deformities can arise that require specific evaluation and management for correction. This article focuses on revision and correction of these soft-tissue–related injuries secondary to facial trauma.

PHASES OF WOUND HEALING

A basic knowledge of the principles of wound healing is critical for surgeons to understand when managing soft-tissue injuries resulting from trauma. An awareness of the intricacies of wound healing enables the surgeon to endeavor to minimize complications that might occur during this process, and helps ensure the best possible postoperative outcome. Wound healing is an extremely

The authors have nothing to disclose.

Dr Kevin L. Rieck is currently at Nebraska Oral and Facial Surgery, 2600 South 56th Street, Suite A, Lincoln, NE 68506, USA.

Division of Oral & Maxillofacial Surgery, Department of Surgery, Mayo College of Medicine, 200 First Street Southwest, Rochester, MN 55905, USA

* Corresponding author. Nebraska Oral and Facial Surgery, 2600 South 56th Street, Suite A, Lincoln, NE 68506, USA.

E-mail address: klrieckddsmd@alumni.mayo.edu

complex process of overlapping phases whereby numerous cell types are responsible for executing a multitude of cellular functions, and can be organized into the 4 following phases:

- Immediate response
- Inflammatory phase
- Proliferative phase
- Remodeling/maturation

Prolongation of any one of these phases can result in delayed or compromised healing of a wound and can eventually lead to suboptimal outcomes from a clinical standpoint.

Immediate Response

The immediate response to an injury in which there is a violation of tissue integrity is a rapid alteration in cell-signaling pathways that modify cellular gene expression, metabolism, and cell survival.[1] Pathways leading to hemostasis are triggered and lead to local vasoconstriction of damaged blood vessels, platelet activation, platelet aggregation, and formation of a provisional fibrin matrix that also serves as a medium through which cells are recruited to participate in wound repair.[2] Activated platelets are also responsible for the secretion of multiple cytokines, growth factors, and chemotactic agents needed for progression of the healing process, such as vascular endothelial growth factor (VEGF), platelet-derived growth factor (PDGF), fibroblast growth factor, transforming growth factor β (TGF-β), CXCL4, and RANTES.[1]

Inflammatory Phase

The inflammatory phase is typified by the passive ingress of circulating leukocytes (predominantly neutrophils) from damaged blood vessels coupled with activation of immune cells present within the damaged tissues (mast cells, T cells, and Langerhans cells).[1] This ingress of phagocytic cells represents the transition of the wound into a state of active repair, and is facilitated by an increase in vascular permeability secondary to locally released factors such as nitric oxide (NO), mast cell–derived histamine, and tissue plasminogen activator.[1] Neutrophils are recruited to the site of injury to cleanse the wound through phagocytosis of invading microorganisms and removal of cellular debris. Monocytes are slowly recruited to the site of injury, and will peak in numbers approximately 24 hours after the initial injury.[1] Monocytes further the efforts set forth by the neutrophils, and will clear additional cellular debris along with nonviable neutrophils in preparation for the next phase of wound healing. In noncontaminated wounds the presence of neutrophils and monocytes is relatively short lived; however, in contaminated wounds the presence of phagocytic cells can persist, leading to a prolongation of the inflammatory phase and compromised outcomes in terms of wound healing and scar formation.

Proliferative Phase

The second phase of wound healing is the proliferative phase, during which the processes of reepithelialization, angiogenesis, collagen deposition, and wound contraction predominate. Reepithelialization will occur through the migration and proliferation of epithelial stem cells present at the wound margins and in deeper adnexal structures such as the hair-follicle bulge.[2] The provisional fibrin matrix that was deposited during the inflammatory phase will be replaced with granulation tissue within about 72 hours following initial injury, and will persist for approximately 14 days.[2] Fibroblast proliferation in response to TGF-β, PDGF, and fibroblast growth factor leads to synthesis of extracellular matrix components including glycosaminoglycans, proteoglycans, and collagen (predominantly type III).[2] Angiogenesis leads to extension of capillaries from the wound edge into the zone of injury.[3] This process is critical for providing the oxygen and nutrients necessary for continuation of healing. Collagen deposition will increase wound strength, while fibroblasts in close proximity to the wound edges will begin producing weakly contractile actin bundles to facilitate contraction of the wound.[1] The proliferative phase culminates with restoration of tissue integrity via newly formed epithelial barrier and reapproximation of deeper layers through the process of wound contracture and synthesis of new extracellular matrix: essentially, formation of a scar.

Remodeling and Maturation

The final phase of wound healing is the longest of the 3 phases, and can take anywhere from several months to several years depending on the patient, the integrity of their immune system, and overall systemic health. This phase is essential for modification of tissue integrity and the normalization of tissue appearance. The hallmark of this phase is the reorganization of the collagenous matrix created during the proliferative phase, and involves the sequential replacement of type III collagen fibrils with stronger and more robust type I collagen. Larger collagen bundles with a higher proportion of intermolecular cross-linking are created,[2] and the microvascular network within the scar is also revised to become a more functional network of blood vessels.[1] The extracellular matrix that was formed in the dermis will undergo additional maturation involving the deposition of collagen fibers in a more parallel fashion, improving both the overall appearance and tensile strength of the scar. However, it is noteworthy that the tensile strength of the healed wound will never reach more than 80% of the original tensile strength of healthy unwounded skin.[2]

OPTIMIZING WOUND HEALING

Optimizing the conditions for wound healing is essential for ensuring a positive clinical outcome when dealing with soft-tissue injuries in facial trauma. Many surgeons are familiar with the traditional Halstedian principles of surgical technique and tissue management, and these principles have subsequently been expanded on by other investigators.[4] Combined principles of wound management are presented in **Box 1**.

Close adherence to the aforementioned principles during the primary repair of soft-tissue injuries will help to minimize the possibility of delayed or aberrant wound healing; however, multiple factors must be considered when prognosticating the necessity for future revisions. Wound contamination,

---

Box 1
Traditional Halstedian principles and expanded surgical principles

Halstedian Principles

- Gentle handling of tissue
- Aseptic technique
- Sharp anatomic dissection of tissue
- Obtaining adequate hemostasis
- Obliteration of dead space
- Avoidance of tension in wound closure
- Reliance on rest

Expanded Principles

- Removal and debridement of foreign bodies
- Control and prevention of infection
- Diversion of salivary secretions
- Diversion of excess exudates with the use of drains
- Creation of fresh wound edges to promote reepithelialization
- Coverage of tissue defects with skin grafts when appropriate

Adapted from Hom D, Sun GH, Elluru RG. A contemporary review of wound healing in otolaryngology: current state and future promise. Laryngoscope 2009;119(11):2100; with permission.

---

the presence of foreign bodies, compromised blood supply, presence of devitalized tissue, irregularity of wound margins, and tissue avulsion can all contribute to the need for secondary procedures despite the skillfulness and quality of the primary repair. Even with meticulous wound irrigation, adequate dermal suturing for wound-edge eversion, and minimization of skin tension during the primary repair, poor aesthetics following wound healing are sometimes unavoidable, and the late revision of soft-tissue injuries inevitable.

HYPERTROPHIC SCARS AND KELOIDS

Because of their many similarities, the terms hypertrophic scar and keloid are often used interchangeably; however, this represents an incorrect assumption that the two processes are one in the same. There are in fact multiple distinctions between a hypertrophic scar and a keloid in terms of their clinical, biochemical, and histopathologic presentation. In generating a treatment plan for management of hypertrophic scars and keloids, the appropriate diagnosis of the correct clinical entity is paramount; this is particularly true in the early stages of keloid formation, when it may visually appear very similar to a hypertrophic scar. The pathogenesis of both disease processes represents an abnormal fibroproliferation during healing, which leads to excessive disorganized collagen deposition within the skin.[5] Of importance is that neither keloids nor hypertrophic scars are known to occur spontaneously and will always follow some form of tissue insult, whether from surgery or from trauma. Histopathologic review can be helpful in determining which clinical entity is present, although it should be noted that the histologic distinction between these entities continues to evolve.[6] The salient differences between hypertrophic scars and keloids are presented in **Table 1**.

Treatment of Hypertrophic Scars and Keloids

Perhaps the best possible treatment for hypertrophic scars and keloids is to take an early preventive mindset, with specific attention being given to minimizing the inciting factors that may lead to their formation. Wound contracture and excessive skin tension have been implicated in the formation of both hypertrophic scars and keloids, although this theory is still subject to debate.[7] Nevertheless, when planning revision procedures it is important to orient surgical incisions parallel to relaxed skin-tension lines so that the vector of wound closure parallels the lines of maximum extensibility and minimizes wound-closure tension. Unfortunately, keloid and hypertrophic scar

Table 1
Salient differences between hypertrophic scars and keloids

	Hypertrophic Scars	Keloids
Timing of onset	Follows progression similar to normal wound healing, but with prolongation of the proliferative and maturation phases	Variable; can occur during initial wound healing but also can occur spontaneously years after stable scar formation has completed
Progression	Rapid intense enlargement of scar for several months followed by spontaneous entrance into regressive phase	Persistent growth potential and low likelihood of quiescence. Will not spontaneously enter into a regressive phase
Lesion extension	Remains contained to initial boundaries of injury	Extension beyond boundaries of initial injury (defining feature of keloids)
Clinical presentation	Raised pink or red scar that may or may not be pruritic	Raised erythematous scar with greater propensity to be extremely painful and pruritic
Recurrence	Rare following surgical excision	Almost 100% following surgical excision alone
Associated skin type	None	Predilection for darker-skinned individuals
Hormonal influence	None	Known to worsen during pregnancy and puberty
Histopathologic features	Type III collagen oriented parallel to epidermal surface Abundant nodules containing myofibroblasts Large extracellular collagen filaments No invasion of surrounding dermis	Disorganized type I and type III collagen Nodules lacking myofibroblasts Presence of hyalinized collagen Acellular core with thick collagen bundles Prominent fascia-like fibrous bands Invasion into normal surrounding dermis

Data from Refs.[7–9]

formation may sometimes be unavoidable, given the nature of a patient's injury and the underlying predisposition to excessive scarring. In general, management of keloids is more troubling than that of hypertrophic scars, given their indefinite growth potential and propensity for recurrence even with treatment, whereas surgical excision of hypertrophic scars is often curative.[7] Several therapeutic options have been suggested, which encompass surgery, local injection of steroids, compression therapy, silicone sheeting, radiation, and chemotherapy.

Surgery

Surgical excision of keloids and hypertrophic scars has traditionally been a mainstay of treatment. In the case of hypertrophic scars, surgical excision alone is often sufficient in providing improvement of scar cosmesis. This point is particularly true if the hypertrophic scar is the end result of a complicated (infected) wound or a wound that has undergone delayed closure, as the appearance of the wound is not necessarily the direct product of an underlying predisposition toward aberrant scarring. Surgical principles

detailing the excision, reorientation, and camouflage of simple hypertrophic scars are outlined in later sections of this article.

Surgical excision of hypertrophic scars and keloids arising from uncomplicated wounds is often fraught with difficulty, and recurrence rates of 50% to 100% following excision alone are often reported.[8,9] The surrounding tissue disruption created by the surgical procedure can also lead to increased collagen deposition and the recurrence of a keloid larger than the lesion initially excised.[10] Accordingly, use of adjuvant therapies in addition to surgery is a prerequisite to effectively managing refractory hypertrophic scars and keloids.

Intralesional steroids

Given the high recurrence rate of keloids treated with surgical excision alone, adjuvant therapies are often required to obtain adequate control. Intralesional corticosteroids have become a mainstay of treatment of both hypertrophic scars and keloids. Intralesional steroids work by reducing collagen synthesis, decreasing fibroblast proliferation, inhibiting glycosaminoglycan synthesis, and suppressing proinflammatory mediators such as TGF-β and VEGF.[11,12] Patients should be counseled on both the possible side effects of the corticosteroid injection and the need for serial treatments. Steroids can soften and flatten the appearance hypertrophic scars and keloids; however, they will not narrow the scar or result in complete resolution of the lesion[11]; hence the need for multimodal treatment. Possible side effects of injected corticosteroids include skin and subcutaneous tissue atrophy, depigmentation, telangiectasias, skin necrosis and ulceration, and, in extreme cases, development of Cushingoid features.[9] Triamcinolone acetonide (TA) is the most commonly used steroid in the treatment of keloids and hypertrophic scars. Multiple investigators advocate mixing TA with equal parts lidocaine and epinephrine to improve patient comfort during injections.[9,11,13] Recommendations on dosing strength and frequency vary in the literature, but treatment schedule will largely be predicated on the response to the injections. Doses of 10 mg/mL to 40 mg/mL of TA are reported by numerous investigators.[9,11,13] The injection should be oriented to infiltrate the dermal layer, which will ease the injection and dispersement of the solution. Multiple injections interspersed over several months are often required to obtain adequate improvement in the appearance of the keloid/scar. The injections should be discontinued once the scar/keloid becomes stable or when adverse side effects begin to develop.

Compression therapy

The use of pressure dressings for reduction of scar formation was first reported in 1835, and has been used in prophylaxis against excessive scarring from burns since the 1970s.[9,11] Unfortunately, application of compression therapy to scars resulting from facial trauma is often exceedingly difficult from both practical and patient-compliance standpoints. Owing to the long durations of treatment (6–12 months), the use of compression therapy for the head and neck region has largely been relegated to applications specifically involving keloids of the earlobes, and thus are not covered in any further detail here.

Silicone-gel sheeting

The use of topical silicone-gel sheeting for scar treatment was first reported in the 1980s and has gained in popularity over the subsequent decades. It is one of the few scar treatment modalities that has been evaluated in randomized controlled trials, and has thus been recommended by some investigators as a first-line treatment before consideration of surgery and intralesional steroid injections.[12] Silicone-gel sheeting can also be used as a prophylactic measure if patients are known to be hypertrophic scar formers or have a known history of keloid formation. It is recommended that the silicone gel be applied soon after wound epithelialization has completed, and it should remain in place for a minimum of 12 hours per day for at least 2 months.[11,12] Although the exact mechanism whereby silicone sheeting reduces scar formation is not yet well understood,[9,11] it represents an effective and minimally invasive treatment strategy that is generally well tolerated by patients.

Radiation and chemotherapy

The use of radiation therapy and chemotherapeutics in the treatment of keloids has been well documented within the literature.[9,11–13] Incorporation of these modalities is generally not considered until keloids have failed to respond to initial attempts with more conservative treatment strategies. Accordingly the specifics of radiation and immunotherapy, being beyond the scope of this article, are not presented here.

ATROPHIC SCARS

Atrophic scars are another common complication of aberrant wound healing, and represent clinical entity distinct from hypertrophic scars and keloids. Rather than forming from an excess of fibroproliferation, as is the case for hypertrophic scars and keloids, atrophic scars result from an underfunctioning of fibroproliferative mechanisms. Impaired collagen deposition and dermal atrophy lead to topographic depressions within the skin, a hallmark of the atrophic scar. Surgery, skin trauma, acne, and wound contracture are just some of the potential causes of atrophic scar formation. These scars can initially appear erythematous, but with continued wound maturation they will often become more fibrotic, hypopigmented, and depressed relative to the surrounding tissue.

SCAR REVISION BY LASER

At present there are several different laser-resurfacing options at the disposal of the surgeon for applications in scar revision. The basic principle of laser resurfacing involves selective tissue ablation followed by subsequent induction of endogenous repair mechanisms, leading to collagen reorganization and improved appearance of scarred tissue. The varying properties of each laser system will largely depend on the wavelength of emitted light and the respective tissue chromophore absorbing the light within the desired range. It is this principle that allows different laser systems to preferentially affect specific molecular targets within tissue and cause discrete areas of tissue damage while leaving other components of tissue unaffected. With several different laser systems currently available on the market, it is important for the surgeon to have a basic understanding of the properties of each system so that the correct laser-resurfacing modality is applied for the appropriate clinical scenario.

CO_2 Laser

The CO_2 laser has the longest track record of any laser-resurfacing system available on the market today, and still possesses utility in a multitude of applications beyond delayed treatment of scarred tissue. The wavelength of light emitted by CO_2 lasers ranges from 9400 to 10,600 nm. At this wavelength the principle chromophore is water, and the mechanism of selective tissue ablation is through intracellular and extracellular water vaporization.[14,15] CO_2 lasers induce thermal coagulation in the dermal layer of the skin, and can stimulate tissue remodeling and robust neocollagenesis (**Fig. 1**).[15] Accordingly, CO_2 lasers have applications in the treatment of atrophic scars whereby the induction of fibroproliferation is desirable to regain dermal tissue volume, whereas use in the treatment of keloids almost always invariably results in recurrence for the very same reason.[16] The primary disadvantage of CO_2 lasers is the greater level of tissue damage produced relative to other laser systems. The deeper penetration of the zone of thermal damage can lead to persistent postoperative erythema that can last anywhere from 2 to 6 months following a resurfacing procedure.[14,15] Additional complications of CO_2 laser treatments include edema, oozing, crusting, infection, scarring, acne flares, pruritus, and delayed or immediate onset of skin-pigment alteration.[15]

Er:YAG Lasers

The erbium-doped yttrium-aluminum-garnet (Er: YAG) laser is another ablative laser that was introduced in the mid-1990s. Er:YAG lasers have an emitted wavelength of 2940 nm and also target water as the primary tissue chromophore. The Er:YAG lasers were touted for having a water-absorption coefficient 16 times greater than that of CO_2 lasers and a concomitant capability to reduce thermal damage to tissue.[17] Higher affinity for water and decreased thermal damage of tissue correlates with reduced postoperative morbidity, shortened recovery times, and reduced anesthesia requirements in comparison with traditional CO_2 laser therapy.[18] However, reduced penetration depth of the emitted wavelength along with reduced thermal injury also correlates with diminished clinical efficacy in tissue remodeling when compared with the CO_2 laser.[17,18] Nevertheless, the more superficial penetration of the Er:YAG laser also renders it less likely to cause hypopigmentation of the skin, and is thus considered to be safer in the application of scar revision for darker-skinned individuals.[17,18]

Nonablative Lasers

In contrast to the previously discussed ablative laser technologies, nonablative lasers are able to induce dermal remodeling without concomitantly ablating the epidermal surface. Lasers using this technology include the pulsed-dye laser (PDL) and the neodymium-doped yttrium-aluminum-garnet (Nd:YAG) laser.

PDLs generate an emitted wavelength of light ranging from 585 to 595 nm,[14] which is preferentially absorbed by hemoglobin and melanin. This aspect makes this laser system ideal for the treatment of vascular lesions such as port wine stains, telangiectasias, and hemangiomas, but care must be exercised in treatment of darker-skinned individuals, who have a greater risk of dyspigmentation with the use of PDL systems. The nonablative technology of PDLs reduces the likelihood of significant postoperative erythema, which is the primary drawback of ablative CO_2 lasers.[14] PDL technology is suitable for the treatment of red, hyperemic, and hypertrophic scars, and is effective in reducing the pigmentation, vascularity, and bulk of scar tissue.[19]

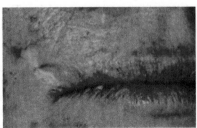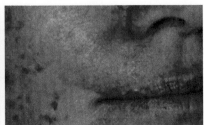

Fig. 1. Preoperative and postoperative CO_2 laser resurfacing of scar on right upper lip.

Nd:YAG nonablative laser technology relies on light energy emitted in the near-infrared and mid-infrared regions (1064–1320 nm), and is weakly absorbed by melanin. Early trials of 1230-nm Nd:YAG lasers demonstrated a propensity to induce epidermal blistering and necrosis, which is why these laser systems are often coupled with adjunctive cryogen spray-cooling technology.[20] This technology relies on a millisecond of cryogen spurt delivered to the skin surface to cool the epidermis while simultaneously leaving the dermal structures susceptible to the thermal injury.[21] By effectively controlling skin-surface temperature, one of the primary benefits of the Nd:YAG laser systems is that it can be used in the treatment of patients with darker skin types with less likelihood of inducing posttreatment dyspigmentation.[22,23]

Fractional Photothermolysis

Fractional photothermolysis (FP) was first introduced in 2004,[24] and has become the most advanced form of laser therapy on the market today. FP has been used in both ablative and non-ablative laser applications, and represents a unique and discrete method of laser delivery to scarred tissues. This technology relies on splitting the laser beam into an array of smaller beams, which create focal columns of tissue necrosis referred to as microscopic treatment zones (MTZs). These MTZs are surrounded by areas of undisturbed tissue, which facilitate rapid healing of the intervening necrotic zones.[25] The MTZs created by ablative fractional lasers (fractionated CO_2 and Er:YAG lasers) involve both epidermal and dermal layers, whereas nonablative fractional lasers only create a dermal column of necrosis. In addition, nonablative fractional lasers will not violate the stratum corneum, which preserves epidermal barrier function postoperatively, whereas ablative fractional lasers will vaporize the stratum corneum.[25] Clinically, skin treated with ablative fractional lasers has an appearance similar to that treated by older ablative laser technology because the columns of necrosis lack a protective epithelial cap, resulting in a similar postoperative erythema and serosanguinous drainage in the treated area. However, reepithelialization will rapidly ensue as a result of ingress of fibroblasts and epithelial cells from the intact tissue surrounding the MTZs. Thus, posttreatment erythema with fractional lasers will resolve in a period of 6 to 7 days, whereas erythema from older ablative laser systems typically persists for 2 to 6 months.[25]

Patients with fairer skin types (Fitzpatrick types I–III) are considered to be more ideal for treatment with fractional laser systems, although treatment of darker skin tones (Fitzpatrick types IV–V) can be safely treated as well. Fractional laser systems have gained popularity because of their shortened postoperative recovery periods and their reduced side-effect profiles in comparison with purely ablative laser technologies. It should be noted that with all laser systems, those that are capable of generating higher levels of thermal injury to tissue (ablative systems) will generally be capable of reaching greater levels of clinical efficacy; however, higher risks of adverse events (dyspigmentation, erythema, pain, infection, and so forth) may occur as well. **Fig. 2** illustrates facial scar revision with use of the Fraxel laser. Three treatments were performed using topical anesthesia over the course of 8 months. Significant resolution of the irregular scar was noted.

DERMABRASION AND CHEMICAL PEELS

Dermabrasion and chemical peeling are additional forms of skin resurfacing that can be useful in the management of scarring secondary to facial trauma. The principles of dermabrasion are similar to those of scar revision by laser, in that it results in the selective removal of the epidermis and partial removal of the underlying dermal layers. Dermabrasion is typically carried out with diamond fraises or wire brushes attached to rotary hand pieces capable of variable speeds. Dermabrasion is effective in treating both atrophic and hypertrophic scars, in addition to being used in several other applications including treatment of rhytides, rhinophyma, and superficial premalignant and malignant skin lesions.[26] During preoperative evaluation before dermabrasion, it is important for the surgeon to specifically ask about current or previous use of isotretinoin (Accutane), as this has been linked to formation hypertrophic scars and keloids following dermabrasion treatment.[26,27] Accordingly, patients should have this medication discontinued for 6 to 12 months before undergoing a dermabrasion procedure.[28] Patients with darker skin complexion should be thoroughly counseled on the risk of hyperpigmentation following the procedure, as well as the increased likelihood of this complication with concomitant estrogen and sun exposure.[27]

Peeling techniques use chemical ablative agents to selectively disrupt epithelial and dermal tissues of the skin, which results in collagen reorganization and improvement in the appearance of scarred tissues. Agents used for chemical peels are classified based on their depth of penetration into the skin, and can broadly be categorized as superficial, medium, and deep peeling agents.

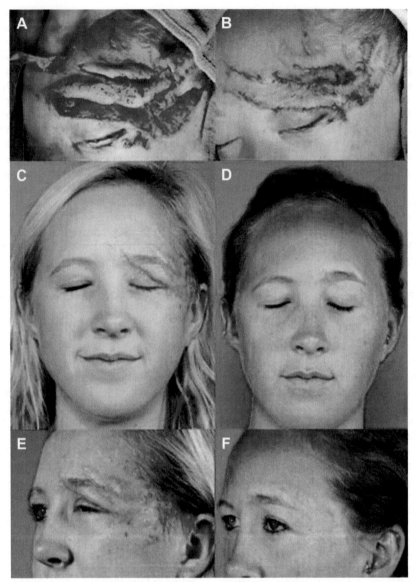

Fig. 2. (*A, B*) Initial injury from motor vehicle collision and initial primary repair. (*C, E*) One month after repair. (*D, F*) Ten months postoperatively after 3 Fraxel laser skin-resurfacing procedures.

However, the depth of penetration of these agents will also depend on their concentration, duration of application, and number of times they are applied. **Table 2** highlights the various agents commonly used for facial resurfacing, and their level of penetration into the dermis.

Superficial peels can often be applied and tolerated by patients without the need for local anesthesia or intravenous sedation. Increasing the depth of chemical penetration will necessitate additional endeavors to control pain during the application. Regional blocks and intravenous sedation are often required to increase comfort during application of medium and deep peels. It

should be noted that increasing the depth of chemical peel will also be positively correlated with a higher degree of morbidity, including textural and pigmentary changes in the skin. It is also important for the surgeon to be aware of the potential cardiotoxicity associated with phenol-based peel solutions, and that intraoperative cardiac monitoring is essential for avoiding potentially life-threatening arrhythmias.

SURGICAL TECHNIQUES FOR SCAR REVISION

Several different surgical scar-revision techniques are available to aid in camouflage, reorientation, or

Table 2
Common chemical peeling agents

Superficial Peels	Medium Peels	Deep Peels
Penetration: Stratum Corneum to Papillary Dermis	Penetration: Upper Reticular Dermis	Penetration: Mid Reticular Dermis
Low-concentration glycolic acid 10%–20% Trichloroacetic acid Jessner solution Tretinoin 5-Fluorouracil Salicylic acid β-Hydroxy acid	35% Trichloroacetic acid combined with Jessner solution 70% Glycolic acid 88% Phenol	Baker solution (88% phenol, septisol, croton oil, and distilled water)

excision of unaesthetic scars resulting from facial fractures. These techniques can help to hide scars within boundaries between anatomic subunits of the face, and can also conceal scars within the relaxed skin-tension lines. Reorienting scars to run parallel with relaxed skin-tension lines also aids in decreasing wound tension, and reduces mechanical stresses that contribute to aberrant wound healing and scar formation. This section discusses various surgical techniques of scar revision commonly used in clinical practice.

Simple Excision and Serial Excision

Under ideal circumstances, simple reexcision of a scar can be an effective treatment modality for obtaining an aesthetic result. Small scars already oriented parallel to relaxed skin-tension lines can be excised in an elliptical fashion, peripherally undermined to facilitate closure, and then reapproximated with sufficient dermal suturing to ensure wound-edge eversion. Peripheral undermining of tissue will aid in reducing wound tension and subsequent widening of the scar, while adequate eversion will help prevent formation of a depressed scar following wound contracture during healing. Wide scars that are already optimally oriented relative to relaxed skin-tension lines can also be treated with serial excision to take advantage of mechanical creep inherent to tissues. Partial scar excision followed by periods of healing allows the surgeon to take advantage of the viscoelastic properties of the skin, and allows a broad scar to be reduced over multiple treatments that would otherwise be impossible to revise in a single procedure alone.

Z-Plasty

The use of Z-plasty in scar revision serves 3 primary purposes in terms of altering the characteristics of a scar: it can be used to reorient the

directionality of a scar; it can interrupt scar linearity to aid in scar camouflage; and it can also lengthen a scar, which is beneficial when scars create undesirable contracture of the surrounding tissues. Z-plasty is particularly useful in reorienting scars to fall within natural relaxed skin-tension lines of the face or to move scars to fall between anatomic subunits of the face where they will be less conspicuous. Z-plasty is also advantageous in that it requires minimal excision of tissue, which is a prerequisite for other types of revision procedures (ie, W-plasty or geometric broken-line closure).[29] A drawback of Z-plasty is the production of 2 new scars, increasing the length of the original scar by a factor of 3. In addition, at least 1 limb of the newly created scar will generally fall outside of relaxed skin-tension lines. Nevertheless, with appropriate clinical application and meticulous surgical technique, Z-plasty is an effective method of increasing scar cosmesis.

W-Plasty and Geometric Broken-Line Closure

The primary consideration for the use of a W-plasty revision is a wide linear scar running perpendicular to relaxed skin-tension lines in a convex area of the face such as the brow, temples, or malar regions. The use of this technique requires excision of both scar tissue and normal adjacent tissue, and should only be used in areas of sufficient tissue laxity to allow for the necessary advancement of the wound edges. When designing a W-plasty it is critical to ensure that at least 50% of the limbs are oriented parallel to the relaxed skin-tension lines, to reduce the likelihood of excessive wound tension during closure and rewidening of the scar with contracture during healing (**Figs. 3** and **4**).

The geometric broken-line closure is similar to the W-plasty in that it is also indicated for linear scars running parallel to relaxed skin-tension lines in convex areas of the face. It follows the same

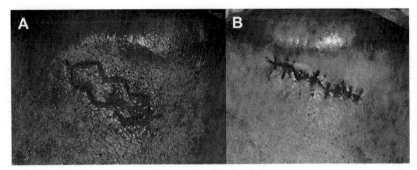

Fig. 3. W-plasty for a depressed scar. (*A*) Initial incision. (*B*) Final closure.

principles of the W-plasty in that it is a geometric bilateral advancement flap; however, it substitutes irregular geometric shapes for the cross-linking triangular limbs used in the W-plasty. This geometric broken-line closure is better suited for the treatment of long scars that are not optimally revised with the W-plasty. The repetitive closure pattern produced by the W-plasty becomes more easily noticeable when scar length increases, and the geometric broken-line closure circumvents this issue by breaking up the linearity of the scar in a more randomized pattern.

Subcision

Subcision is a useful technique in the management of depressed scars that may have resulted from insufficient wound-edge eversion or excessive scar contraction during healing. Subcision relies on the principle of severing subcutaneous fibrotic attachments tethering down a depressed scar and subsequent induction of neocollagenesis, which elevates the scar following reparative healing (**Fig. 5**). The procedure is typically carried out with circumferential insertion of a hypodermic needle into a depressed scar, followed by a gentle

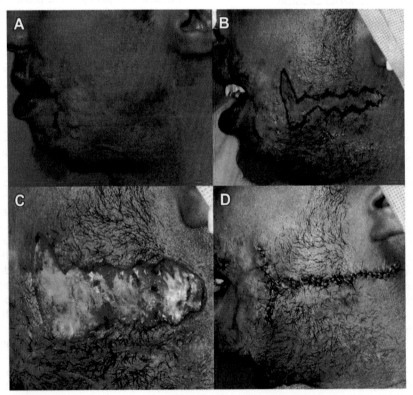

Fig. 4. Modified W-plasty for complex posttraumatic facial scar. (*A, B*) Initial presentation with outline. (*C, D*) Excised tissue and final closure.

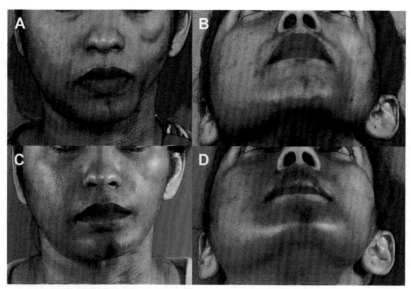

Fig. 5. Subcision of adherent tissue causing clefting in the chin. (*A, B*) Preoperative anterior and bird's-eye views. (*C, D*) The same views showing improvement in the early postoperative stage.

lifting maneuver to elevate the overlying epidermal tissue from the underlying dermis. Multiple modifications can be made to the hypodermic needle, with the use of various forceps to facilitate ease of use and accommodate surgeon preference.[30,31] The technique is easily performed and has minimal postoperative morbidity owing to the minimally invasive nature of the procedure; however, pain, swelling, bruising, hyperpigmentation, and hematoma formation can occur if the procedure is carried out too vigorously or if needle penetration traverses too deeply.[31]

POSTTRAUMATIC FACIAL SOFT-TISSUE VOLUME DEFICIENCY

A challenging aspect of posttraumatic facial reconstruction is accounting for volume loss. Traumatic avulsion of simple or composite tissues may occur acutely, as in dog bites or gunshot wounds. Alternatively, facial volume loss may be secondary to surgical intervention intended to treat the original trauma. For example, a patient may experience atrophy of the temporal fat pad following a coronal surgical approach. Denervation may also induce fat and muscular atrophy.[32] Other patients may suffer from what appears to be volume loss secondary to failure to resuspend the tissues after surgery that has detached musculofascial attachments to the facial skeleton.

Types of Volume Abnormalities

Following wound repair, soft tissues undergo contracture, and subcutaneous fat and muscular tissues may atrophy, causing irregularity and thinning of soft tissues. Fat atrophy occurs in the setting of trauma when subcutaneous tissues or fat collections (ie, periorbital fat, superficial temporal fat pad, or buccal fat pad) lose their blood supply or innervation.[32] This process begins within weeks after the initial trauma, but may require several months to realize its full extent. In addition, structural fat collections may be displaced or ptotic secondary to initial trauma or surgical intervention, with failure to resuspend them. Finally, after definitive reconstruction, some flaps may provide excess soft tissue and require debulking. When considering restoration of volume in the posttraumatic period, one must account for timing of treatment, what is possible, and what is both practical and reasonable in consultation with the patient.

Timing of Repair and Revision

In general, volume-restorative techniques include adjacent transfer of tissue, free transfer of tissue, and prosthetic or alloplastic volume replacement. These interventions must be timed appropriately to maximize the benefit of treatment and avoid inadequate restoration. In general, restoration before full manifestation of the defect may result in inadequate reconstitution of proper form. In some cases, when skin and subcutaneous tissues are lost, allowing weeks until full granulation may yield acceptable initial results while rendering the eventual required reconstruction less sizable; this is particularly true in the upper forehead, but may also meet with success in areas with more complex anatomy, such as the lips.[33] Alternatively, a biological coverage such as Integra bilayer matrix wound dressing may be used. The wound may be freshened at a later date when definitive coverage is to be achieved. Presuturing, or providing mechanical creep, may also improve soft-tissue outcomes prior to definitive late closure.[34]

In other circumstances when reconstruction is not as clearly staged, defects require a certain amount of time to fully manifest before proper reconstruction. In cases of tissue atrophy, volume restoration by any means should be withheld until the extent of the atrophy declares itself. This situation may require up to 6 months to a year to occur in some cases, but the surgeon should monitor for stability on examination prior to intervention. Where tissue ptosis is implicated, early intervention is often acceptable, and even advisable, before scarring and contracture render corrective suspension more difficult. In cases of large avulsive defects and composite defects, staging of reconstruction may involve microvascular surgery, and is summarized here.

Timing of Large or Composite Defects Requiring Microvascular Free Tissue Transfer

When possible, reconstruction of large or composite defects should be planned in a staged fashion. After initial management and stabilization, the first steps are establishment of the soft-tissue envelope with the best possible soft-tissue closure. Part of this is establishing as much bony framework for soft-tissue draping as possible, as this minimizes contracture of the tissues for later intervention. Initial soft-tissue draping occurs concomitant with debridement as necessary and establishment of occlusion. At this stage, if it is clear that free composite tissue will be required, initial management will be altered. For example, early rotational or other flaps may alter anatomy and render definitive reconstruction more difficult. Also, in the interim, a segmental bony defect may be maintained with a reconstruction plate or other prosthesis until the second phase of reconstruction.

After tissue transfer and adequate healing has taken place, debulking and commissuroplasty as well as other cosmetic procedures can finalize the reconstruction in the late phase.[35] Debulking and vestibuloplasty may take place 6 weeks or later following the initial flap placement. If a second debulking is required, the surgeon should wait at least 6 months, and up to a year, after the first procedure to allow for full contracture and atrophy, of both subcutaneous fat and any accompanying muscle. Excluding staging, details of free

flap and major reconstruction is beyond the scope of this article.

LOCAL ROTATIONAL AND ADVANCEMENT FLAPS

When tissue is required to augment or reconstruct a volume deficit, local transfer of adjacent tissue may often result in good outcomes. Local flaps may be vascularized by specific vessels (ie, the supratrochlear artery for the paramedian forehead flap) or randomly (ie, most flaps of the cheeks and chin). In general, the thickness and quality of the tissue adjacent to an avulsed defect is similar to that of the missing tissue, which is beneficial from a surgical and aesthetic standpoint. An example for local flaps is treatment of an avulsed nasal tip via a paramedian forehead flap. Understanding of basic design techniques and principles of flaps is not covered here, but should be within the scope of the practitioner to maximize flap success.[36] The lips and oral aperture are another location amenable to this type of treatment when tissue is avulsed or necessarily surgically debrided early on. In some cases, for example with cheek defects, a facial artery musculomucosal flap may be indicated. Finally, in cases where sufficient local tissue is unavailable, such as for large scalp defects, tissue expanders may be drawn on to generate tissue for full coverage.

FREE TISSUE TRANSFER

Within the spectrum of free tissue transfer are circumscribed many modalities of reconstruction, ranging from skin grafts to fat transfer to composite free flaps. When viable tissue is needed and local tissue is insufficient, not indicated, or undesirable, free tissue may often restore volume and structure in a lasting way. In some cases, such as in radial forearm flaps for lip reconstruction, these techniques may also restore function, in this case lip competence and sensation.[37]

Full-Thickness Skin Grafting

Grafting of free tissue may also take the form of full-thickness skin grafts and fat grafting. Full-thickness skin grafting provides a good match for soft-tissue tone, quality, and thickness. For skin replacement, if rotational flaps are not available or provide incomplete coverage, a skin graft may be obtained. Excellent graft may be obtained from the preauricular and postauricular areas in many individuals. Alternatively, excess tissue from rotational flaps may also be used when excised and trimmed appropriately.[38] There is some initial contracture, but with proper sizing, bolstering, and aftercare, graft viability and final results are excellent and reliable.

Structural Fat Transfer

Whereas free skin grafts may aid in soft-tissue coverage, intermediate-level soft-tissue volume may be regained via fat transfer. Fat grafting, first described by Neuber[39] in 1893 but more recently popularized by Coleman[40,41] and others in the 1990s, is an effective means of adding bulk to atrophied areas as well as smoothing out irregularities. It may be used in conjunction with subcision of depressed scars or in recontouring larger defects, such as temporal hollowing (**Figs. 6** and **7**).[42] Fat grafting is also thought to rejuvenate the overlying skin,[43] possibly with the help of stem cells.[44]

Fat harvest and grafting may require more than 1 procedure to achieve adequate results, owing to the less than 100% take of the graft. This amount is technique dependent, and investigators have reported retention of the initially transplanted volume of between 20% and 100%.[40,45–50] Traumatized or scarred tissue may retain less transplanted fat because vascular supply is diminished from virgin tissue.[51] It is generally well tolerated by patients, and the benefits endure beyond common fillers that may also be used for small volume replacements. Complications of structural fat grafting include overcorrection, undercorrection, surface irregularity, graft migration, and infection. In addition to injection of fat for grafting, dermal fat grafting has been found to be helpful for restoration of defects in facial volume.[42] In the case of dermal fat grafting, the size of the harvest can be tailored to the size of the defect in question, and reconstruction may less often require repeat augmentation because of the more robust vascularization of the dermal fat graft. Still other surgeons prefer vascularized adipose for large defects.[35]

Soft-Tissue Fillers

The past several years have seen a virtual explosion of available fillers for facial augmentation.

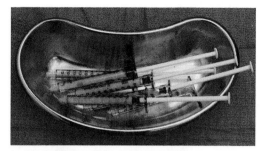

Fig. 7. Syringes of fat harvested for the patient in **Fig. 6**.

No longer are we having to skin-test our patients for allergen sensitivity to such products. Contemporary materials available for facial augmentation include the nonanimal stabilized hyaluronic acids, such as Restylane and Juvederm. These products are readily available and well tolerated by patients, and can be useful for replacing volume deficiencies secondary to facial trauma or for enhancing the outcomes of certain scars. Use of these products can certainly help improve the appearance of scars, but may also be a transition to a more permanent type of filler in the long term. The materials are supplied sterile, and can be injected at various levels in the dermis and subdermal level for the desired effect. Surgeons should consider these materials as adjuncts available for use when contemplating minor revisional procedures for late effects of soft-tissue injuries or defects secondary to facial trauma (**Fig. 8**).

Vascularized Free Tissue Transfer

Free tissue transfer has enabled reconstruction of simple or composite defects with vascularized tissue. As mentioned previously, this is best accomplished in a staged manner. Composite volume deficit more commonly occurs secondary to high-velocity ballistic injuries or high-energy trauma. In this case, skin as well as muscle and/or bone may be lost. Local tissue advancement

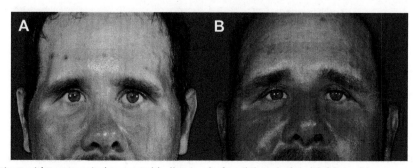

Fig. 6. A patient with postsurgical temporal hollowing before (*A*) and after (*B*) fat grafting.

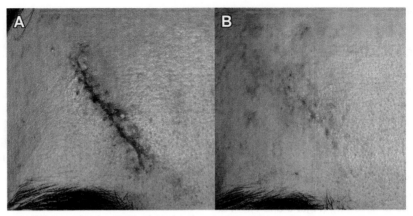

Fig. 8. (*A*) Frontal scar that became depressed after healing. Treatment was injection of hyaluronic acid (*B*).

or rotation is an excellent choice in many cases, but for larger defects or those requiring bone, free tissue transfer may offer the most definitive solution. This type of composite reconstruction and revision is beyond the scope of this article.

Free tissue transfer may be used only for soft tissue. Free flaps may be used to reconstruct the lips, especially the lower lip. The radial forearm flap with palmaris longus tendon transfer may be used to create a new lower lip and restore oral

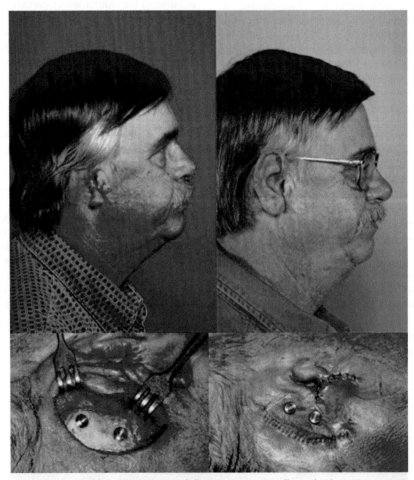

Fig. 9. Auricular prosthesis used for reconstruction following traumatically avulsed ear. Preoperative and postoperative views showing the defect and the prosthesis in place. The prosthesis is retained by 2 craniofacial implants.

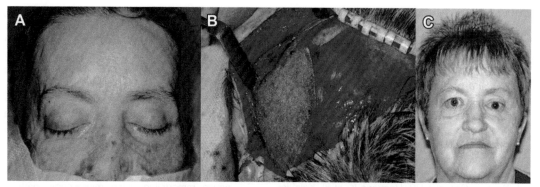

Fig. 10. Postsurgical temporal hollowing treated with Medpor implant. (*A*) Preoperative view. (*B*) Intraoperative placement of the implant. (*C*) Postoperative view.

competence. Radial forearm flaps may also provide definitive orbital coverage following enucleation. Similarly, anterolateral thigh flaps may be used when a larger amount of soft tissue is required for coverage. All of these flaps may require later debulking and reshaping, the timing of which is described in a previous section.

ALLOPLASTIC AND PROSTHETIC RECONSTRUCTION OF SOFT-TISSUE DEFECTS

In some cases, where grafting is not possible or undesirable to the patient, or where the surgeon requires a greater degree of customization of the result, alloplastic materials and prosthetics may be used to improve soft-tissue appearance in the posttraumatic patient. Prosthetics are ideal in some cases where tissues are completely avulsed or missing, such as ears or noses. The oral and maxillofacial surgeon is in an ideal position to help in reconstruction of these defects by anchoring a prosthetic with osseointegrated craniofacial implants (**Fig. 9**).[52]

Ptosis of tissues may result secondary to traumatic facial nerve damage or failure to resuspend tissues appropriately, or from disruption of fascial and dermal attachments to the facial skeleton. In both the midface and the forehead, this problem is readily approached with Endotine-type devices or similar lifting procedures,[53] which may be applied using transoral and transcutaneous approaches familiar to practitioners of maxillofacial surgery. Endoscopic techniques may be used in some cases. Conversely, resuspension with sutures or bone anchors may also be used in some cases with good results, although larger dissection and exposure may be required.

For deep facial contour defects in general and temporal hollowing in particular, multiple materials have been advocated for reconstruction, from titanium mesh[54] to porous polyethylene (ie, Medpor)

to custom PEEK (poly ether ether ketone) prostheses (**Fig. 10**), all of which have proven track records, with variable degrees of customizability. Whereas stock Medpor may be adjusted in situ,[55] implants such as Medpor, silicone, and PEEK may be custom-modeled from computed tomography scans to match the patient's individual bony contours and provide a facial profile mirroring the contralateral side. All of these implants carry an increased risk of infection, with the eventual possibility of explantation. In general, however, they are well tolerated and produce good results. In some cases, additional fat grafting over the prosthesis in the subcutaneous space may soften the appearance and feel of the restored area.[45]

SUMMARY

The contemporary maxillofacial surgeon has continued to expand on the historical management of facial fractures established by pioneers in our specialty. Advances in understanding the biological aspects of wound healing and surgical options to rectify acute and delayed facial soft-tissue deformities, combined with current technological techniques, facilitate improved outcomes. This article serves as a basis to understand these concepts and treatment options for the betterment of patients.

REFERENCES

1. Shaw T, Martin P. Wound repair at a glance. J Cell Sci 2009;122(18):3209–13.
2. Sgonc R, Gruber J. Age-related aspects of cutaneous wound healing: a mini-review. Gerontology 2013;59(2):159–64.
3. Tonnensen M, Feng X, Clark RA. Angiogenesis in wound healing. J Investig Dermatol Symp Proc 2000;5:40–6.

4. Hom D, Sun GH, Elluru RG. A contemporary review of wound healing in otolaryngology: current state and future promise. Laryngoscope 2009;119(11): 2099–110.

5. Chen M, Davidson TM. Scar management: prevention and treatment strategies. Curr Opin Otolaryngol Head Neck Surg 2005;13(4):242–7.

6. Huang C, Akaishi S, Hyakusoku H, et al. Are keloid and hypertrophic scar different forms of the same disorder? A fibroproliferative skin disorder hypothesis based on keloid findings. Int Wound J 2012. [Epub ahead of print].

7. Bran G, Goessler UR, Hormann K, et al. Keloids: current concepts of pathogenesis (review). Int J Mol Med 2009;24(3):283–93.

8. Slemp A, Kirschner RE. Keloids and scars: a review of keloids and scars, their pathogenesis, risk factors, and management. Curr Opin Pediatr 2006;18(4):396–402.

9. Sidle D, Kim H. Keloids: prevention and management. Facial Plast Surg Clin North Am 2011;19(3): 505–15.

10. Datubo-Brown D. Keloids: a review of the literature. Br J Plast Surg 1990;43(1):70–7.

11. Wolfram D, Tzankov A, Pülzl P, et al. Hypertrophic scars and keloids—a review of their pathophysiology, risk factors, and therapeutic management. Dermatol Surg 2009;35(2):171–81.

12. Mustoe T, Cooter RD, Gold MH, et al. International clinical recommendations on scar management. Plast Reconstr Surg 2002;110(2):560–71.

13. Kelly A. Update on the management of keloids. Semin Cutan Med Surg 2009;28(2):71–6.

14. Oliaei S, Nelson JS, Fitzpatrick R, et al. Use of lasers in acute management of surgical and traumatic incisions on the face. Facial Plast Surg Clin North Am 2011;19(3):543–50.

15. Weiss E, Chapas A, Brightman L, et al. Successful treatment of atrophic postoperative and traumatic scarring with carbon dioxide ablative fractional resurfacing: quantitative volumetric scar improvement. Arch Dermatol 2010;146(2):133–40.

16. Apfelberg D, Maser MR, White DN, et al. Failure of carbon dioxide laser excision of keloids. Lasers Surg Med 1989;9(4):382–8.

17. Papadavid E, Katsambas A. Lasers for facial rejuvenation: a review. Int J Dermatol 2003;42(6):480–7.

18. Alster T, Lupton JR. Erbium:YAG cutaneous laser resurfacing. Dermatol Clin 2001;19(3):453–6.

19. Alster T, Handrick C. Laser treatment of hypertrophic scars, keloids, and striae. Semin Cutan Med Surg 2000;19(4):287–92.

20. Nelson J, Milner TE, Anvari B, et al. Dynamic epidermal cooling during pulsed laser treatment of port-wine stain. A new methodology with preliminary clinical evaluation. Arch Dermatol 1995; 131(6):695–700.

21. Kelly K, Nelson JS, Lask GP, et al. Cryogen spray cooling in combination with nonablative laser treatment of facial rhytides. Arch Dermatol 1999;135(6): 691–4.

22. Pham R. Nonablative laser resurfacing. Facial Plast Surg Clin North Am 2001;9(2):303–10.

23. Pham R. Treatment of vascular lesions with combined dynamic precooling, postcooling thermal quenching, and ND: YAG 1,064-nm laser. Facial Plast Surg 2001;17(3):203–8.

24. Manstein D, Herron GS, Sink RK, et al. Fractional photothermolysis: a new concept for cutaneous remodeling using microscopic patterns of thermal injury. Lasers Surg Med 2004;34(5): 426–38.

25. Sobanko J, Alster TS. Laser treatment for improvement and minimization of facial scars. Facial Plast Surg Clin North Am 2011;19(3):527–42.

26. Kim E, Hovsepian RV, Mathew P, et al. Dermabrasion. Clin Plast Surg 2011;38(3):391–5.

27. Surowitz J, Shockley WW. Enhancement of facial scars with dermabrasion. Facial Plast Surg Clin North Am 2011;19(3):517–25.

28. Rivera A. Acne scarring: a review and current treatment modalities. J Am Acad Dermatol 2008;59(4): 659–76.

29. Shockley W. Scar revision techniques: z-plasty, w-plasty, and geometric broken line closure. Facial Plast Surg Clin North Am 2011;19(3):455–63.

30. Alsufyani M, Alsufyani MA. Subcision: a further modification, an ever continuing process. Dermatol Res Pract 2012;2012:685347.

31. Khunger N, Khunger M. Subcision for depressed facial scars made easy using a simple modification. Dermatol Surg 2011;37(4):514–7.

32. Kim S, Matic DB. The anatomy of temporal hollowing: the superficial temporal fat pad. J Craniofac Surg 2005;16:651–4.

33. Rhee ST, Colville C, Buchman SR. Conservative management of large avulsions of the lip and local landmarks. Pediatr Emerg Care 2004;20:40–2.

34. Zide MF. Pexing and presuturing for closure of traumatic soft tissue injuries. J Oral Maxillofac Surg 1994;52:698–703.

35. Futran ND. Maxillofacial trauma reconstruction. Facial Plast Surg Clin North Am 2009;17:239–51.

36. Zide MF, Topper D. Pivot point and secondary defect problems with rotation flaps. J Oral Maxillofac Surg 2004;62:1069–75.

37. Odell MJ, Varvares MA. Microvascular reconstruction of major lip defects. Facial Plast Surg Clin North Am 2009;17:203–9.

38. Johnson T, Zide MF. Freehand full-thickness grafting for facial defects: a review of methods. J Oral Maxillofac Surg 1997;55:1050–6.

39. Neuber F. Fet transplantation. Chir Kongr Verhandl Dtsch Ges Chir 1893;22:66–8.

40. Coleman SR. Long term survival of fat transplants: controlled demonstration. Aesthetic Plast Surg 1995;19:421–5.

41. Coleman SR. Techniques of periorbital infiltration. Oper Tech Plast Reconstr Surg 1994;1:120–6.

42. McNichols CH, Hatef DA, Cole P, et al. Contemporary techniques for the correction of temporal hollowing: augmentation temporoplasty with the classic dermal fat graft. J Craniofac Surg 2012;23:e234–8.

43. Coleman SR. Fat grafting: more than a permanent filler. Plast Reconstr Surg 2006;118:108–11.

44. Clauser LC, Tieghi R, Galiè M, et al. Structural fat grafting: facial volumetric restoration in complex reconstructive surgery. J Craniofac Surg 2011;22: 1695–701.

45. Ducic Y, Pontius AT, Smith JE. Lipotransfer as an adjunct in head and neck reconstruction. Laryngoscope 2003;113:1600–4.

46. Pinski KS, Roenigk HH Jr. Autologous fat transplantation: long-term follow-up. J Dermatol Surg Oncol 1992;18:179–83.

47. Chajchir A, Benzaquen I. Fat-grafting injection for soft-tissue augmentation. Plast Reconstr Surg 1989;84:921–5.

48. Niechajev I, Sevćuk O. Long-term results of fat transplantation: clinical and histologic studies. Plast Reconstr Surg 1994;94:496–506.

49. Illouz YG. The fat cell graft: a new technique to fill depressions. Plast Reconstr Surg 1986;78:122–6.

50. Peer LA. Loss of weight and volume in human fat grafts. Plast Reconstr Surg 1950;5:217–30.

51. Ducic Y. Fat grafting in trauma and reconstructive surgery. Facial Plast Surg Clin North Am 2008;16: 409–16.

52. Sharma A, Rahul GR, Poduval ST, et al. Implant-supported auricular prosthesis—an overview. J Oral Implantol 2012. [Epub ahead of print].

53. Boehmler JH 4th, Judson BL, Davison SP. Reconstructive application of the Endotine suspension devices. Arch Facial Plast Surg 2007;9: 328–32.

54. Guo J, Tian W, Long J, et al. A retrospective study of traumatic temporal hollowing and treatment with titanium mesh. Ann Plast Surg 2012; 68:279–85.

55. Yaremchuk MJ. Facial skeletal reconstruction using porous polyethylene implants. Plast Reconstr Surg 2003;111:1818–27.

Index

Note: Page numbers of article titles are in **boldface** type.

Oral Maxillofacial Surg Clin N Am 25 (2013) 715–721
http://dx.doi.org/10.1016/S1042-3699(13)00128-3
1042-3699/13/$ – see front matter © 2013 Elsevier Inc. All rights reserved.

United States Postal Service

Statement of Ownership, Management, and Circulation
(All Periodicals Publications Except Requestor Publications)

1. Publication Title	2. Publication Number	3. Filing Date
Oral and Maxillofacial Surgery Clinics of North America	0 0 6 - 3 6 2	9/14/13

4. Issue Frequency	5. Number of Issues Published Annually	6. Annual Subscription Price
Feb, May, Aug, Nov	4	$369.00

7. Complete Mailing Address of Known Office of Publication (Not printer) (Street, city, county, state, and ZIP+4®)

Elsevier Inc.
360 Park Avenue South
New York, NY 10010-1710

Contact Person
Stephen R. Bushing
Telephone (Include area code)
215-239-3688

8. Complete Mailing Address of Headquarters or General Business Office of Publisher (Not printer)

Elsevier Inc., 360 Park Avenue South, New York, NY 10010-1710

9. Full Names and Complete Mailing Addresses of Publisher, Editor, and Managing Editor (Do not leave blank)

Publisher (Name and complete mailing address)

Linda Belfus, Elsevier, Inc., 1600 John F. Kennedy Blvd. Suite 1800, Philadelphia, PA 19103-2899

Editor (Name and complete mailing address)

John Vassallo, Elsevier, Inc., 1600 John F. Kennedy Blvd. Suite 1800, Philadelphia, PA 19103-2899

Managing Editor (Name and complete mailing address)

Barbara Cohen-Kligerman, Elsevier, Inc., 1600 John F. Kennedy Blvd. Suite 1800, Philadelphia, PA 19103-2899

10. Owner (Do not leave blank. If the publication is owned by a corporation, give the name and address of the corporation immediately followed by the names and addresses of all stockholders owning or holding 1 percent or more of the total amount of stock. If not owned by a corporation, give the names and addresses of the individual owners. If owned by a partnership or other unincorporated firm, give its name and address as well as those of each individual owner. If the publication is published by a nonprofit organization, give its name and address.)

Full Name	Complete Mailing Address
Wholly owned subsidiary of	1600 John F. Kennedy Blvd., Ste. 1800
Reed/Elsevier, US holdings	Philadelphia, PA 19103-2899

11. Known Bondholders, Mortgagees, and Other Security Holders Owning or Holding 1 Percent or More of Total Amount of Bonds, Mortgages, or Other Securities. If none, check box ▸ ☐ None

Full Name	Complete Mailing Address
N/A	

12. Tax Status (For completion by nonprofit organizations authorized to mail at nonprofit rates) (Check one)
The purpose, function, and nonprofit status of this organization and the exempt status for federal income tax purposes:
☐ Has Not Changed During Preceding 12 Months
☐ Has Changed During Preceding 12 Months (Publisher must submit explanation of change with this statement)

13. Publication Title	14. Issue Date for Circulation Data Below
Oral and Maxillofacial Surgery Clinics of North America	August 2013

15. Extent and Nature of Circulation		Average No. Copies Each Issue During Preceding 12 Months	No. Copies of Single Issue Published Nearest to Filing Date
a. Total Number of Copies (Net press run)		1,591	1,465
b. Paid Circulation (By Mail and Outside the Mail)	(1) Mailed Outside-County Paid Subscriptions Stated on PS Form 3541. (Include paid distribution above nominal rate, advertiser's proof copies, and exchange copies)	1,138	1,055
	(2) Mailed In-County Paid Subscriptions Stated on PS Form 3541 (Include paid distribution above nominal rate, advertiser's proof copies, and exchange copies)		
	(3) Paid Distribution Outside the Mails Including Sales Through Dealers and Carriers, Street Vendors, Counter Sales, and Other Paid Distribution Outside USPS®	183	189
	(4) Paid Distribution by Other Classes Mailed Through the USPS (e.g. First-Class Mail®)		
c. Total Paid Distribution (Sum of 15b (1), (2), (3), and (4))	▸	1,321	1,244
d. Free or Nominal Rate Distribution (By Mail and Outside the Mail)	(1) Free or Nominal Rate Outside-County Copies Included on PS Form 3541	65	61
	(2) Free or Nominal Rate In-County Copies Included on PS Form 3541		
	(3) Free or Nominal Rate Copies Mailed at Other Classes Through the USPS (e.g. First-Class Mail)		
	(4) Free or Nominal Rate Distribution Outside the Mail (Carriers or other means)		
e. Total Free or Nominal Rate Distribution (Sum of 15d (1), (2), (3) and (4))	▸	65	61
f. Total Distribution (Sum of 15c and 15e)	▸	1,386	1,305
g. Copies not Distributed (See instructions to publishers #4 (page #3))	▸	205	160
h. Total (Sum of 15f and g)	▸	1,591	1,465
i. Percent Paid (15c divided by 15f times 100)		95.31%	95.33%

16. Publication of Statement of Ownership
☐ If the publication is a general publication, publication of this statement is required. Will be printed in the November 2013 issue of this publication.
☐ Publication not required

17. Signature and Title of Editor, Publisher, Business Manager, or Owner

Stephen R. Bushing [signature]

Stephen R. Bushing – Inventory Distribution Coordinator

Date: September 14, 2013

I certify that all information furnished on this form is true and complete. I understand that anyone who furnishes false or misleading information on this form or who omits material or information requested on the form may be subject to criminal sanctions (including fines and imprisonment) and/or civil sanctions (including civil penalties).

PS Form 3526, September 2007 (Page 2 of 3)

PS Form 3526, September 2007 (Page 1 of 3 (Instructions Page 3)) PSN 7530-01-000-9931 PRIVACY NOTICE: See our Privacy policy in www.usps.com

Moving?

Make sure your subscription moves with you!

To notify us of your new address, find your **Clinics Account Number** (located on your mailing label above your name), and contact customer service at:

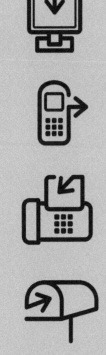

Email: journalscustomerservice-usa@elsevier.com

800-654-2452 (subscribers in the U.S. & Canada)
314-447-8871 (subscribers outside of the U.S. & Canada)

Fax number: 314-447-8029

Elsevier Health Sciences Division
Subscription Customer Service
3251 Riverport Lane
Maryland Heights, MO 63043

ELSEVIER

Moving?

Make sure your subscription moves with you!

To notify us of your new address, find your Clinics Account Number (located on your mailing label above your name), and contact customer service at:

Email: journalscustomerservice-usa@elsevier.com

800-654-2452 (subscribers in the U.S. & Canada)
314-447-8871 (subscribers outside of the U.S. & Canada)

Fax number: 314-447-8029

Elsevier Health Sciences Division
Subscription Customer Service
3251 Riverport Lane
Maryland Heights, MO 63043

*To ensure uninterrupted delivery of your subscription, please notify us at least 4 weeks in advance of move.

Printed and bound by CPI Group (UK) Ltd, Croydon, CR0 4YY

03/10/2024

01040309-0014